MW01701651

AMERICAN ACADEMY™
OF OPHTHALMOLOGY

4

Ophthalmic Pathology and Intraocular Tumors

2016–2017
BCSC
Basic and Clinical Science Course™

Protecting Sight. Empowering Lives.™

EB
Published after collaborative review with the European Board of Ophthalmology subcommittee

The American Academy of Ophthalmology is accredited by the Accreditation Council for Continuing Medical Education to provide continuing medical education for physicians.

The American Academy of Ophthalmology designates this enduring material for a maximum of 10 *AMA PRA Category 1 Credits*™. Physicians should claim only the credit commensurate with the extent of their participation in the activity.

CME expiration date: June 1, 2019. *AMA PRA Category 1 Credits*™ may be claimed only once between June 1, 2016, and the expiration date.

BCSC® volumes are designed to increase the physician's ophthalmic knowledge through study and review. Users of this activity are encouraged to read the text and then answer the study questions provided at the back of the book.

To claim *AMA PRA Category 1 Credits*™ upon completion of this activity, learners must demonstrate appropriate knowledge and participation in the activity by taking the posttest for Section 4 and achieving a score of 80% or higher. For further details, please see the instructions for requesting CME credit at the back of the book.

The Academy provides this material for educational purposes only. It is not intended to represent the only or best method or procedure in every case, nor to replace a physician's own judgment or give specific advice for case management. Including all indications, contraindications, side effects, and alternative agents for each drug or treatment is beyond the scope of this material. All information and recommendations should be verified, prior to use, with current information included in the manufacturers' package inserts or other independent sources, and considered in light of the patient's condition and history. Reference to certain drugs, instruments, and other products in this course is made for illustrative purposes only and is not intended to constitute an endorsement of such. Some material may include information on applications that are not considered community standard, that reflect indications not included in approved FDA labeling, or that are approved for use only in restricted research settings. **The FDA has stated that it is the responsibility of the physician to determine the FDA status of each drug or device he or she wishes to use, and to use them with appropriate, informed patient consent in compliance with applicable law.** The Academy specifically disclaims any and all liability for injury or other damages of any kind, from negligence or otherwise, for any and all claims that may arise from the use of any recommendations or other information contained herein.

Cover image: From BCSC Section 10, *Glaucoma*. Typical gonioscopic appearance of angle recession. *Courtesy of Steven T. Simmons, MD.*

FSC
www.fsc.org
MIX
Paper from responsible sources
FSC® C103061

Basic and Clinical Science Course

Louis B. Cantor, MD, Indianapolis, Indiana, *Senior Secretary for Clinical Education*
Christopher J. Rapuano, MD, Philadelphia, Pennsylvania, *Secretary for Ophthalmic Knowledge*
George A. Cioffi, MD, New York, New York, *BCSC Course Chair*

Section 4

Faculty

Robert H. Rosa Jr, MD, *Chair,* Temple, Texas
Michele M. Bloomer, MD, San Francisco, California
Dan S. Gombos, MD, Houston, Texas
Tatyana Milman, MD, Philadelphia, Pennsylvania
Heather A.D. Potter, MD, Madison, Wisconsin
Nasreen A. Syed, MD, Iowa City, Iowa
Tero T. Kivelä, MD, *Consultant,* Helsinki, Finland

The Academy wishes to acknowledge the *American Association of Ophthalmic Oncologists and Pathologists* for recommending faculty members to the BCSC Section 4 committee.

The Academy also wishes to acknowledge the following committees for review of this edition:

Committee on Aging: Patricia Chévez-Barrios, MD, Houston, Texas

Vision Rehabilitation Committee: Joseph L. Fontenot, MD, Daphne, Alabama

Practicing Ophthalmologists Advisory Committee for Education: Robert G. Fante, MD, *Primary Reviewer,* Denver, CO; Edward K. Isbey III, *Chair,* Asheville, North Carolina; Alice Bashinsky, MD, Asheville, North Carolina; David Browning, MD, PhD, Charlotte, North Carolina; Bradley Fouraker, MD, Tampa, Florida; Dasa Gangadhar, MD, Wichita, Kansas; Steven J. Grosser, MD, Golden Valley, Minnesota; Stephen R. Klapper, MD, Carmel, Indiana

EB

European Board of Ophthalmology: Tero T. Kivelä, MD, *Chair,* Helsinki, Finland; Edoardo Midena, MD, PhD, *Liaison,* Padua, Italy; Nikolaos E. Bechrakis, MD, FEBO, Innsbruck, Austria; Sarah E. Coupland, MBBS, PhD, FRCPath, Liverpool, United Kingdom; Laurence Desjardins, MD, Paris, France; Steffen Heegaard, MD, DMSc, Copenhagen, Denmark; Elisabeth M. Messmer, MD, PhD, FEBO, Munich, Germany; Fiona Roberts, MBChB, MD, FRCPath, Glasgow, United Kingdom

Financial Disclosures

Academy staff members who contributed to the development of this product state that within the 12 months prior to their contributions to this CME activity and for the duration of development, they have had no financial interest in or other relationship with any entity discussed in this course that produces, markets, resells, or distributes ophthalmic health care goods or services consumed by or used in patients, or with any competing commercial product or service.

The authors and reviewers state that within the 12 months prior to their contributions to this CME activity and for the duration of development, they have had the following financial relationships:*

Dr Bechrakis: Alcon Laboratories (C, S), Bayer (C, S), HOYA (S), Novartis Pharmaceuticals (C)

Dr Browning: Aerpio Therapeutics (S), Alimera Sciences (C), Genentech (S), Novartis Pharmaceuticals (S), Pfizer (S), Regeneron Pharmaceuticals (S)

Dr Fouraker: Addition Technology (C, L), Alcon Laboratories (C, L), KeraVision (C, L), OASIS Medical (C, L)

Dr Grosser: Ivantis (O)

Dr Heegaard: Santen (L), Théa (L)

Dr Messmer: Alcon Pharmaceuticals (C, L), Allergan (C, L), CROMA-PHARMA (C, L), Dompé (C), Théa (C, L), URSAPHARM (L)

The other authors and reviewers state that within the past 12 months prior to their contributions to this CME activity and for the duration of development, they have had no financial interest in or other relationship with any entity discussed in this course that produces, markets, resells, or distributes ophthalmic health care goods or services consumed by or used in patients, or with any competing commercial product or service.

*C = consultant fees, paid advisory boards, or fees for attending a meeting; L = lecture fees (honoraria), travel fees, or reimbursements when speaking at the invitation of a commercial sponsor; O = equity ownership/stock options of publicly or privately traded firms (excluding mutual funds) with manufacturers of commercial ophthalmic products or commercial ophthalmic services; P = patents and/or royalties that might be viewed as creating a potential conflict of interest; S = grant support for the past year (all sources) and all sources used for a specific talk or manuscript with no time limitation

Recent Past Faculty

Ronald Buggage, MD
George J. Harocopos, MD
Theresa Retue Kramer, MD
Jacob Pe'er, MD
Ron W. Pelton, MD, PhD
Matthew W. Wilson, MD

In addition, the Academy gratefully acknowledges the contributions of numerous past faculty and advisory committee members who have played an important role in the development of previous editions of the Basic and Clinical Science Course.

American Academy of Ophthalmology Staff

Dale E. Fajardo, *Vice President, Education*
Beth Wilson, *Director, Continuing Professional Development*
Ann McGuire, *Acquisitions and Development Manager*
Stephanie Tanaka, *Publications Manager*
D. Jean Ray, *Production Manager*
Beth Collins, *Medical Editor*
Naomi Ruiz, *Editorial Assistant*

American Academy of Ophthalmology
655 Beach Street
Box 7424
San Francisco, CA 94120-7424

Contents

General Introduction

The Basic and Clinical Science Course (BCSC) is designed to meet the needs of residents and practitioners for a comprehensive yet concise curriculum of the field of ophthalmology. The BCSC has developed from its original brief outline format, which relied heavily on outside readings, to a more convenient and educationally useful self-contained text. The Academy updates and revises the course annually, with the goals of integrating the basic science and clinical practice of ophthalmology and of keeping ophthalmologists current with new developments in the various subspecialties.

The BCSC incorporates the effort and expertise of more than 80 ophthalmologists, organized into 13 Section faculties, working with Academy editorial staff. In addition, the course continues to benefit from many lasting contributions made by the faculties of previous editions. Members of the Academy's Practicing Ophthalmologists Advisory Committee for Education, Committee on Aging, and Vision Rehabilitation Committee review every volume before major revisions. Members of the European Board of Ophthalmology, organized into Section faculties, also review each volume before major revisions, focusing primarily on differences between American and European ophthalmology practice.

Organization of the Course

The Basic and Clinical Science Course comprises 13 volumes, incorporating fundamental ophthalmic knowledge, subspecialty areas, and special topics:

1 Update on General Medicine
2 Fundamentals and Principles of Ophthalmology
3 Clinical Optics
4 Ophthalmic Pathology and Intraocular Tumors
5 Neuro-Ophthalmology
6 Pediatric Ophthalmology and Strabismus
7 Orbit, Eyelids, and Lacrimal System
8 External Disease and Cornea
9 Intraocular Inflammation and Uveitis
10 Glaucoma
11 Lens and Cataract
12 Retina and Vitreous
13 Refractive Surgery

In addition, a comprehensive Master Index allows the reader to easily locate subjects throughout the entire series.

References

Readers who wish to explore specific topics in greater detail may consult the references cited within each chapter and listed in the Basic Texts section at the back of the book.

These references are intended to be selective rather than exhaustive, chosen by the BCSC faculty as being important, current, and readily available to residents and practitioners.

Videos

This edition of Section 4, *Ophthalmic Pathology and Intraocular Tumors,* includes videos related to topics covered in the book. The videos were selected by members of the BCSC faculty and are available to readers of the print and electronic versions of Section 4 (www.aao.org/bcscvideo_section04). Mobile-device users can scan the QR code below (a QR-code reader must already be installed on the device) to access the video content.

Study Questions and CME Credit

Each volume of the BCSC is designed as an independent study activity for ophthalmology residents and practitioners. The learning objectives for this volume are given on page 1. The text, illustrations, and references provide the information necessary to achieve the objectives; the study questions allow readers to test their understanding of the material and their mastery of the objectives. Physicians who wish to claim CME credit for this educational activity may do so by following the instructions given at the end of the book.

Conclusion

The Basic and Clinical Science Course has expanded greatly over the years, with the addition of much new text and numerous illustrations. Recent editions have sought to place a greater emphasis on clinical applicability while maintaining a solid foundation in basic science. As with any educational program, it reflects the experience of its authors. As its faculties change and as medicine progresses, new viewpoints are always emerging on controversial subjects and techniques. Not all alternate approaches can be included in this series; as with any educational endeavor, the learner should seek additional sources, including such carefully balanced opinions as the Academy's Preferred Practice Patterns.

The BCSC faculty and staff are continually striving to improve the educational usefulness of the course; you, the reader, can contribute to this ongoing process. If you have any suggestions or questions about the series, please do not hesitate to contact the faculty or the editors.

The authors, editors, and reviewers hope that your study of the BCSC will be of lasting value and that each Section will serve as a practical resource for quality patient care.

Objectives

Upon completion of BCSC Section 4, *Ophthalmic Pathology and Intraocular Tumors,* the reader should be able to

- describe a structured approach to understanding major ocular conditions based on a hierarchical framework of topography, disease process, general diagnosis, and differential diagnosis
- list the steps for handling ocular specimens for pathologic study, including obtaining, dissecting, processing, and staining tissues
- explain the basic principles of special procedures used in ophthalmic pathology, including immunohistochemistry, flow cytometry, molecular pathology, and diagnostic electron microscopy
- discuss the types of specimens, processing, and techniques appropriate to the clinical situation
- describe the histopathology of common ocular conditions
- discuss the relationship between clinical and pathologic findings in various ocular conditions
- list the steps in wound healing in ocular tissues
- state current information about the most common primary tumors of the eye
- identify those ophthalmic lesions that indicate systemic disease and are potentially life threatening
- discuss genetic information that would be useful to provide to families affected by retinoblastoma
- describe current treatment modalities for ocular tumors in terms of patient prognosis and ocular function

PART I

Ophthalmic Pathology

CHAPTER 1

Introduction to Part I

BCSC Section 4, *Ophthalmic Pathology and Intraocular Tumors,* provides a general overview of the fields of ophthalmic pathology and ocular oncology. This book contains numerous illustrations of entities commonly encountered in an ophthalmic pathology laboratory and in the practice of ocular oncology. In addition, important but less common entities are included for teaching purposes. For more comprehensive reviews of ophthalmic pathology and ocular oncology, please refer to the excellent textbooks listed in Basic Texts at the end of this volume.

Ophthalmic pathology is recognized as a subspecialty by the American Academy of Ophthalmology, the American Board of Ophthalmology, the Association of University Professors of Ophthalmology, and the International Council of Ophthalmology. The study of ophthalmic pathology has contributed significantly to understanding the pathogenesis of diseases of the eye and ocular adnexa. The Accreditation Council for Graduate Medical Education (ACGME) requires that resident education in ophthalmic pathology be directed by faculty members with expertise in that field, and the residency training curriculum of the International Council of Ophthalmology stipulates "engage[ment] with an ophthalmic pathologist." In the United States, ophthalmologists and pathologists may receive subspecialty fellowship training in ophthalmic pathology after completion of an ACGME-accredited training program in ophthalmology or pathology; some ophthalmic pathologists are board certified in both ophthalmology and pathology.

Part I of this text provides a framework for the study of ophthalmic pathology according to the following hierarchical organizational paradigm (explained in detail in the next section): topography, disease process, general diagnosis, and differential diagnosis. Chapter 2 briefly covers basic principles and specific aspects of wound repair as it applies to ophthalmic tissues, which exhibit distinct responses to trauma. Chapter 3 discusses specimen handling, including orientation and dissection, and emphasizes the critical communication between the ophthalmologist and the pathologist. Most ophthalmic pathology specimens are routinely processed, and slides are stained with hematoxylin-eosin. Special procedures such as immunohistochemical staining, flow cytometry, polymerase chain reaction (PCR), and frozen sections are used in selected cases, which will be discussed in Chapter 4. Chapters 5 through 15 apply the organizational paradigm to specific anatomical locations.

Organization

As mentioned, Chapters 5 through 15 are each devoted to a particular ocular structure. Within these chapters, the text is organized from general to specific, according to the following hierarchical framework:

- topography
- disease process
- general diagnosis
- differential diagnosis

Topography

A microscopic evaluation of a specimen should begin with a description of any normal tissue. For instance, the topography of the cornea features nonkeratinized stratified squamous epithelium, Bowman layer, stroma, Descemet membrane, and endothelium. By recognizing a particular structure in a biopsy specimen, such as Bowman layer or Descemet membrane, an examiner might be able to identify the specimen in question as cornea. Similarly, the presence of a tarsal plate in a specimen showing the topographic features of keratinized stratified squamous epithelium overlying dermis with dermal appendages may be identified as eyelid skin. See BCSC Section 2, *Fundamentals and Principles of Ophthalmology,* for a review of ophthalmic anatomy.

Disease Process

After identifying a tissue source, the examiner should attempt to categorize the general disease process. These processes include

- congenital anomaly
- inflammation
- degeneration and dystrophy
- neoplasia

Congenital anomaly

Congenital anomalies usually involve abnormalities in size, location, organization, or amount of tissue. One example is congenital hypertrophy of the retinal pigment epithelium (CHRPE) (see Chapter 11, Fig 11-6; and Chapter 17, Fig 17-10). Many congenital abnormalities may be classified as choristomas or hamartomas.

A *choristoma* consists of normal, mature tissue (up to 1 or 2 embryonic germ layers) at an abnormal location. An example of a choristoma is a *dermoid:* skin that is otherwise normal and mature present in an abnormal location, the limbus. A tumor made up of tissue derived from all 3 embryonic germ layers is called a *teratoma* (Fig 1-1).

In contrast, the term *hamartoma* describes hypertrophy and hyperplasia (abnormal amount) of mature tissue at a normal location. An example of a hamartoma is a *cavernous hemangioma,* an encapsulated mass of mature venous channels in the orbit.

Inflammation

The next disease process in the schema, inflammation, can be classified in several ways. It may be acute or chronic in onset and focal or diffuse in location. Chronic inflammation

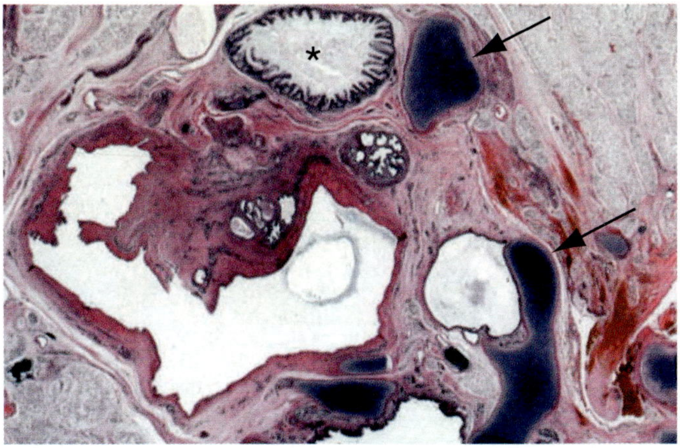

Figure 1-1 Orbital teratoma with tissue from 3 germ layers. Note gastrointestinal mucosa *(asterisk)* and cartilage *(arrows)* in the tumor. *(Courtesy of Hans E. Grossniklaus, MD.)*

is classified further as either granulomatous or nongranulomatous. For example, a bacterial corneal ulcer is generally an acute, focal, nongranulomatous inflammation, whereas sympathetic ophthalmia is a chronic, diffuse, granulomatous inflammation.

Polymorphonuclear leukocytes (PMNs), including neutrophils, eosinophils, and basophils, circulate in the blood and may be present in tissue in early phases of the inflammatory process (Figs 1-2, 1-3, and 1-4). *Neutrophils* typify acute inflammatory cells and can be recognized by a multisegmented nucleus and intracytoplasmic granules. They are associated with bacterial infection and may be found in the walls of blood vessels in some forms of vasculitis. *Eosinophils* have bilobed nuclei and prominent intracytoplasmic eosinophilic granules. They are commonly found in allergic reactions, although they may also be present in chronic inflammatory processes such as sympathetic ophthalmia. *Basophils* contain basophilic intracytoplasmic granules. *Mast cells* are the tissue-bound equivalent of the blood-borne basophils.

Inflammatory cells that are characteristic of chronic inflammatory processes include monocytes (Fig 1-5) and lymphocytes (Fig 1-6). *Monocytes* that migrate from the intravascular space into tissue are classified as *histiocytes* or *macrophages.* Histiocytes have eccentric nuclei and abundant eosinophilic cytoplasm. Some histiocytes, known as *epithelioid histiocytes,* may take on the appearance of epithelial cells, with abundant eosinophilic cytoplasm and sharp cell borders. Epithelioid histiocytes may form a ball-like aggregate known as a *granuloma,* the hallmark of granulomatous inflammation. Granulomas may contain only histologically intact cells ("hard" tubercles, Fig 1-7), or they may exhibit necrotic centers ("caseating" granulomas, Fig 1-8). Epithelioid histiocytes may merge to form a *multinucleated giant cell.* Giant cells formed from histiocytes come in several varieties, including

- Langhans cells, characterized by a horseshoe arrangement of the nuclei (Fig 1-9)
- Touton giant cells, which have an annulus of nuclei surrounded by a lipid-filled clear zone (Fig 1-10)
- foreign body giant cells, with haphazardly arranged nuclei (Fig 1-11)

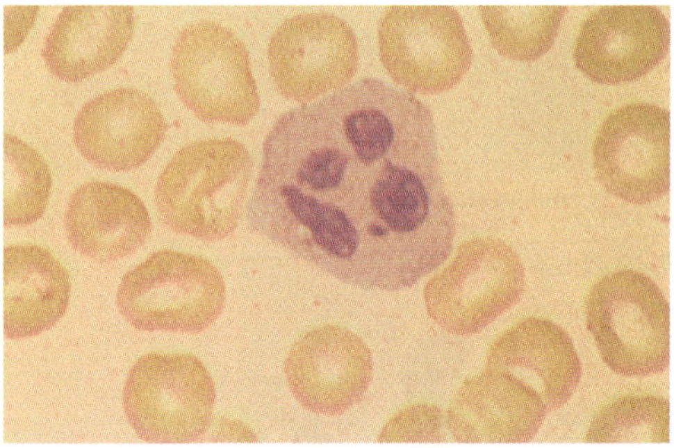

Figure 1-2 Polymorphonuclear leukocyte with multisegmented nucleus. *(Courtesy of Hans E. Grossniklaus, MD.)*

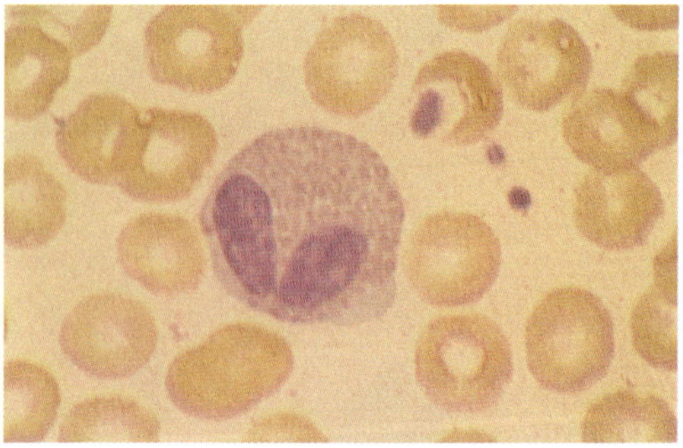

Figure 1-3 Eosinophil with bilobed nucleus and intracytoplasmic eosinophilic granules. *(Courtesy of Hans E. Grossniklaus, MD.)*

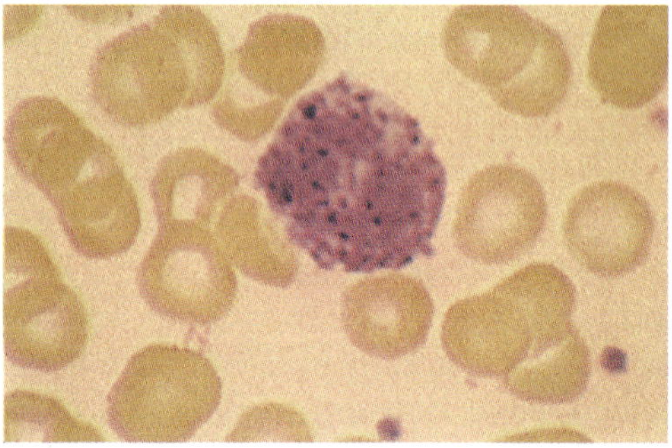

Figure 1-4 Basophil with intracytoplasmic basophilic granules. *(Courtesy of Hans E. Grossniklaus, MD.)*

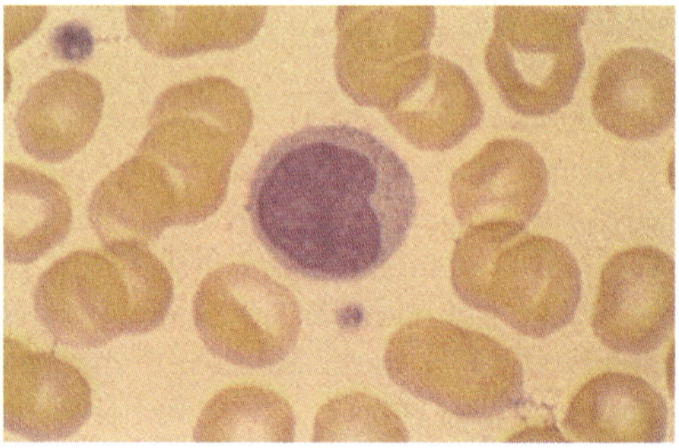

Figure 1-5 Monocyte with indented nucleus. *(Courtesy of Hans E. Grossniklaus, MD.)*

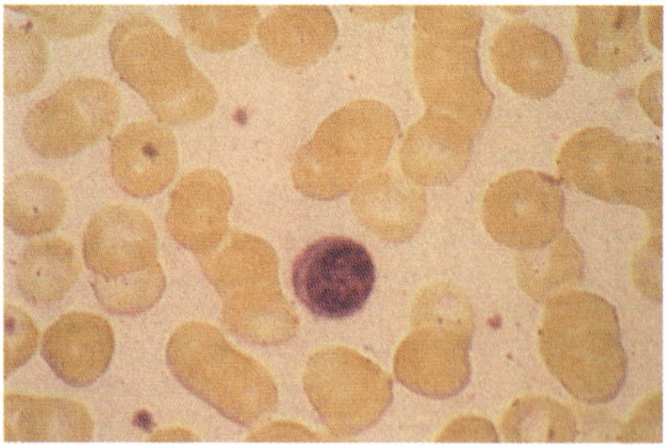

Figure 1-6 Lymphocyte with small, hyperchromatic nucleus and scant cytoplasm. *(Courtesy of Hans E. Grossniklaus, MD.)*

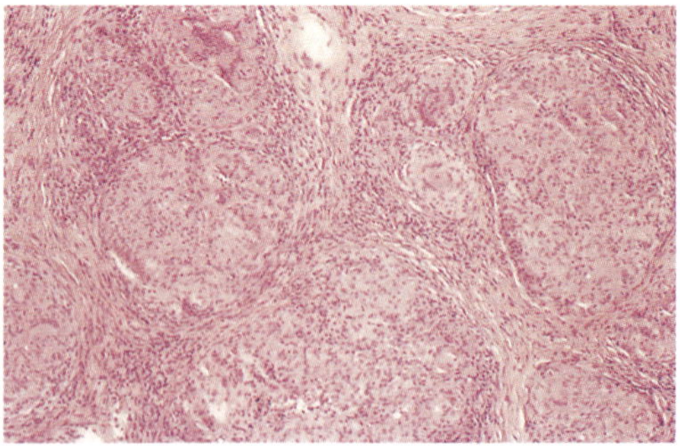

Figure 1-7 Noncaseating granulomas, or "hard" tubercles, are formed by aggregates of epithelioid histiocytes. *(Courtesy of Hans E. Grossniklaus, MD.)*

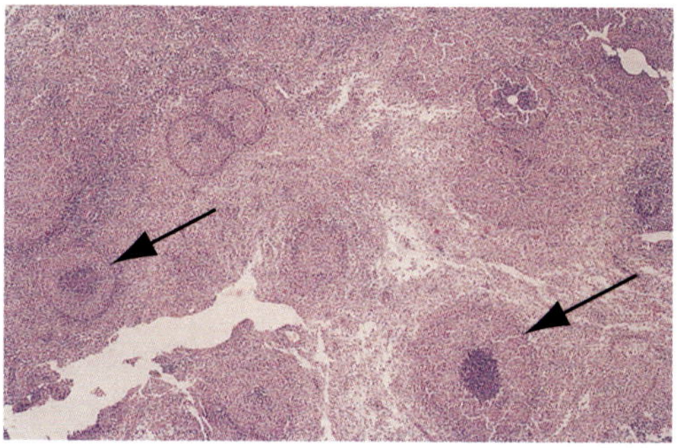

Figure 1-8 Granulomas with necrotic centers *(arrows)* are classified as caseating granulomas. *(Courtesy of Hans E. Grossniklaus, MD.)*

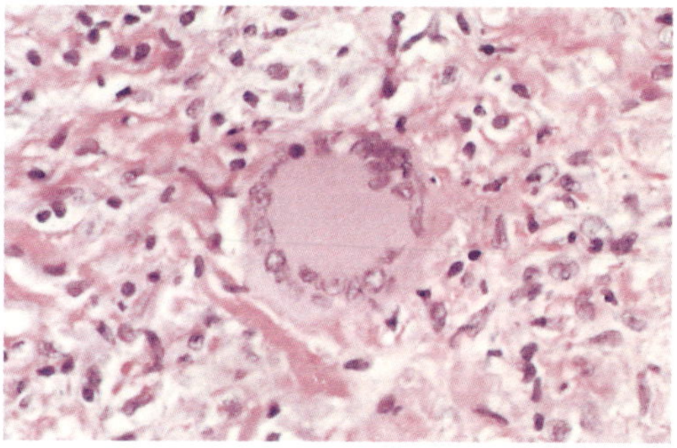

Figure 1-9 Langhans giant cell. Note peripheral arrangement of nuclei.

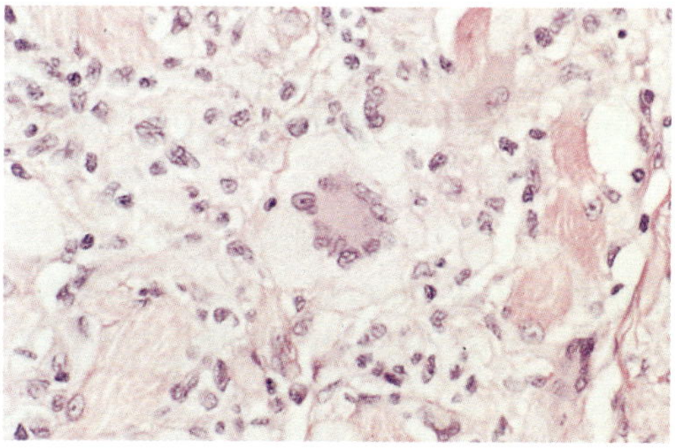

Figure 1-10 Touton giant cell. Note central eosinophilic cytoplasm and annulus of nuclei surrounded by lipid-filled clear zone.

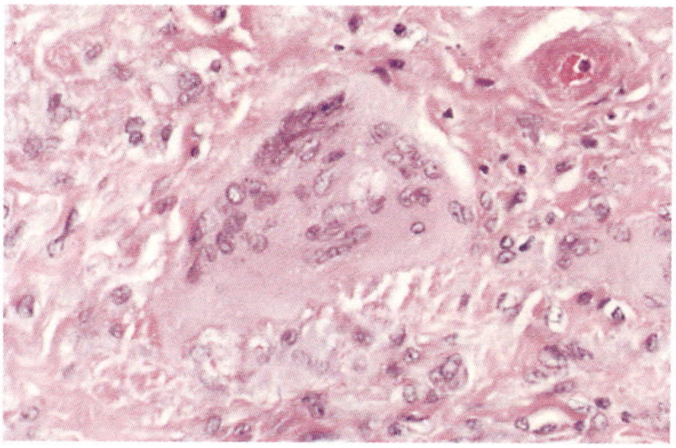

Figure 1-11 Foreign body giant cell. Note haphazardly arranged nuclei.

Lymphocytes are small cells with round, hyperchromatic nuclei and scant cytoplasm. Circulating lymphocytes infiltrate tissue in all types of chronic inflammatory processes. These cells terminally differentiate in the thymus *(T cells)* or bursa equivalent *(B cells)*. It is not possible to distinguish between B and T lymphocytes with routine histologic stains. B cells may produce immunoglobulin and differentiate into *plasma cells,* with eccentric "cartwheel," or "clockface," nuclei and a perinuclear halo corresponding to the Golgi apparatus. These cells may become completely distended with immunoglobulin and form *Russell bodies.* BCSC Section 9, *Intraocular Inflammation and Uveitis,* discusses the cells involved in the inflammatory process in depth in Part I, Ocular Immunology.

Degeneration and dystrophy

The term *degeneration* refers to a wide variety of tissue changes that may occur over time. Degenerative processes are not usually associated with a proliferation of cells; rather, there is often an accumulation of acellular material or a loss of tissue mass. Extracellular deposits may result from cellular overproduction of normal material or metabolically abnormal material. These processes may occur in response to an injury or an inflammatory process.

As used in this book, "degeneration" is an artificial category used to encompass a wide variety of disease processes. Various categories of diseases, such as those due to vascular causes, normal aging, and trauma, could be considered separately. However, in order to efficiently convey the hierarchical scheme used in this book, these causes are lumped under the rubric of "degeneration." *Dystrophies* are defined as usually bilateral, symmetric, inherited conditions that appear to have little or no relationship to environmental or systemic factors.

Degeneration of tissue may be seen in conjunction with other general disease processes. Examples include calcification of the lens (degeneration) in association with a congenital cataract (congenital anomaly); corneal amyloid (degeneration) in association with trachoma (inflammation); and orbital amyloid (degeneration) in association with lymphoma (neoplasm). The ophthalmic manifestations of diabetes mellitus can be classified as degenerative changes associated with a metabolic disease.

Neoplasia

A *neoplasm* is a stereotypic, monotonous new growth of a specific tissue phenotype. Neoplasms can occur in either benign or malignant forms. Examples found in particular tissues include

- adenoma (benign) versus adenocarcinoma (malignant) in glandular epithelium
- topography + *oma* (benign) versus topography + *sarcoma* (malignant) in soft tissue
- hyperplasia/infiltrate (benign) versus leukemia/lymphoma (malignant) in hematopoietic tissue

Some neoplastic proliferations are called *borderline* or *indeterminate,* because they are difficult to classify histologically as benign or malignant. Although most of the neoplasms illustrated and discussed in this text are classified as benign or malignant, the reader should be aware that tissue evaluation in a particular disease can give only a static portrait of a dynamic process. Table 1-1 summarizes the origin, general classification of benign versus malignant, and growth pattern of neoplasms found in various tissues.

The growth patterns described in Table 1-1 are shown in Figure 1-12. General histologic signs of malignancy include nuclear hyperchromasia and pleomorphism, necrosis, hemorrhage, and mitotic activity.

Table 1-1 Classification of Neoplasia

Tissue Origin	Benign	Malignant	Growth Pattern
Epithelium	Hyperplasia/adenoma	Carcinoma Adenocarcinoma	Cords Tubules
Soft tissue	Topography + *oma*	Topography + *sarcoma*	Coherent sheets
Hematopoietic tissue	Hyperplasia/infiltrate	Leukemia Lymphoma	Loosely arranged

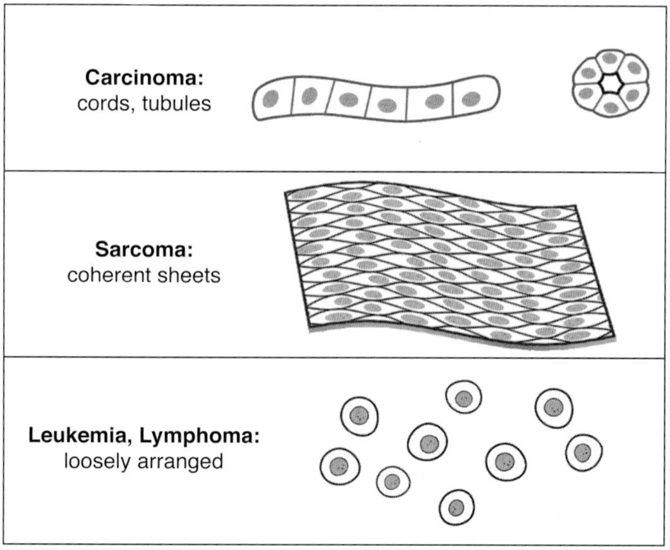

Figure 1-12 General classification and growth patterns of malignant tumors. *(Illustration by Christine Gralapp.)*

General Diagnosis

After considering the topography and disease process, the examiner formulates the general diagnosis. Recognizing a tissue *index feature* is a critical step in arriving at the general diagnosis. Index features are morphologic identifiers that help to define the disease process more specifically. Examples include the presence of pigment in a pigmented neoplasm and necrosis in a necrotizing granulomatous inflammation. The index feature should differentiate the particular specimen from others demonstrating the same general disease process. For instance, retinoblastoma and uveal melanoma are both intraocular malignant neoplasms; the former is a retinal malignancy, and the latter is a uveal tract malignancy. Other index features for distinguishing between these lesions could be "small, round, blue cell tumors" for the retinoblastoma and "melanocytic proliferation" for the melanoma. Although the most basic index features can be recognized without great difficulty, it takes experience and practice to identify subtle index features.

Differential Diagnosis

After the examiner has distinguished a key index feature and formulated a general diagnosis, developing a differential diagnosis is the next step before establishing a definitive or specific diagnosis. The differential diagnosis is a limited list of specific conditions resulting from pathologic processes that were identified in the general diagnosis. For instance, the differential diagnosis based on the features of noncaseating granulomatous inflammation of the conjunctiva includes sarcoidosis, foreign body, and fungal and mycobacterial infections. The differential diagnosis of melanocytic proliferation of the conjunctiva includes nevus, primary acquired melanosis, and melanoma.

Readers are encouraged to practice working through the hierarchical framework by verbalizing each step in sequence while examining a pathologic specimen. Chapters 5 through 15 of this book provide tissue-specific examples of the differential diagnoses for each of the 4 disease process categories. The expanded organizational paradigm is shown in Table 1-2.

Table 1-2 Organizational Paradigm for Ophthalmic Pathology

Topography
- Conjunctiva
- Cornea
- Anterior chamber/trabecular meshwork
- Sclera
- Lens
- Vitreous
- Retina
- Uveal tract
- Eyelids
- Orbit
- Optic nerve

Disease process
- Congenital anomaly
  - Choristoma versus hamartoma
- Inflammation
  - Acute versus chronic
  - Focal versus diffuse
  - Granulomatous versus nongranulomatous
- Degeneration (includes dystrophy)
- Neoplasia
  - Benign versus malignant
  - Epithelial versus soft tissue versus hematopoietic

General diagnosis
- Index feature

Differential diagnosis
- Limited list of conditions resulting from pathologic processes identified above

CHAPTER **2**

Wound Repair

General Aspects of Wound Repair

Wound healing, though a common physiologic process, requires a complicated sequence of tissue events. The purpose of wound healing is to restore the anatomical and functional integrity of an organ or tissue as quickly and perfectly as possible. The process may take many months, and the end result is typically a scar (Fig 2-1). A series of responses occurs following a wound:

- The *acute inflammatory phase* may last from minutes to hours. Blood clots quickly in adjacent vessels in response to tissue activators. Neutrophils and fluid enter the extravascular space. *Macrophages* remove debris from the damaged tissues, new vessels form, and fibroblasts begin to produce collagen.
- *Regeneration,* the replacement of lost cells, occurs only in tissues composed of cells capable of undergoing mitosis throughout life (eg, epithelial cells, fibroblasts). *Repair* is the process of restructuring of tissues that leads to a fibrous scar.
- In the final phase, *contraction* causes the reparative tissues to shrink so that the scar is smaller than the surrounding uninjured tissues.

Healing in Specific Ocular Tissues

Wound healing has variable mechanisms and consequences in different ocular tissues. The processes summarized in the following sections are also discussed in other volumes of the BCSC; to find more information on a particular topic, consult the *Master Index.* Also see the appropriate chapters in this volume for a specific topography.

Cornea

A corneal *abrasion,* or corneal (epithelial) erosion, refers to a wound that is limited to the surface corneal epithelium, although Bowman layer and superficial stroma may also be involved. Within an hour of injury, the parabasilar epithelial cells begin to migrate across the denuded area until they touch other migrating cells; then *contact inhibition* stops further migration. Simultaneously, the surrounding basal cells undergo mitosis to supply additional cells to cover the defect. Although a large corneal abrasion is usually covered by migrating epithelial cells within 24–48 hours, complete healing, which includes restoration of the full thickness of epithelium (5–7 layers) and re-formation of the anchoring

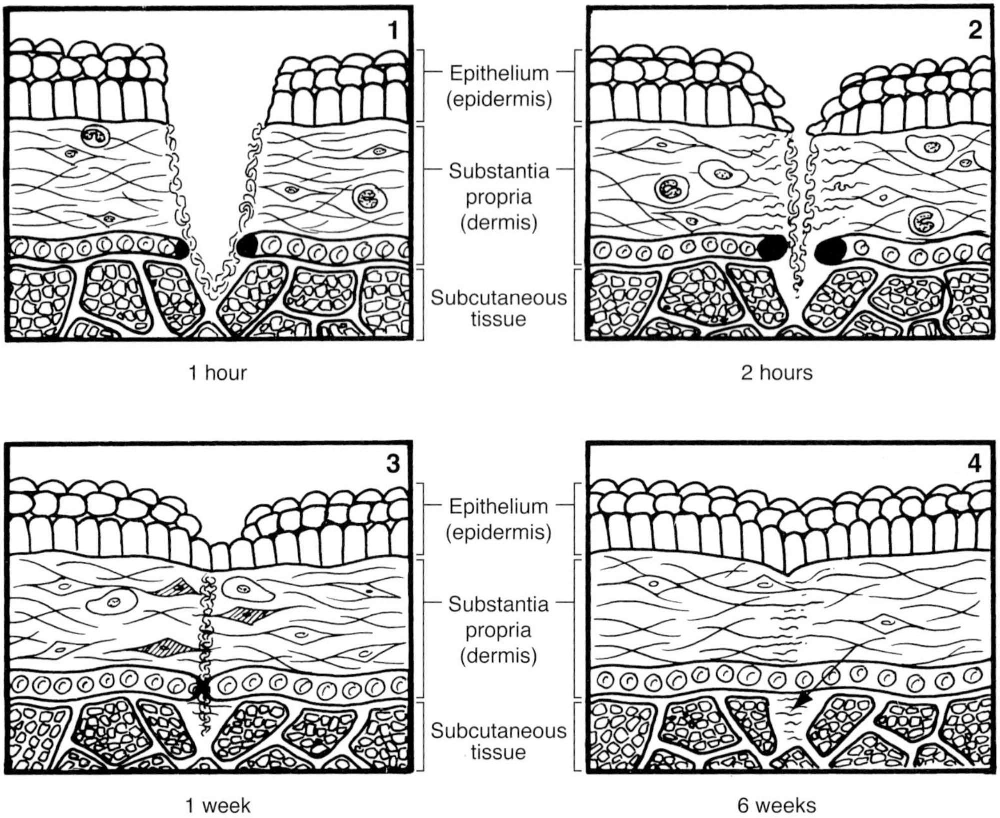

Figure 2-1 Sequence of general wound healing with an epithelial surface. **1,** The wound is created. Blood clots in the vessels; neutrophils migrate to the wound; the wounded edges begin to disintegrate. **2,** The wound edges are reapposed with the various tissue planes in good alignment. The epithelium is lost over the wound but starts to migrate. The stromal/dermal fibroblasts enlarge and become activated. Fibronectin is deposited at the wound edges. The blood vessels begin to produce buds. **3,** The epithelium seals the surface. Fibroblasts and blood vessels enter the wound and lay down new collagen. Much of the debris is removed by macrophages. **4,** As the scar matures, the fibroblasts subside. Newly formed blood vessels canalize. New collagen strengthens the wound, which contracts. Note that the striated muscle cells in the subcutaneous tissue do not regenerate and are replaced by a scar *(arrow).*

fibrils, takes 4–6 weeks. If a thin layer of anterior corneal stroma is lost with the abrasion, epithelium will fill the shallow crater, forming a facet.

Corneal stromal healing is avascular. Healing in the corneal stroma occurs via the process of fibrosis rather than the fibrovascular proliferation seen in other tissues (Fig 2-2). The avascular aspect of corneal wound healing is critical to the success of penetrating keratoplasty as well as the various forms of refractive surgery.

Following a central corneal wound, neutrophils arrive at the site via the tears (Fig 2-3), and the edges of the wound swell. Serum-derived healing factors are not present. The corneal matrix glycosaminoglycans, keratan sulfate and chondroitin sulfate, disintegrate at the edge of the wound. The stromal keratocytes, fibroblast-like cells (also known as fibrocytes), are activated and eventually migrate across the wound, laying down collagen

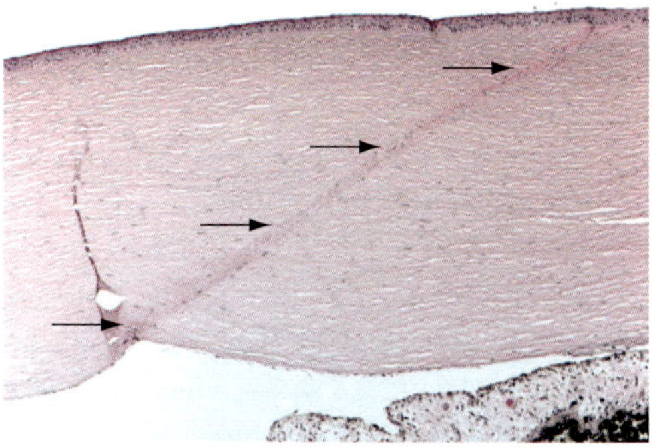

Figure 2-2 Full-thickness corneal wound *(arrows)* from cataract surgery. Note the mild hypercellularity of the wound due to fibrosis. There are no blood vessels in or around the wound. *(Courtesy of Nasreen A. Syed, MD.)*

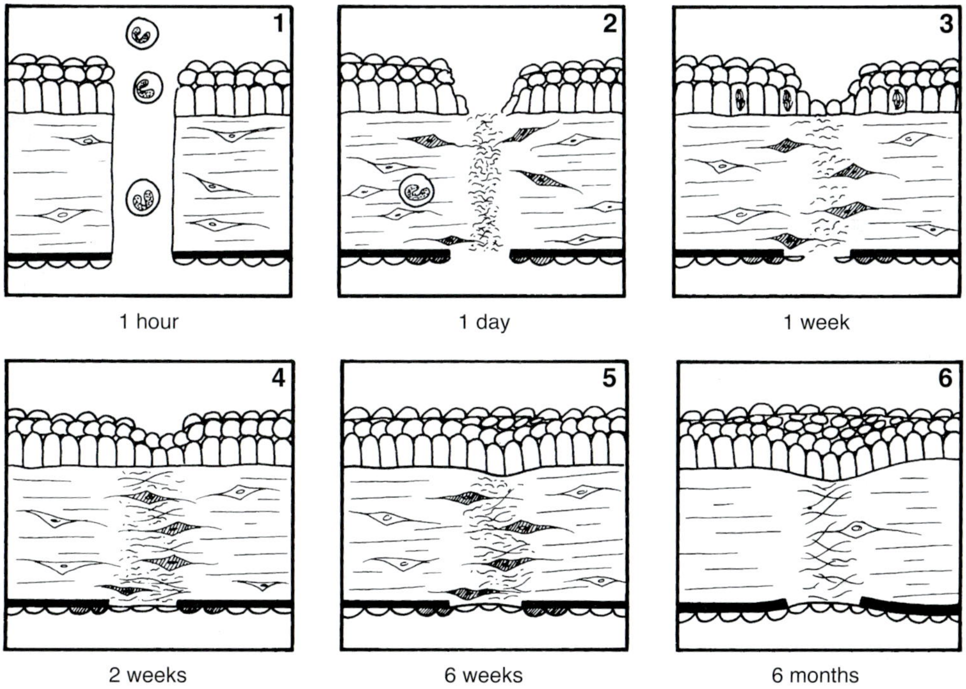

Figure 2-3 Clear corneal wound. **1,** Tears carry neutrophils with lysozymes to the wound within an hour. **2,** Immediately after closure of the incision, the wound edge shows early disintegration and edema. The glycosaminoglycans at the edge are degraded. The nearby fibrocytes are activated. **3,** At 1 week, migrating epithelial and endothelial cells partially seal the wound; fibrocytes begin to migrate and supply collagen. **4,** Fibrocyte activity and collagen and matrix deposition continue. The endothelium, sealing the inner wound, lays down new Descemet membrane. **5,** Epithelial regeneration is complete. Fibrocytes fill the wound with type I collagen and repair slows. **6,** The final wound contracts. The collagen fibers are not parallel with the surrounding lamellae. The number of fibrocytes decreases.

and fibronectin. The direction of the keratocytes and collagen is not parallel to the stromal lamellae. Hence, cells are directed anteriorly and posteriorly across a wound that will always be visible microscopically as an irregularity in the stroma and clinically as an opacity. If the wound edges are not well-apposed, the gap will not be completely filled by the proliferating keratocytes, resulting in focal stromal thinning.

Both the epithelium and the endothelium are critical to good central wound healing. If the epithelium does not cover the wound within days, the subjacent stromal healing will be limited, and the wound will be weak. Growth factors from the epithelium stimulate and sustain healing. The endothelial cells adjacent to the wound slide across the posterior cornea; a few cells are replaced through mitosis. The endothelium lays down a new thin layer of Descemet membrane. If the internal aspect of the wound is not covered by Descemet membrane, stromal fibrocytes may continue to proliferate into the anterior chamber as fibrous ingrowth, or the posterior wound may permanently remain open. In the late months of healing, the initial fibrillar collagen is replaced by stronger collagen. Bowman layer is not replaced when it is incised or destroyed. For example, the surface of a healed ulceration is covered by epithelium, but little of its lost stroma is replaced by fibrous tissue.

Sclera

The sclera differs from the cornea in that its collagen fibers are randomly distributed rather than laid down in orderly lamellae, and dermatan sulfate is its glycosaminoglycan. The sclera is relatively avascular and hypocellular. When stimulated by wounding, the episclera migrates into the scleral wound, supplying vessels, fibroblasts, and activated macrophages. The final wound contracts, creating a puckered appearance. If the adjacent uvea is damaged, uveal fibrovascular tissue may enter the scleral wound, resulting in a scar with dense adhesion between the uvea and the sclera. Indolent episcleral fibrosis produces a dense coat around an extrascleral foreign body such as an encircling scleral buckling element or a glaucoma tube shunt. Because the wound healing processes in the cornea and sclera are relatively avascular, the tensile strength of wounds is less than that of the native, undisturbed tissue. In certain clinical situations, modifying the healing process through the use of topical chemotherapy, such as 5-fluorouracil or mitomycin C, or via collagen cross-linking, may be desirable (see BCSC Section 10, *Glaucoma,* Chapter 8).

Uvea

In most circumstances, wounds of the iris do not stimulate a healing response in either the stroma or the epithelium. Though richly endowed with blood vessels and fibroblasts, the iris stroma does not produce granulation tissue to close a defect. In some circumstances, the pigmented epithelium may be stimulated to migrate, but that migration is usually limited to the subjacent surface of the lens capsule, where subsequent adhesion of epithelial cells occurs (posterior synechia). When fibrovascular tissue forms, it usually does so on the anterior surface of the iris as a neovascular membrane that may cover iridectomy or pupillary openings. This fibrovascular tissue may arise from the iris, the chamber angle, or the peripheral cornea.

The stroma and melanocytes of the ciliary body and choroid do not regenerate after injury. Macrophages remove debris, and a thin fibrous scar, which appears white and atrophic clinically, develops.

Dunn SP. Iris repair: putting the pieces back together. *Focal Points: Clinical Modules for Ophthalmologists.* San Francisco: American Academy of Ophthalmology; 2002, module 11.

Lens

Small tears in the anterior lens capsule are sealed by nearby lenticular epithelial cells. In circumstances that make the lenticular epithelium anoxic or hypoxic, such as posterior synechiae or markedly elevated intraocular pressure (IOP), a metaplastic response may occur, producing fibrous plaques intermixed with basement membrane.

Retina

The retina is made of terminally differentiated cells that typically do not regenerate when injured. Because the retina is part of the CNS, glial cells (eg, Müller cells, fibrous astrocytes), rather than fibroblasts, proliferate in response to retinal trauma. Surgical techniques to close openings in the neurosensory retina are successful when the retina and retinal pigment epithelium (RPE) are intentionally injured (eg, as a result of cryotherapy, photocoagulation) forming an adhesive, atrophic scar (see Chapter 11, Fig 11-28). Adhesion between the neurosensory retina and Bruch membrane develops according to the size of the original wound and the type of injury. The internal limiting membrane (ILM) and Bruch membrane provide the architectural planes for glial scarring; adhesions from the ILM to Bruch membrane may incorporate a rare residual glial cell, and variable numbers of retinal and RPE cells may be present between the membranes. If the wound has damaged Bruch membrane, choroidal fibroblasts and vessels may participate in the formation of the final scar. The end result is a metaplastic fibrous or fibrovascular plaque in the sub–neurosensory retina and sub-RPE areas. The RPE usually undergoes hyperplasia in such scars, causing the dense black clumps seen clinically in scars of the fundus.

Vitreous

The vitreous has few cells and no blood vessels. However, the collagen fibrils of the vitreous can provide a scaffold for glial and fibrovascular tissue from the retina and uveal tract to grow and extend into the vitreous to proliferate as membranes. These membranes usually have a contractile component, which can lead to retinal traction.

Eyelid, Orbit, and Lacrimal Tissues

The rich blood supply to the skin of the eyelids supports rapid healing. Approximately the third day after an injury to the skin, myofibroblasts derived from vascular pericytes migrate around the wound and actively contract, decreasing the size of the wound. The eyelid and orbit are compartmentalized by intertwining fascial membranes that enclose muscular, tendinous, fatty, lacrimal, and ocular tissues; these tissues can become distorted by scarring. Exuberant contraction distorts the muscle action, producing dysfunctional scars. The striated muscles of the orbicularis oculi and extraocular muscles are made of terminally differentiated cells that do not regenerate, but the viable cells may hypertrophy.

Histologic Sequelae of Ocular Trauma

Rupture of Descemet membrane may occur after minor trauma (eg, in keratoconus; Fig 2-4) or major trauma (eg, after forceps injury; Fig 2-5).

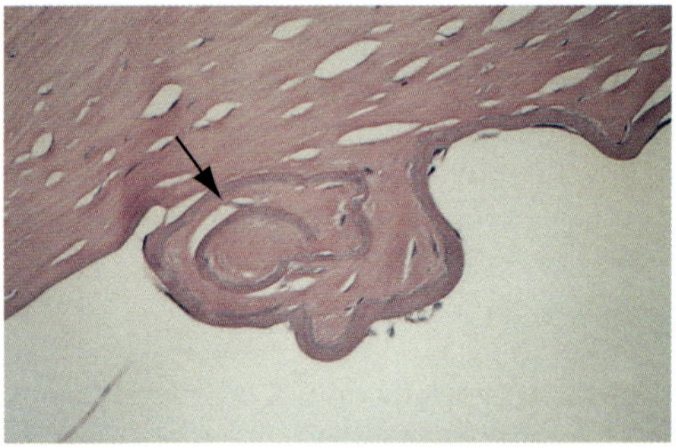

Figure 2-4 A break in Descemet membrane in keratoconus shows anterior curling of Descemet membrane toward the corneal stroma *(arrow)*. *(Courtesy of Hans E. Grossniklaus, MD.)*

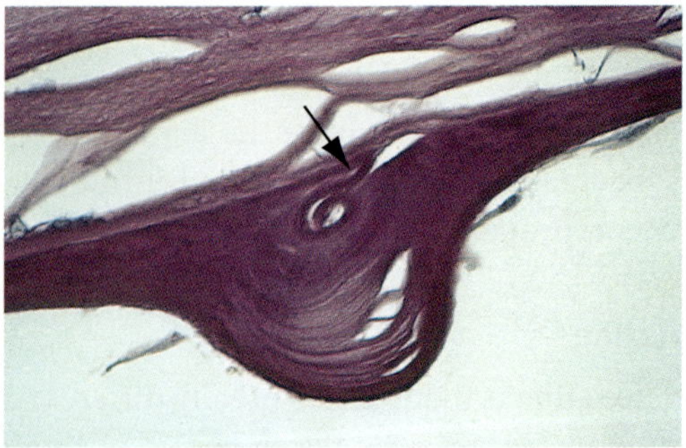

Figure 2-5 A break in Descemet membrane as a result of forceps injury shows anterior curling of the original membrane *(arrow)* and production of a secondary thickened membrane. *(Courtesy of Hans E. Grossniklaus, MD.)*

The anterior chamber angle structures, especially the trabecular beams, are vulnerable to distortion of the anterior globe. *Traumatic recession of the anterior chamber angle* occurs when there is a tear in the ciliary body between the longitudinal and circular muscles with posterior displacement of the iris root (Fig 2-6). Concurrent damage to the trabecular meshwork may lead to glaucoma.

Cyclodialysis results from disinsertion of the longitudinal muscle of the ciliary body from the scleral spur (Fig 2-7). This condition can lead to hypotony because the aqueous of the anterior chamber now has free access to the suprachoroidal space; in addition, because the blood supply to the ciliary body is diminished, the production of aqueous is decreased.

The uveal tract is attached to the sclera at 3 points: the scleral spur, the internal ostia of the vortex veins, and the peripapillary tissue. This anatomical arrangement is the basis of the evisceration technique and explains the vulnerability of the eye to expulsive choroidal hemorrhage. The borders of a dome-shaped suprachoroidal hemorrhage are defined by the position of the vortex veins and the scleral spur (Fig 2-8).

An *iridodialysis* is a tear in the iris at the thinnest portion of the diaphragm, the iris root, where it inserts into the supportive tissue of the ciliary body (Fig 2-9). Only a small amount of supporting tissue surrounds the iris sphincter. If that sphincter muscle is torn, the contraction of the remaining muscle will create a notch at the pupillary border.

A *Vossius ring* appears when iris pigment epithelial cells are compressed against the anterior surface of the lens, depositing a ring of melanin pigment concentric with the pupil.

If the lens capsule is disrupted, a *cataract* may form immediately. The capsule is thinnest at the posterior pole, the point farthest away from the lens epithelial cells. The epithelium of the lens may be stimulated by trauma to form an anterior fibrous plaque just inside the capsule. The lens zonular fibers are points of relative weakness; if they rupture, lens displacement occurs, either partial (subluxation) or complete (luxation). Focal areas of zonular rupture may allow formed vitreous to enter the anterior chamber.

Commotio retinae (Berlin edema) often complicates blunt trauma to the eye. Although it is most prominent in the macula, commotio retinae can affect any portion of the retina.

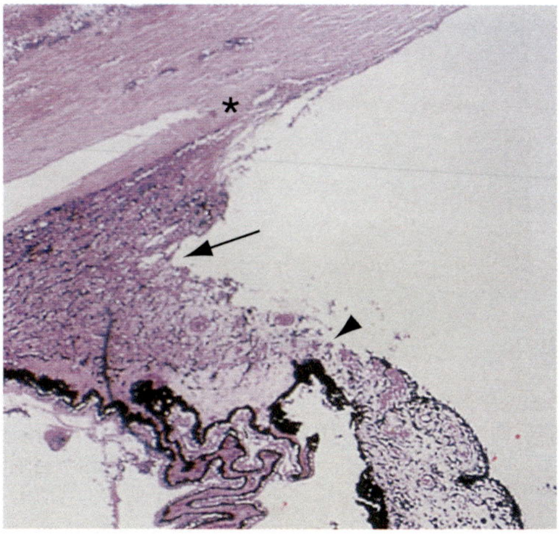

Figure 2-6 Angle recession due to a tear in the ciliary body in the plane between the external longitudinal muscle fibers and the internal circular and oblique fibers *(arrow);* the iris root is displaced posteriorly *(arrowhead).* Note the scleral spur *(asterisk).*

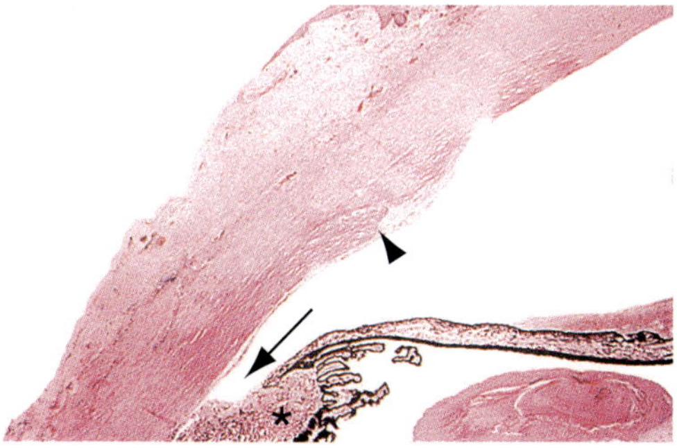

Figure 2-7 Cyclodialysis *(arrow)* resulting from the disinsertion of the ciliary body muscle *(asterisk)* from the scleral spur *(arrowhead). (Courtesy of Hans E. Grossniklaus, MD.)*

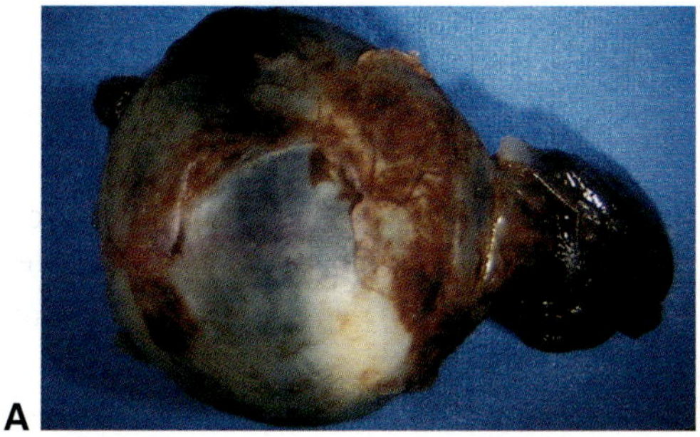

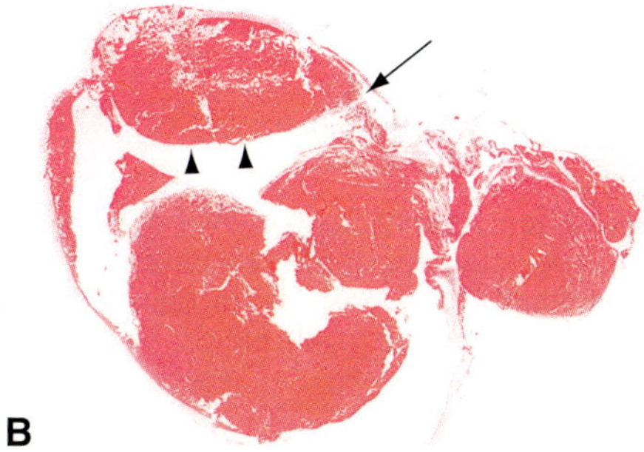

Figure 2-8 Suprachoroidal hemorrhage. **A,** This eye developed an expulsive hemorrhage after a corneal perforation. **B,** The intraocular suprachoroidal hemorrhage is dome shaped *(arrowheads),* delineated anteriorly by the insertion of the choroid at the scleral spur *(arrow). (Courtesy of Hans E. Grossniklaus, MD.)*

The retinal opacification seen clinically results from disruption in the architecture of the inner and outer segments of the photoreceptors.

Retinal dialysis is most likely to develop in the inferotemporal or superonasal quadrant. The retina is anchored anteriorly to the nonpigmented epithelium of the pars plana. This union is reinforced by the attachment of the vitreous base, which straddles the ora

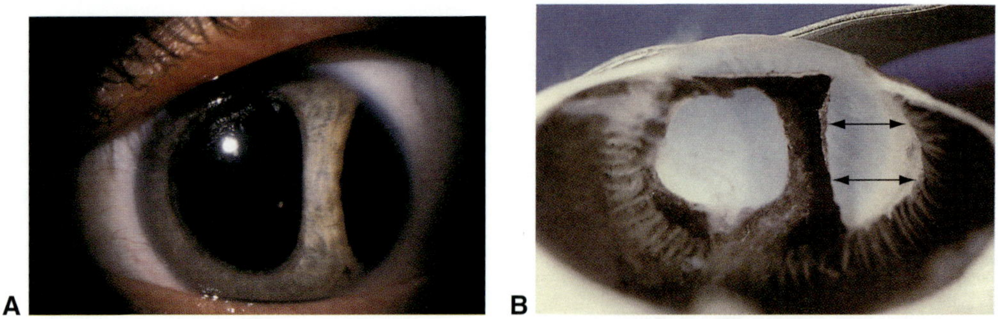

Figure 2-9 Iridodialysis. **A,** Clinical photograph of an eye showing iridodialysis, a disinsertion of the iris root from the ciliary body. **B,** Gross photograph showing a posterior view of iridodialysis *(arrows)*. *(Part A courtesy of Hans E. Grossniklaus, MD.)*

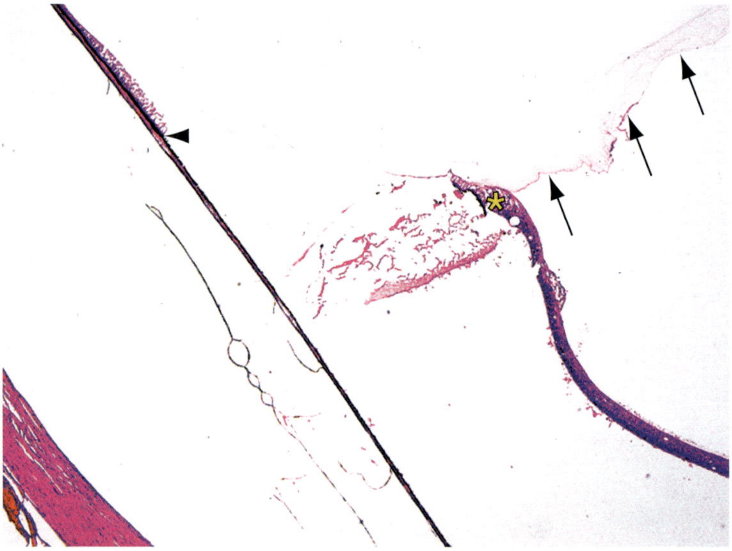

Figure 2-10 Retinal dialysis. This photomicrograph illustrates the separation of the retina from its normal attachment to the posterior edge of the nonpigmented epithelium of the pars plana *(arrowhead)* at the ora serrata *(asterisk)*. The vitreous base is still attached to the ora serrata *(arrows)*. *(Courtesy of Tatyana Milman, MD.)*

serrata. Deformation of the eye can result in a circumferential retinal tear at the point of attachment of the ora serrata or immediately posterior to the point of attachment of the vitreous base (Fig 2-10). The interface between necrotic and normal neurosensory retina is also vulnerable to retinal tears.

After a penetrating injury, intraocular *fibrocellular proliferation* may occur. This proliferation may lead to vitreous/subretinal/choroidal hemorrhage; tractional retinal detachment; proliferative vitreoretinopathy (PVR), including anterior PVR (Fig 2-11); hypotony; and ultimately phthisis bulbi (discussed later in this section). Formation of

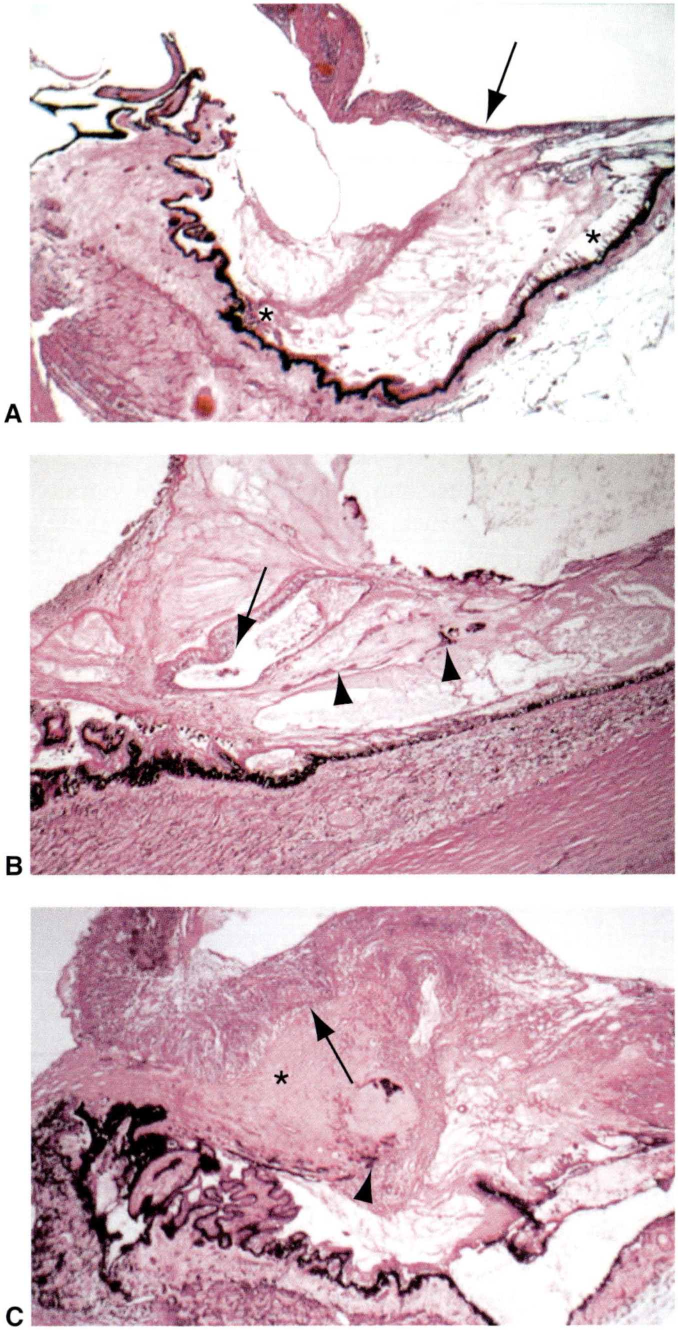

Figure 2-11 Anterior proliferative vitreoretinopathy (PVR). **A,** Traction of the vitreous base on the peripheral retina *(arrow)* and ciliary body epithelium *(asterisks)*. **B,** Incorporation of peripheral retinal *(arrow)* and ciliary body tissue *(arrowheads)* into the vitreous base. **C,** A condensed vitreous base *(asterisk)*, adherent retina *(arrow)*, and RPE hyperplasia *(arrowhead)*. *(Courtesy of Hans E. Grossniklaus, MD.)*

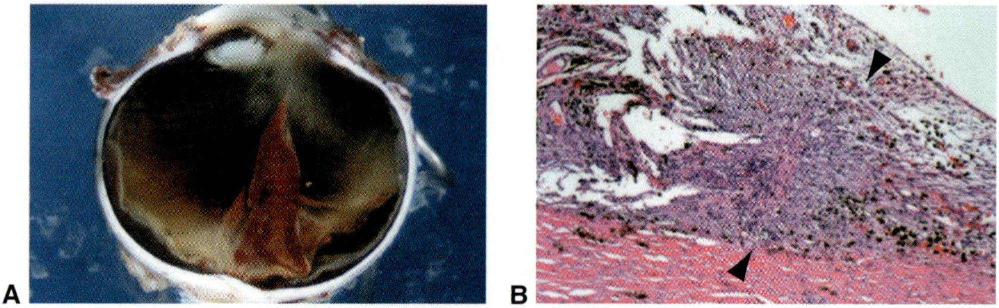

Figure 2-12 Focal posttraumatic choroidal granulomatous inflammation. **A,** An enucleated eye in which a projectile caused a perforating limbal injury that extends to the posterior choroid. **B,** Microscopic examination shows a focus of choroidal granulomatous inflammation *(between arrowheads).* *(Courtesy of Hans E. Grossniklaus, MD.)*

proliferative intraocular membranes may affect the timing of vitreoretinal surgery. Sequelae of intraocular hemorrhage include hemosiderosis bulbi, cholesterolosis, and hemoglobin spherulosis.

Rupture of Bruch membrane or a *choroidal rupture* may occur after direct or indirect injury to the globe. Choroidal neovascularization, granulation tissue proliferation, and scar formation may occur in areas where the choroid has ruptured or where there are disruptions in Bruch membrane. A subset of direct choroidal ruptures, those usually occurring after a projectile injury, may result in *focal posttraumatic choroidal granulomatous inflammation* (Fig 2-12). This inflammation may be related to foreign material introduced into the choroid. A chorioretinal rupture and necrosis is known as *chorioretinitis sclopetaria.*

Phthisis bulbi is defined as atrophy, shrinkage, and disorganization of the eye and intraocular contents. Not all eyes rendered sightless by trauma become phthisical. If the nutritional status of the eye and near-normal IOP are maintained during the repair process, the globe will remain clinically stable. However, blind eyes are at high risk for repeated trauma with cumulative destructive effects. Slow, progressive functional decompensation may also prevail. Many blind eyes pass through several stages of atrophy and disorganization before progressing to the end stage of phthisis bulbi:

- *Atrophia bulbi without shrinkage.* In this initial stage, the size and shape of the eye are maintained despite the atrophy of intraocular tissues. The following structures are most sensitive to loss of nutrition: the lens, which becomes cataractous; the retina, which atrophies and becomes separated from the RPE by serous fluid accumulation; and the aqueous outflow tract, where anterior and posterior synechiae develop.
- *Atrophia bulbi with shrinkage.* In this stage, the eye becomes soft because of ciliary body dysfunction and the progressive diminution of IOP. The globe becomes smaller and assumes a squared-off configuration as a result of the influence of the 4 rectus muscles. The anterior chamber collapses. Associated corneal endothelial cell damage initially results in corneal edema, followed by opacification from degenerative pannus, stromal scarring, and vascularization. Most of the remaining internal structures of the eye will be atrophic but recognizable histologically.

- *Phthisis bulbi* (Fig 2-13). In this end stage, the size of the globe shrinks from a normal average diameter of 24–26 mm to an average diameter of 16–19 mm. Most of the ocular contents become disorganized. In areas of preserved uvea, the RPE proliferates, and drusen may develop. In addition, extensive dystrophic calcification of Bowman layer, lens, retina, and drusen usually occurs. Osseous metaplasia of the RPE with bone formation may be a prominent feature. Finally, the sclera becomes markedly thickened, particularly posteriorly.

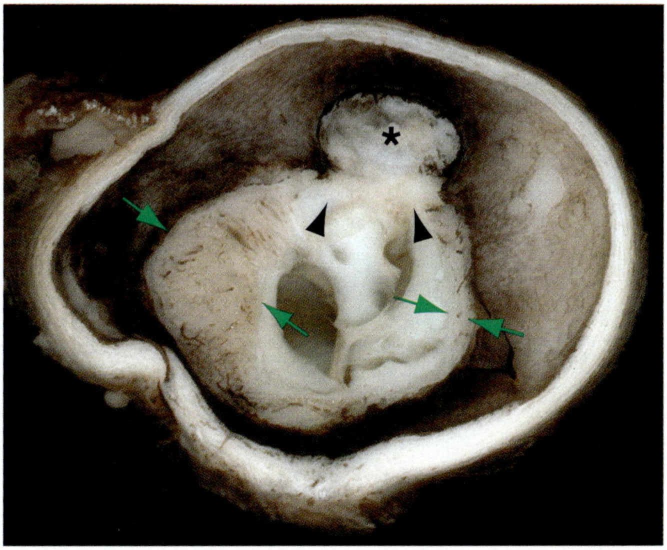

A

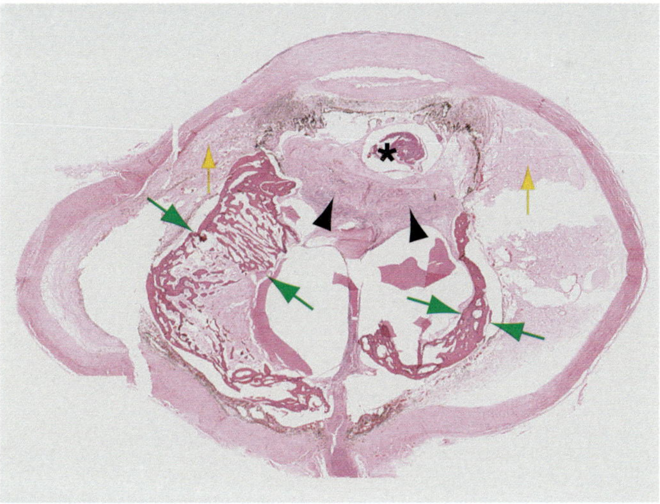

B

Figure 2-13 Phthisis bulbi. **A,** Gross photograph showing a globe with irregular contour, cataractous lens with calcification *(asterisk)*, cyclitic membrane with adherent retina *(arrowheads)*, and bone formation *(between green arrows)*. **B,** Photomicrograph demonstrating the histopathologic correlation with the gross photograph shown in part **A.** In addition, organized ciliochoroidal effusions are apparent histologically *(yellow arrows)*. *(Courtesy of Robert H. Rosa, Jr, MD.)*

CHAPTER 3

Specimen Handling

This chapter includes related videos, which can be accessed by scanning the QR codes provided in the text or going to www.aao.org/bcscvideo_section04.

Communication

Communication with the pathologist before, during, and after surgical procedures is an essential aspect of quality patient care. Standards for the technical handling of specimens and reporting of results have been developed; a few are available online at no cost. The ophthalmologist should provide a relevant and reasonably detailed clinical history when submitting the specimen to the laboratory. This history facilitates clinicopathologic correlation and enables the pathologist to provide the most accurate interpretation of the specimen. The final histologic diagnosis reflects successful collaborative work between clinician and pathologist.

If the pathologist and the ophthalmologist have an ongoing relationship, communication can usually be accomplished via the pathology request form and the pathology report. However, if malignancy is suspected or if the biopsy will be used to establish a critical diagnosis, direct and personal preoperative communication between the surgeon and the pathologist can be essential. This consultation allows the physicians to discuss the best way to submit a specimen. For example, the pathologist may wish to have fresh tissue for immunofluorescence staining and molecular diagnostic studies, glutaraldehyde-fixed tissue for electron microscopy, and formalin-fixed tissue for routine paraffin embedding. If the tissue is simply submitted in formalin, the opportunity to perform certain studies may be lost, resulting in a less definitive diagnosis. Communication between clinician and pathologist is especially important in ophthalmic pathology, in which specimens are often very small and require very careful handling. In some cases, careful selection of the surgical facility is necessary to ensure proper specimen handling. See Chapter 4, Table 4-1, for a preoperative checklist addressing the handling of ophthalmic pathology specimens.

Anytime a previous biopsy has been performed at the site of the present pathology, the clinician should request the sections of the previous biopsy and review them with the pathologist who will interpret the second biopsy. The surgical plan may be altered substantially if the initial biopsy was thought to represent, for example, a basal cell carcinoma when in fact the disease was a sebaceous carcinoma. In addition, when the case has been reviewed in advance, the pathologist will be able to interpret intraoperative frozen sections more accurately.

If substantial disagreement arises between the clinical diagnosis and the histologic diagnosis, the ophthalmologist should promptly contact the pathologist directly to resolve the discrepancy. For example, merely correcting the patient age on the pathology request form may change the interpretation of melanotic lesions of the conjunctiva from benign to malignant, or vice versa.

College of American Pathologists. Cancer protocol templates. www.cap.org/web/home/resources/cancer-reporting-tools/cancer-protocol-templates. Accessed March 7, 2016.

Jain D, Pernick N. Eye. PathologyOutlines.com. www.pathologyoutlines.com/eye.html. Accessed March 7, 2016.

Fixatives for Tissue Preservation

The most commonly used fixative is 10% neutral-buffered formalin. Formalin is a 40% solution of formaldehyde that stabilizes proteins, lipids, and carbohydrates and prevents enzymatic destruction of the tissue (autolysis). In specific instances, other fixatives may be preferred, such as glutaraldehyde for electron microscopy, ethyl alcohol for cytologic preparations, and Michel medium for immunofluorescence studies. Table 3-1 lists examples of commonly used fixatives.

Formalin diffuses rather quickly through tissue. Because most of the functional tissue of the eye is located within 2–3 mm of the surface, it is not necessary or desirable to open the eye. Opening an eye before fixation may damage or distort sites of pathology, making histologic interpretation difficult or impossible. It is generally desirable to suspend an eye in formalin in a volume of approximately 10:1 for at least 24–48 hours prior to processing to ensure adequate fixation. However, different institutions may use different protocols, so preoperative consultation is critical.

Table 3-1 Fixatives Commonly Used in Ophthalmic Pathology

Fixative	Color	Examples of Use
10% neutral-buffered formalin (NBF)	Clear	Routine fixation of all tissues (eg, eyelid, conjunctiva, globe, orbital)
Bouin solution	Yellow	Small biopsies (eg, gastrointestinal tissue, conjunctiva)
Absolute ethanol or methanol	Clear	Crystals (eg, corneal urate crystals)
Cytology fixatives (ethanol, methanol, or Saccomanno fixative)	Variety of colors	Liquid specimens or smears (eg, vitreous, aqueous, fine-needle aspirates, corneal smears)
Glutaraldehyde	Clear	Electron microscopy (eg, renal biopsy, corneal microsporidia)
Michel or Zeus transport medium*	Clear	Immunofluorescence (eg, conjunctival biopsy for mucous membrane pemphigoid)
Roswell Park Memorial Institute (RPMI) tissue culture medium*	Pink, salmon	Tissue culture (eg, orbital tumor for cytogenetics or flow cytometry)

*Not a true fixative, but prolongs tissue decomposition.

Orientation

Globes may be oriented according to the location of the extraocular muscles and of the long posterior ciliary arteries and nerves, which are located in the horizontal meridian. The medial, inferior, lateral, and superior rectus muscles insert progressively farther from the limbus. Locating the insertion of the inferior oblique muscle is very helpful in distinguishing between a right and a left eye (Fig 3-1). The inferior oblique inserts temporally over the macula, with its fibers running inferiorly. Once the laterality of the eye is determined, accurate location of ocular lesions is possible.

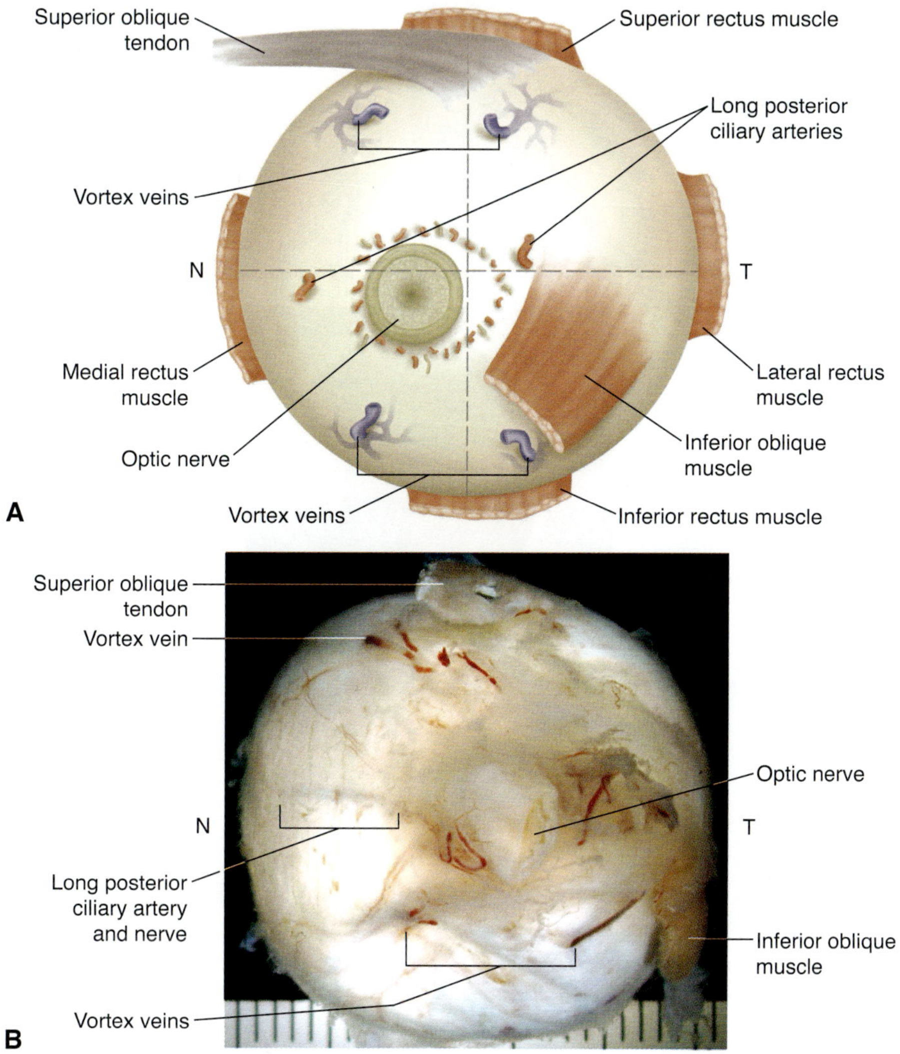

Figure 3-1 Posterior view of right globe. N = nasal, T = temporal. **A,** Diagram. **B,** Macroscopic photograph. Note that the posterior ciliary artery and nerve appear as a subtle blue-gray line as they pass through the sclera. This marks the horizontal meridian of the globe. Also note that the rectus muscle insertions are not present. The rectus muscles are typically incised at their scleral insertion during enucleation so that they may be attached to the orbital implant. *(Part A modified by C.H. Wooley from an illustration by Thomas A. Weingeist, PhD, MD; part B courtesy of Nasreen A. Syed, MD.)*

Gross Dissection

Prior to gross dissection, eyes are *transilluminated* with bright light. This helps to identify intraocular lesions such as tumors, which block the transilluminated light and cast a shadow (Fig 3-2A). The shadow can be outlined with a marking pencil on the sclera

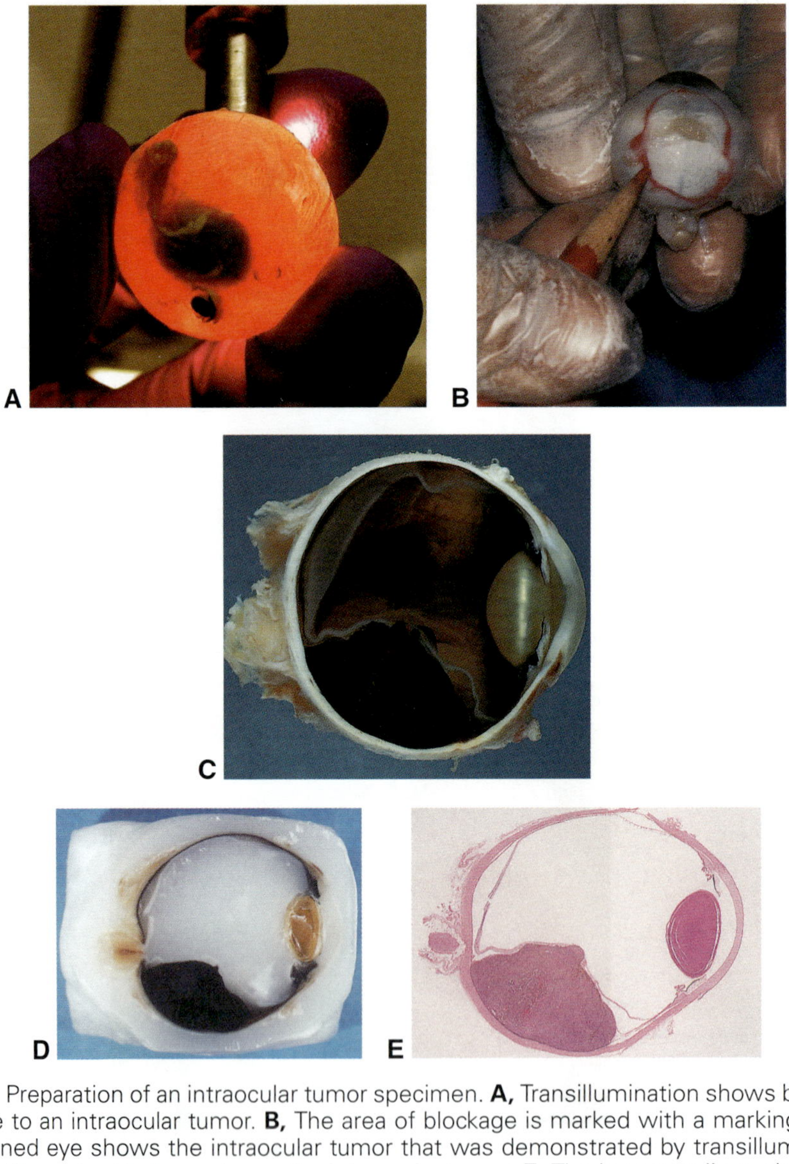

Figure 3-2 Preparation of an intraocular tumor specimen. **A,** Transillumination shows blockage of light due to an intraocular tumor. **B,** The area of blockage is marked with a marking pencil. **C,** The opened eye shows the intraocular tumor that was demonstrated by transillumination. **D,** The paraffin-embedded eye shows the intraocular tumor. **E,** The hematoxylin-eosin (H&E)–stained section shows that the maximum extent of the tumor demonstrated by transillumination is in the center of the section, which includes the pupil and optic nerve. *(Part A courtesy of Nasreen A. Syed, MD; part B courtesy of Hans E. Grossniklaus, MD.)*

(Fig 3-2B). This outline can then be used to guide the gross dissection of the globe so that the center of the section includes the maximum extent of the area of interest (Figs 3-2C to 3-2E).

The objective of gross dissection is to open the globe in such a way as to display as much of the pathologic change as possible on a single slide. The majority of eyes are cut so that the pupil and optic nerve are present in the same section, which is called the *pupil–optic nerve (PO) section.* The meridian, or clock-hour, of the section is determined by the unique features of the case, such as the presence of an intraocular tumor or a history of previous surgery or trauma. In routine cases, eyes with no prior surgery or intraocular neoplasm are typically opened in the horizontal meridian, which includes the macula in the same section as the pupil and optic nerve (Fig 3-3). Globes with a surgical or nonsurgical wound should be opened such that the wound is perpendicular to, and included in,

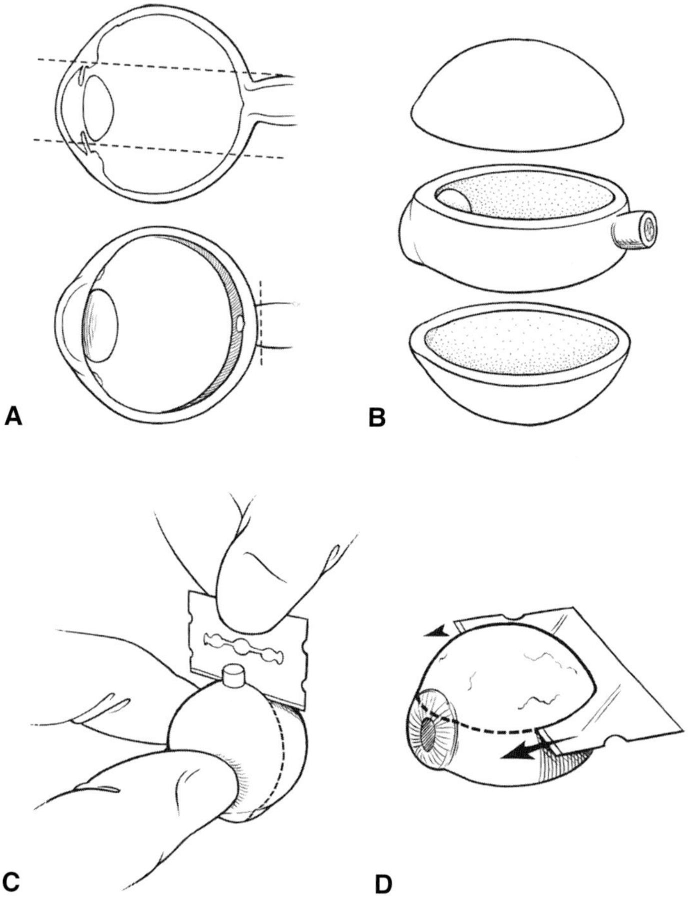

Figure 3-3 Gross dissection of a globe. **A,** The goal of sectioning is to obtain a pupil–optic nerve (PO) section that contains the maximum area of interest. **B,** Two caps, or *calottes,* are removed to obtain a PO section. **C,** The first cut is generally performed from posterior to anterior. **D,** The second cut yields the PO section. *(Illustration by Christine Gralapp.)*

the PO section. Globes with intraocular tumors are opened in a way (horizontal, vertical, or oblique) that places the center of the tumor, as outlined by transillumination, in the PO section (Video 3-1).

VIDEO 3-1 Gross dissection of the eye.
Courtesy of Ralph C. Eagle, Jr, MD.
Access all Section 4 videos at www.aao.org/bcscvideo_section04.

The globe can also be opened coronally with separation of the anterior and posterior segments, allowing a clinician's view of posterior segment pathology.

Processing and Staining

Tissue Processing

The infiltration and embedding process replaces most of the water in the tissue with paraffin. The organic solvents used in this process dissolve lipids and may dissolve some synthetic materials. Routine processing usually dissolves intraocular lenses made of polymethyl methacrylate (PMMA), acrylic, or silicone. Sutures made of silk, nylon, or other synthetic materials do not dissolve during routine processing. Embedding tissue in a paraffin block mechanically stabilizes the tissue, allowing for cutting very thin sections through the tissue.

The processing of even a "routine" specimen usually takes a day. Thus, it is unreasonable for a surgeon to expect an interpretation of a specimen sent for permanent sections to be available on the same day as the biopsy. Techniques for the rapid processing of special surgical pathology material are generally reserved for biopsy specimens that require urgent handling. Because the quality of histologic preparation after rapid processing is usually inferior to that of standard processing, it should not be requested routinely. Surgeons should communicate directly with their pathologists about the availability and shortcomings of these techniques.

Tissue Staining and Slide Preparation

Tissue sections are usually cut at 4–6 μm. The cut section is colorless except for areas of indigenous pigmentation, and various tissue dyes—principally hematoxylin-eosin and periodic acid–Schiff (PAS)—are used to color the tissue for identification. A small amount of resin is placed over the stained section and covered with a thin glass coverslip to protect and preserve it. Table 3-2 lists the histochemical stains commonly used in ophthalmic pathology.

Table 3-2 Stains Commonly Used in Ophthalmic Pathology

Stain	Material Stained: Color	Examples of Use
Hematoxylin-eosin (H&E)	Nucleus: blue Cytoplasm: red	General tissue stain (see Fig 3-2E)
Periodic acid–Schiff (PAS)	Glycogen and proteoglycans: magenta	Descemet membrane (see Fig 6-26E), lens capsule, Bruch membrane, goblet cells
Alcian blue	Acid mucopolysaccharide: blue	Cavernous optic atrophy (see Fig 15-10B)
Alizarin red	Calcium: red	Band keratopathy
Colloidal iron	Acid mucopolysaccharide: blue	Macular dystrophy (see Fig 6-22C)
Congo red	Amyloid: red-orange, apple green with polarized light (dichroism)	Lattice corneal dystrophy (see Fig 6-19C, D)
Crystal violet	Amyloid: magenta (metachromasia)	Lattice corneal dystrophy
Fite-Faraco	Some acid-fast organisms: red	*Mycobacterium leprae*
Giemsa, Wright-Giemsa	Some bacteria and parasites: blue	Conjunctival *Chlamydia* (eg, trachoma), corneal *Acanthamoeba*
Gram stain for tissue (Brown and Brenn [B&B], Brown and Hopps [B&H])	Gram-positive bacteria: blue Gram-negative bacteria: red	Bacterial infection (see Fig 6-7B)
Gomori or Grocott methenamine silver (GMS)	Fungal elements: black	*Fusarium* (see Fig 6-5B)
Masson trichrome	Collagen: blue Muscle: red	Granular dystrophy (see Fig 6-20C) Red deposits
Perls Prussian blue	Iron: blue	Fleischer ring
Thioflavin T (ThT)	Amyloid: fluorescent yellow-white	Lattice corneal dystrophy
Verhoeff–van Gieson (elastic)	Elastic fibers: black	Temporal artery elastic layer (see Fig 15-6B)
von Kossa	Calcium phosphate salts: black	Band keratopathy (see Fig 6-10C)
Ziehl-Neelsen	Acid-fast organisms: red	*Mycobacterium tuberculosis* and most other mycobacteria

CHAPTER 4

Special Procedures

This chapter includes related videos, which can be accessed by scanning the QR codes provided in the text or going to www.aao.org/bcscvideo_section04.

New technologies have contributed to improvements in the diagnosis of infectious agents, dystrophies, degenerations, and neoplasms, as well as to the classification of neoplasms, especially the non-Hodgkin lymphomas and sarcomas. Specifically, refinements in immunohistochemical, flow cytometric, molecular genetic, and cytogenetic techniques allow a more accurate diagnosis and more precise definition of biomarkers of value in risk stratification, prognosis, and targeted therapeutics.

The ophthalmic surgeon is responsible for appropriately obtaining and submitting tissue for evaluation and consulting with the ophthalmic pathologist. See Table 4-1 for a checklist of important considerations when submitting tissue for pathologic consultation.

Immunohistochemistry

A given cell can express specific antigens; pathologists take advantage of this property when making a diagnosis. In the immunohistochemical stains commonly used in ophthalmic pathology, a primary antibody binds to a specific antigen in or on a cell, and a secondary antibody linked to a chromogen then binds to the primary antibody (Fig 4-1). Depending on the chromogen selected for use, the color product of the chromogens generally used in ophthalmic pathology is brown (see Fig 4-1C) or red (see Fig 4-5B) in tissue sections. Red chromogen is especially helpful in working with ocular pigmented tissues and melanomas, because it differs from the brown melanin pigment in the uveal tissue or tumor.

The precise cell or cells that display the specific antigen can be identified using these methods. Many antibodies are used routinely for diagnosis, treatment, and prognosis:

- cytokeratins for diagnosis of lesions composed of epithelial cells (eg, adenoma, carcinoma)
- desmin, myoglobin, or actin for diagnosis of lesions with smooth muscle or skeletal muscle features (eg, leiomyoma, rhabdomyosarcoma)
- S-100 protein for diagnosis of lesions of neuroectodermal origin (eg, schwannoma, neurofibroma, melanoma)

Table 4-1 Checklist for Requesting an Ophthalmic Pathologic Consultation

Routine Specimens (cornea, conjunctiva, eyelid lesions)

1. Fill out requisition form with
   a. Sex and age of patient
   b. Location of lesion (laterality and exact location)
   c. Previous biopsies of the site and diagnosis
   d. Pertinent clinical history
   e. Clinical differential diagnosis
   f. Ophthalmologist phone and fax numbers
2. Submit specimen in adequately sealed container with
   a. Ample amount of 10% formalin (at least 5 times the size of the biopsy specimen)
   b. Label with patient's name and location of biopsy
3. Draw/map the site of biopsy for orientation of margins (eyelid lesions for margins, en bloc resections of conjunctiva, sclera, and ciliary body/iris tumors).

Frozen Sections

1. If possible, initiate communication with ophthalmic pathologist before requesting the section.
2. Fill out frozen section requisition form, specifying the reason for submitting tissue, such as
   a. Margins
   b. Diagnosis
   c. Adequacy of sampling
   d. Obtaining tissue for molecular diagnosis (eg, retinoblastoma, rhabdomyosarcoma, metastatic neuroblastoma) or flow cytometry
3. Map/diagram the lesion, indicating margins and orientation.
4. Label the tissue (ink, sutures) to orient according to the diagram (for margins).

Fine-Needle Aspiration Biopsy and Cytology

1. Initiate communication with ophthalmic pathologist before the biopsy to discuss
   a. Logistics of the biopsy
      i. Possible adequacy check during the biopsy (intraocular tumors)
      ii. Fixative to be used
      iii. Fresh tissue for possible molecular diagnosis
   b. Specific cytology form to be filled out

Flow Cytometry

1. Fresh tissue is critical.
2. Initiate communication with ophthalmic pathologist before the biopsy to discuss
   a. Recommendations on fresh tissue transport (no media versus nutrient media, such as RPMI)
   b. Size of the sample needed
   c. Geographic proximity to the laboratory

Molecular Techniques and Electron Microscopy

1. Initiate communication with ophthalmic pathologist before the biopsy to discuss
   a. Differential diagnosis
   b. Fixative (fresh vs alcohol vs glutaraldehyde vs other)
   c. Logistics of the biopsy
      i. Time and date (availability of specialized personnel)
      ii. Geographic proximity to laboratory

- HMB-45 and Melan A for diagnosis of melanocytic lesions (eg, nevus, melanoma)
- chromogranin and synaptophysin for diagnosis of neuroendocrine lesions (eg, metastatic carcinoid [see Fig 4-1C], small cell carcinoma)
- leukocyte common antigen for diagnosis of lesions of hematopoietic origin (eg, leukemia, lymphoma)

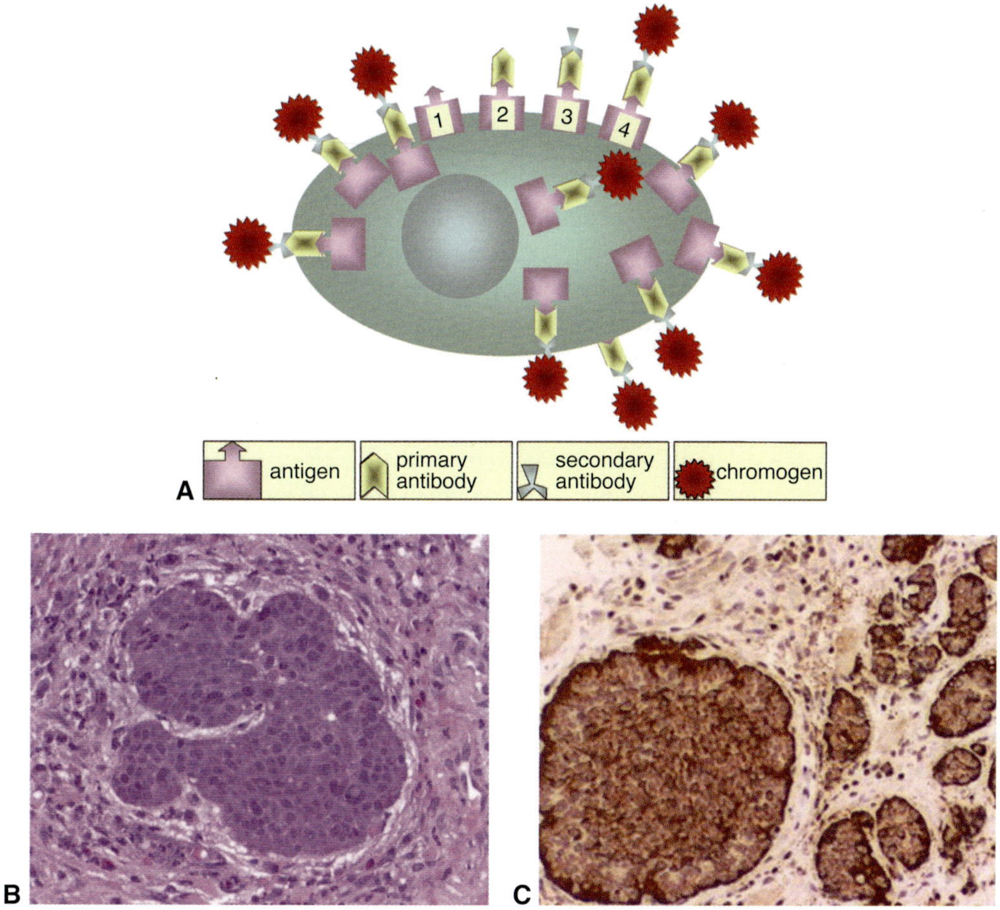

Figure 4-1 Immunohistochemistry. **A,** Schematic representation of the general immunohistochemistry method. (1), The cellular antigen is recognized by the specific primary antibody, (2), A secondary antibody, (3), directed against the primary antibody, reacts with the enzymatic complex to create the chromogen, (4), The final product allows the visualization of the cell containing the antigen. **B and C,** A metastatic carcinoid to the orbit seen by hematoxylin-eosin (H&E) staining **(B)** shows bland epithelial characteristics. In **C,** a chromogranin antibody highlights the neuroendocrine nature of the cells. *(Courtesy of Patricia Chévez-Barrios, MD.)*

- CD antigens for subtyping white blood cells
- BAP1 for prognosis of neoplasia (eg, uveal melanoma)
- Her2Neu (eg, receptor tyrosine-protein kinase erbB-2, also known as CD340 or proto-oncogene Neu) for prognosis and treatment of breast carcinoma
- Estrogen receptors for prognosis and treatment of neoplasia (eg, breast carcinoma)

These antibodies vary in their specificity and sensitivity. The specificities and sensitivities of new antibodies are continually being evaluated. In addition, automated equipment and antigen retrieval techniques are currently used to increase sensitivity and decrease turnaround time.

Flow Cytometry, Molecular Pathology, and Diagnostic Electron Microscopy

Flow Cytometry

Pathologists use flow cytometry (Fig 4-2) to analyze the physical and chemical properties of particles or cells moving in single file in a fluid stream (see Fig 4-2A, *a*). The most common use of flow cytometry in clinical practice is for immunophenotyping hematopoietic proliferations. This procedure may be performed on vitreous, aqueous, or ocular adnexal tissue. One example of flow cytometry is leukocyte immunophenotyping. For this procedure, the cells need to be fresh (unfixed). Fluorochrome-labeled specific antibodies bind to the surface of lymphoid cells, and a suspension of labeled cells is sequentially illuminated by a light source (usually an argon laser) for approximately 10^{-6} second (see Fig 4-2A, *b*). As the excited fluorochrome returns to its resting energy level, a specific wavelength of light is emitted (see Fig 4-2A, *c*), which is sorted by wavelength stream (see Fig 4-2A, *d*) and received by a photodetector (see Fig 4-2A, *e*). The flow cytometer then converts this signal to electronic impulses, which are analyzed by computer software. The results may be represented by a multicolored dot-plot histogram (see Fig 4-2, B and C).

Flow cytometry's advantage is that it actually shows the percentages of particular cells in a specimen. In addition, multiple antibodies and cellular size can be analyzed. For example, CD4 (helper T cells), CD8 (suppressor T cells), both $CD4^+$ and $CD8^+$, or either $CD4^+$ or $CD8^+$ may be displayed for a given lymphocytic infiltrate. Flow cytometry's disadvantages are its failure to show the location and distribution of these cells in tissue and the possibility of sampling errors. Depending on the number of cells in the sample and on clinical information, the flow cytometrist chooses the panel of antibodies to be tested. Flow cytometric data should therefore be used as an adjunct to morphologic hematoxylin-eosin (H&E) staining and immunohistochemistry interpretation.

Molecular Pathology

Molecular biology techniques are used increasingly in diagnostic ophthalmic pathology and extensively in experimental pathology (Table 4-2). More recently, the use of these techniques has expanded to include disease prognostication and treatment determination. Molecular pathology is used to identify tumor-promoting or tumor-inhibiting genes, such as the retinoblastoma gene (eg, via comparative genomic hybridization [CGH], *polymerase chain reaction* [PCR], or array CGH), and viral DNA or RNA strands, such as those seen in herpesviruses and Epstein-Barr virus (eg, via PCR or in situ hybridization [ISH]). Molecular pathology techniques have made it possible not only to recognize the presence or absence of a strand of nucleic acid but also to localize specific DNA sequences within specific cells (eg, via fluorescence in situ hybridization [FISH] or ISH). Two major techniques have markedly advanced our knowledge of developmental biology and tumorigenesis: PCR (and its variations) and microarray (and its subtypes).

Polymerase chain reaction

A common molecular biology technique is the PCR method, which amplifies a single strand of nucleic acid across several orders of magnitude, generating thousands to millions

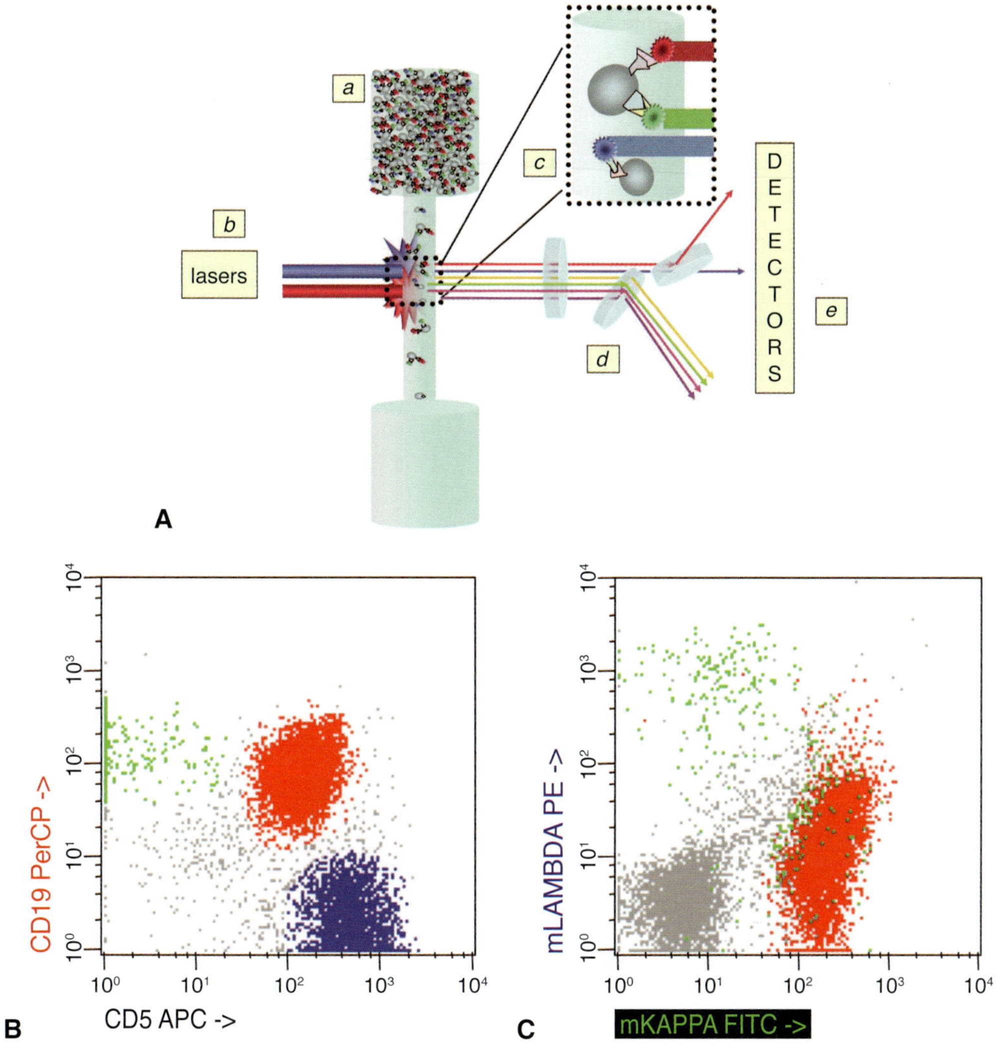

Figure 4-2 Flow cytometry. **A,** Flow cytometry analyzes particles or cells moving in single file in a fluid stream *(a).* Fluorochrome-labeled specific antibodies bind to the surface of cells, and a suspension of labeled cells is sequentially illuminated by a laser *(b).* As the excited fluorochrome returns to its resting energy level, a specific wavelength of light is emitted *(c),* which is sorted by wavelength *(d)* and received by a photodetector *(e).* This signal is then converted to electronic impulses, which are in turn analyzed by computer software. **B and C,** Flow cytometry scatter graphs showing a clonal population of $CD19^+$ kappa-restricted lymphocytes. Note that most of the $CD19^+$ *(red in part **B**)* cells fail to express lambda light chains; however, the cells do exhibit strong kappa expression *(red in part **C**). (Courtesy of Patricia Chévez-Barrios, MD.)*

of copies of a particular DNA sequence (Fig 4-3). This method relies on thermal cycles of repeated heating and cooling of the DNA sample for thermal denaturation (DNA melting) and enzymatic replication. The components required for selective and repeated amplification are *primers,* which are short DNA fragments that contain sequences complementary to the target region, DNA polymerase, and nucleotides. PCR's selectivity is due to the use of primers that are complementary to the DNA region targeted for amplification.

Table 4-2 Summary of Molecular Techniques Used in Diagnostic Pathology

Technique	Method	Advantages	Disadvantages
Comparative genomic hybridization (CGH)	Molecular cytogenetic method for analysis of copy number changes (gains/losses) in the DNA content of an individual, often in tumor cells. Uses epifluorescence and quantitative, regional differences in the fluorescence ratio of gains/losses vs control DNA to identify abnormal regions in the genome at a resolution of 20–80 base pairs	1. Detects and maps alterations in copy number of DNA sequences 2. Analyzes all chromosomes in a single experiment and does not require division of cells	Inability to detect mosaicism, balanced chromosomal translocations, inversions, or whole-genome ploidy changes
Polymerase chain reaction (PCR)	Amplification of a single strand of DNA (nucleic acid) based on thermal cycles of repeated heating and cooling of the sample for DNA melting and enzymatic replication of the DNA. Clinically used for early detection of cancer, hereditary diseases, and infectious diseases	Quality snap-frozen tissue (optimal) and archival paraffin-embedded tissue	1. Variable success rate of DNA extraction 2. Contamination with other nucleic acid material
Fluorescence in situ hybridization (FISH)	Chromosome region-specific, fluorescently labeled DNA probes (cloned pieces of genomic DNA) able to detect their complementary DNA sequences	Microfluidic chip allows automation and clinical use	Known type and location of expected aberrations
Reverse transcriptase-polymerase chain reaction (RT-PCR)	Amplifies DNA from RNA. Clinically used to determine the expression of a gene	Quality snap-frozen tissue (optimal) and archival paraffin-embedded tissue	1. Variable success rate of RNA extraction 2. Contamination with other nucleic acid material

Table 4-2 *(continued)*

Technique	Method	Advantages	Disadvantages
Real-time quantitative PCR (RT-PCR)	Measurement of PCR-product accumulation during the exponential phase of the PCR reaction using a dual-labeled fluorogenic probe	Direct detection of PCR-product formation by measuring the increase in fluorescent emission continuously during the PCR reaction	Variable success rate of RNA extraction
Multiplex ligation-dependent probe amplification (MLPA)	Amplification of multiple targets using only a single primer pair within a single PCR mixture to produce amplicons of varying sizes that are specific to different DNA sequences	Additional information may be gained from a single test run.	Targets must be different enough to form distinct bands when visualized by gel electrophoresis.
Next-generation sequencing (massively parallel sequencing)	Parallelization of the sequencing process, producing thousands or millions of sequences concurrently. Used in genome sequencing and resequencing, transcriptome profiling (RNA-seq), DNA-protein interactions (ChIP-sequencing), and epigenome characterization.	1. Ability to rapidly sequence the entire genome 2. Reduced reagent costs 3. Small amounts of starting material required 4. High precision with some methodologies	1. Short sequencing read lengths and higher error rates with some methodologies 2. Equipment can be expensive
SNP oligonucleotide microarray analysis (SOMA)	Type of DNA microarray used to detect single nucleotide polymorphisms (SNPs), the most frequent type of variation in the genome, within a population. Uses an array containing immobilized nucleic acid sequences and 1 or more labeled allele-specific oligonucleotide probes	1. SNPs, which are highly conserved between species and within a population, serve as a genotypic marker for research. 2. Able to detect copy-neutral loss of heterozygosity to uniparental disomy 3. Has huge potential in cancer diagnostics	Unable to detect mosaicism, balanced chromosomal translocations, inversions, or whole-genome ploidy changes

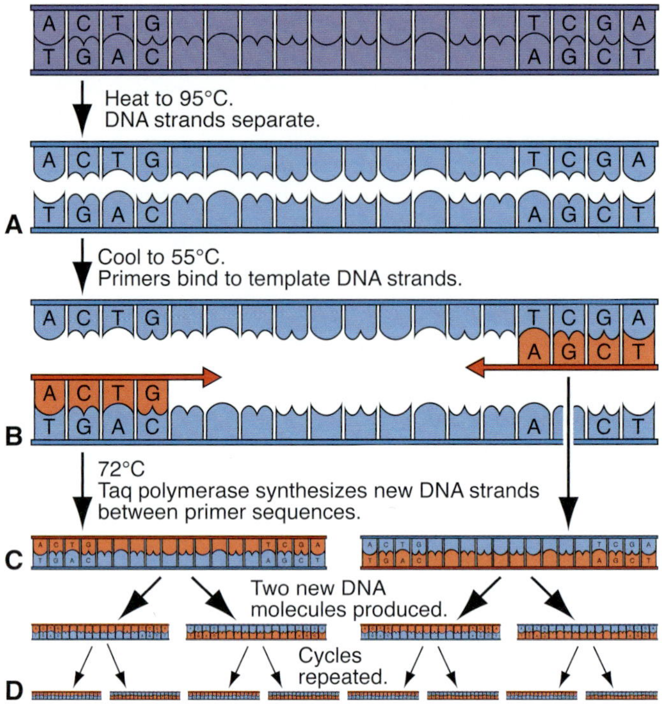

Figure 4-3 Polymerase chain reaction (PCR). **A,** PCR starts with a denaturing step in which DNA samples are heated to 95°C to separate the target DNA into single strands. **B,** The temperature is then lowered to 55°C to allow the primers to anneal to their complementary sequences. The primers are designed to bracket the DNA region to be amplified. **C,** The temperature is raised to 72°C to allow Taq polymerase to attach at each priming site and extend or synthesize a new DNA strand between primer sequences, producing 2 new DNA molecules. **D,** Step C is repeated multiple times to generate thousands to millions of copies. *(Courtesy of Theresa Kramer, MD.)*

PCR techniques have advanced considerably in recent years, and there are now approximately 20 PCR variations (see Table 4-2 for a few of these). The clinical relevance of detecting a PCR product depends on numerous variables, including the primers selected, the laboratory controls, and the demographic considerations. Thus, clinicians making a clinicopathologic diagnosis should use PCR mainly to derive supplementary information. See also Part III, Genetics, in BCSC Section 2, *Fundamentals and Principles of Ophthalmology.*

Microarray

Scientists and clinicians use microarrays to survey the expression of thousands of genes in a single assay, the output of which is called a *gene expression profile.* Microarray technology can help these scientists and clinicians try to understand fundamental aspects of growth and development, to explore the molecular mechanisms underlying normal and dysfunctional biological processes, and to elucidate the genetic causes of many human diseases. Some of the different types of microarrays available are DNA microarrays, microRNA microarrays (MMChips), protein microarrays, tissue microarrays (Fig 4-4), cellular (or transfection) microarrays, antibody microarrays, and carbohydrate (glycoarray) microarrays.

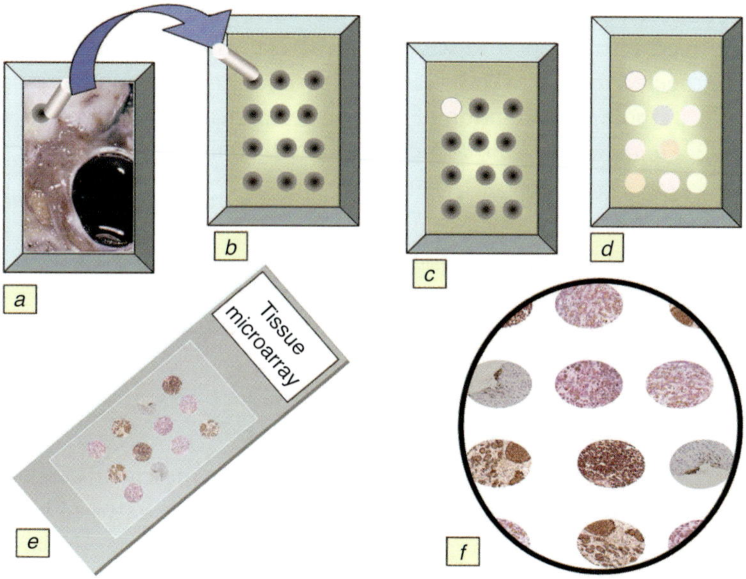

Figure 4-4 Tissue microarrays are constructed with small core biopsies of different tumors/ tissues. A core is obtained from the donor paraffin block of the tumor *(a)*. A recipient paraffin block is prepared, creating empty cores *(b)*. The cores are incorporated into the slots *(c)* until all are occupied *(d)*. Glass slides are prepared and stained with a selected antibody *(e)*. Microscopic examination reveals the different staining patterns of each core *(f)*. *(Courtesy of Patricia Chévez-Barrios, MD.)*

The basic process underlying all of the DNA microarray platforms is straightforward: a glass slide or chip is spotted or "arrayed" with oligonucleotides or DNA fragments (called *probes*) that represent specific gene-coding regions. Fluorescently or chemiluminescently labeled purified cDNA or cRNA (called *target*) is hybridized to the arrayed slide or chip. After the chip is washed, the raw data are obtained by laser scanning, entered into a database (some public, others mined), and analyzed by statistical methods.

An example of one of these microarray platforms is a low-density DNA microarray. Although DNA microarrays were initially developed to quantify the expression of a limited number of genes of clinical relevance, the technology has also been applied to tumor diagnosis and tumor-acquired drug resistance. Validating the results of microarray experiments is a critical step in the analysis of gene expression. Quantitative real-time PCR is the chosen method for validating gene-expression profiling.

Clinical use of PCR and microarray

Routine clinical use of PCR and microarray has been traditionally limited to the diagnosis of leukemias, lymphomas, soft-tissue neoplasms, and tumors with nondiagnostic histopathology results. These methodologies have also been increasingly implemented in the detection of infectious agents (eg, the herpesvirus family), in tumor prognostication (eg, uveal melanoma), and in detection of genetic alterations that are amenable to targeted therapies (eg, cutaneous melanoma and hematologic malignancies). Some current commercial microarray and PCR platforms can now be used to assign biopsy-sized tumor samples to 1 of 2 distinct molecular classes, based on gene expression analysis that distinguishes low-grade tumors from high-grade tumors.

The selection of commercially available microarray and PCR kits is growing rapidly. The continued refinement and wider commercial availability of molecular genetic techniques is expected to lead to progressive integration of these modalities into clinical practice and the pathologic evaluation of biopsy specimens. See also Part III, Genetics, in BCSC Section 2, *Fundamentals and Principles of Ophthalmology.*

Khong JJ, Moore S, Prabhakaran VC, Selva D. Genetic testing in orbital tumors. *Orbit.* 2009; 28(2–3):88–97.

Liu L, Li Y, Li S, et al. Comparison of next-generation sequencing systems [epub ahead of print July 5, 2012]. *J Biomed Biotechnol.* doi: 10.1155/2012/251364.

Vaziri K, Schwartz SG, Kishor K, Flynn HW Jr. Endophthalmitis: state of the art. *Clin Ophthalmol.* 2015;9:95–108.

Diagnostic Electron Microscopy

Diagnostic electron microscopy (DEM) is primarily used to indicate the cell of origin of a tumor of questionable differentiation, rather than to distinguish between benign and malignant processes. Although immunopathologic studies are less expensive and performed more rapidly than DEM, DEM complements immunopathologic studies in some cases. The surgeon should consult with the pathologist before surgery to determine whether DEM should play a role in the study of a particular tissue specimen.

Special Techniques

Fine-Needle Aspiration Biopsy

Intraocular fine-needle aspiration biopsy (FNAB) may be useful in distinguishing between primary uveal tumors and metastases. In cases of suspected uveal melanoma, biopsy specimens can undergo genetic analysis to identify prognostic chromosomal abnormalities and gene expression profiling patterns. Intraocular FNAB has also been utilized in the diagnosis of primary intraocular lymphoma. The biopsy specimens can undergo flow cytometric analysis, immunocytologic analysis, cytokine analysis, or molecular biological analysis (using PCR on both fixed and nonfixed material). Special fixatives are used for cytology specimens. See also Chapters 17 and 20 in this volume.

The procedure is performed under direct visualization through a dilated pupil, transvitreally (Video 4-1) or transclerally (Video 4-2). Iris tumors may be accessible for FNAB during slit-lamp biomicroscopy. FNAB alone may reliably predict the prognosis of a uveal melanoma. Intraocular FNAB may also enable tumor cells to escape the eye; this possibility is a controversial topic. In general, properly performed, FNAB does not pose a significant risk for seeding a tumor; however, retinoblastoma is a notable exception. FNAB of a possible retinoblastoma lesion, if indicated, should be performed by an *ophthalmic oncologist* with experience in making the diagnosis and performing the procedure.

VIDEO 4-1 Transvitreal fine-needle aspiration biopsy.
Courtesy of Thomas Aaberg, Jr, MD.
Access all Section 4 videos at www.aao.org/bcscvideo_section04.

VIDEO 4-2 Transscleral fine-needle aspiration biopsy.
Courtesy of Thomas Aaberg, Jr, MD.

The cells obtained through FNAB can be processed through cytospin of fluid or preparation of a cell block (Fig 4-5). A cell block allows the pathologist to employ special stains, immunohistochemistry, ISH, microarray, and gene expression profiling, if needed.

Some orbital surgeons have used FNAB when diagnosing orbital lesions, especially presumed metastases to the orbit and optic nerve tumors (Video 4-3). However, FNAB of orbital masses may not adequately sample all representative areas of the tumor, because it is difficult to make several passes at different angles through an intraorbital tumor. Specific indications for when to perform intraocular or intraorbital FNAB are beyond the scope of this discussion, but some of these indications are discussed in Chapters 16 and 20 in Part II of this book, Intraocular Tumors: Clinical Aspects. Ophthalmic FNAB should be performed only when an ophthalmic pathologist or cytologist experienced in preparing and interpreting the specimens is available.

VIDEO 4-3 Orbital fine-needle aspiration biopsy.
Courtesy of Jasmine Francis, MD.

Eide N, Walaas L. Fine-needle aspiration biopsy and other biopsies in suspected intraocular malignant disease: a review. *Acta Ophthalmol.* 2009;87(6):588–601.

Frozen Section

Permanent sections (tissue that is processed through alcohols and xylenes after fixation, embedded in paraffin, and sectioned) are always preferred in ophthalmic pathology because of the inherent small size of the samples. If the lesion is too small, it could be lost during frozen sectioning. A frozen section (tissue that is snap-frozen and immediately sectioned in a cryostat) is indicated when the results of the study will affect management of the patient

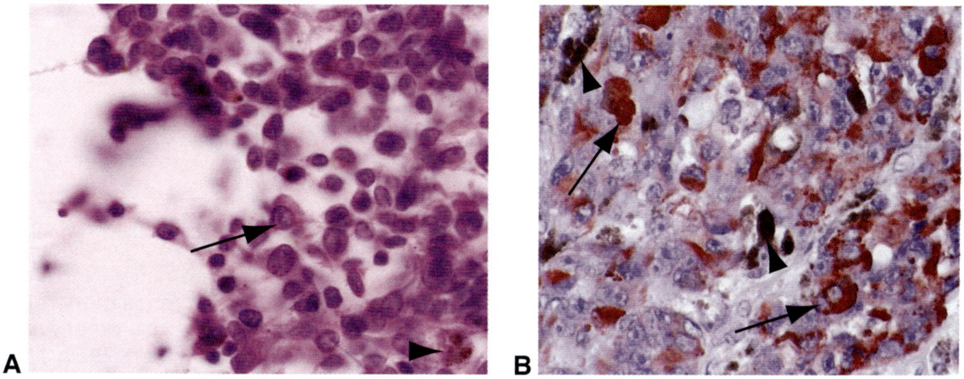

Figure 4-5 Fine-needle aspiration biopsy (FNAB) of choroidal tumor. **A,** Cytologic liquid-based preparation displays prominent nucleoli *(arrow)* and some brown pigment *(arrowhead)* suggestive of melanoma. **B,** Cell block of the aspirated cells, stained with HMB-45 using a red chromogen, is positive, confirming the diagnosis of melanoma. Notice the difference between the red chromogen *(arrows)* and the brown melanin *(arrowheads)*. *(Courtesy of Patricia Chévez-Barrios, MD.)*

in the operating room. For example, the most frequent indication for a frozen section is to determine whether the resection margins are free of tumor, especially in eyelid carcinomas. When tissue is submitted for margin evaluation, appropriate orientation of the specimen, correlated with documentation (through drawings of the excision site, labeled margins, or margins of the excised tissue that are tagged with sutures or other markers) is crucial.

Two techniques can be used for assessing the margins in eyelid carcinomas (eg, basal cell carcinoma, squamous cell carcinoma, and sebaceous carcinoma): routine frozen sections (as discussed previously) and Mohs micrographic surgery (Fig 4-6). Mohs surgery

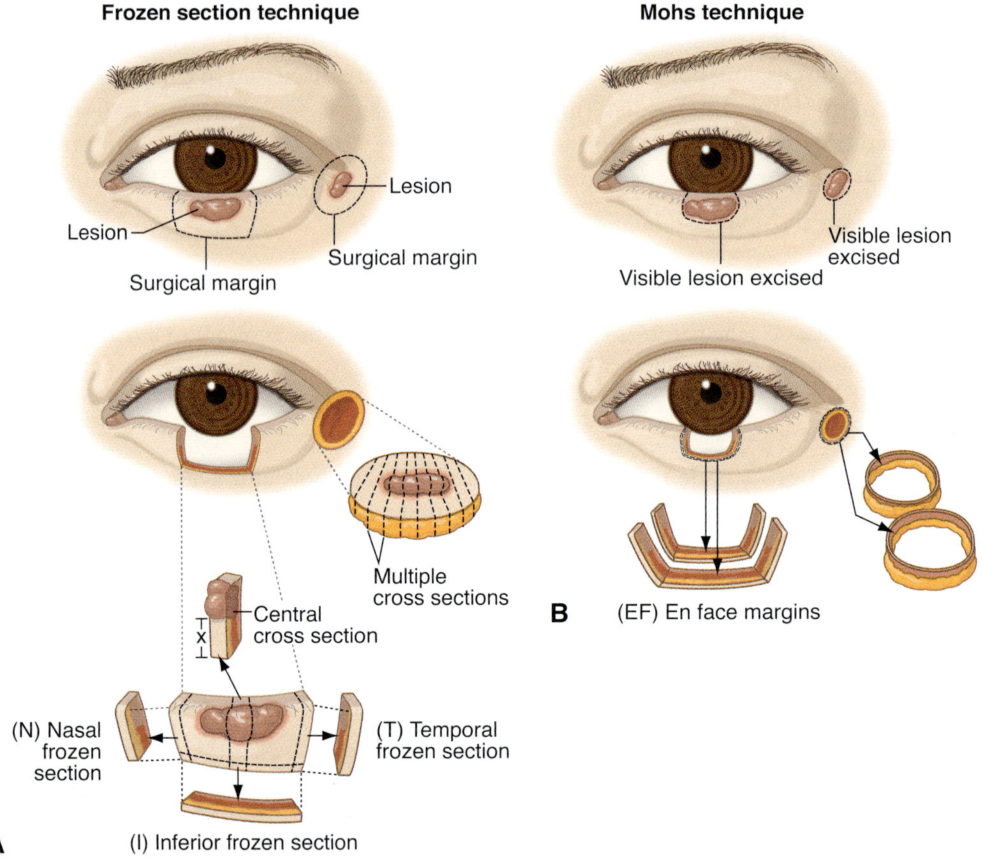

Figure 4-6 Frozen section and Mohs micrographic surgery techniques. **A,** To prepare a frozen section, the surgeon excises lesions with a surgical margin. For an eyelid margin lesion, the surgeon performs a wedge eyelid resection. The pathologist samples the nasal (N), temporal (T), and inferior margins. A central cross section (C) demonstrates the distance of the tumor from the inferior surgical margin. Similarly, an elliptical excision of the tumor can be evaluated by the bread-loaf technique in which multiple cross sections (C) are prepared. **B,** In Mohs micrographic surgery performed on an eyelid margin tumor, the surgeon excises the visible lesion. Then, additional thin shavings of tissue are prepared from the bed of the residual defect, allowing the surgeon to evaluate en face margins (EF). In another variation of Mohs surgery, the surgeon performs an elliptical excision of the visible tumor. Frozen en face (EF) sections are obtained from the undersurface and the edges of the excised lesion. The tumor locations are marked on a map for a subsequent second-stage excision. *(Illustration developed by Tatyana Milman, MD, and rendered by Mark Miller.)*

preserves tissue while obtaining free margins. Eyelid lesions, especially those located in the canthal areas, require tissue conservation to maintain adequate cosmetic and functional results.

Other frequent indications for frozen sections are to determine whether the surgeon has obtained, through biopsy, enough representative material for diagnosis (especially of metastasis) and to submit fresh tissue for flow cytometry and molecular genetics (eg, cancers). Frozen sections are a time-intensive and costly process and should be used with discretion.

See the section on eyelid disorders in BCSC Section 7, *Orbit, Eyelids, and Lacrimal System,* for more information.

Chévez-Barrios P. Frozen section diagnosis and indications in ophthalmic pathology. *Arch Pathol Lab Med.* 2005;129(12):1626–1634.

CHAPTER 5

Conjunctiva

Topography

The conjunctiva is a mucous membrane that lines the posterior surface of the eyelids and the anterior surface of the globe as far as the limbus. It can be divided into 3 regions: *palpebral, forniceal,* and *bulbar.* The conjunctiva consists of nonkeratinized stratified squamous epithelium with goblet cells and a delicate basement membrane, which rests on the underlying stroma *(substantia propria)* (Fig 5-1A–D). Elements of the stroma include loosely arranged collagen fibers; blood vessels and lymphatic channels; nerves; occasional accessory lacrimal glands; and resident lymphocytes, plasma cells, macrophages, and mast cells. In places, the lymphocytes are organized into lymphoid follicles, referred to as *conjunctiva-associated lymphoid tissue (CALT),* which is a subtype of *mucosa-associated lymphoid tissue (MALT)* (see the section Lymphoid Lesions in this chapter). The stroma of the caruncle is the only part of the conjunctiva that, like skin, also contains sebaceous glands and hair follicles (Fig 5-1E). See BCSC Section 2, *Fundamentals and Principles of Ophthalmology,* and Section 8, *External Disease and Cornea,* for further discussion of the conjunctiva.

Congenital Anomalies

Choristomas

Choristomatous lesions of the ocular surface range from limbal dermoid to complex choristoma. A *choristoma* is a benign, congenital proliferation of histologically mature tissue that is abnormal for a given topographic location.

Dermoids are firm, dome-shaped, white-yellow nodules typically found at or straddling the limbus, most commonly in the inferotemporal quadrant (Fig 5-2A, B). Dermoids may occur in isolation or, particularly when bilateral, as a manifestation of a congenital complex such as Goldenhar syndrome (oculoauriculovertebral dysgenesis, characterized by epibulbar dermoid, upper eyelid coloboma, preauricular skin tags, and vertebral anomalies) or linear nevus sebaceous syndrome (an oculoneurocutaneous disorder). Dermoids often contain dermal adnexal structures. The surface epithelium may or may not be keratinized (Fig 5-2C).

In contrast with dermoids, *lipodermoids* (or *dermolipomas*) occur more commonly in the superotemporal quadrant, toward the fornix; they may extend posteriorly into

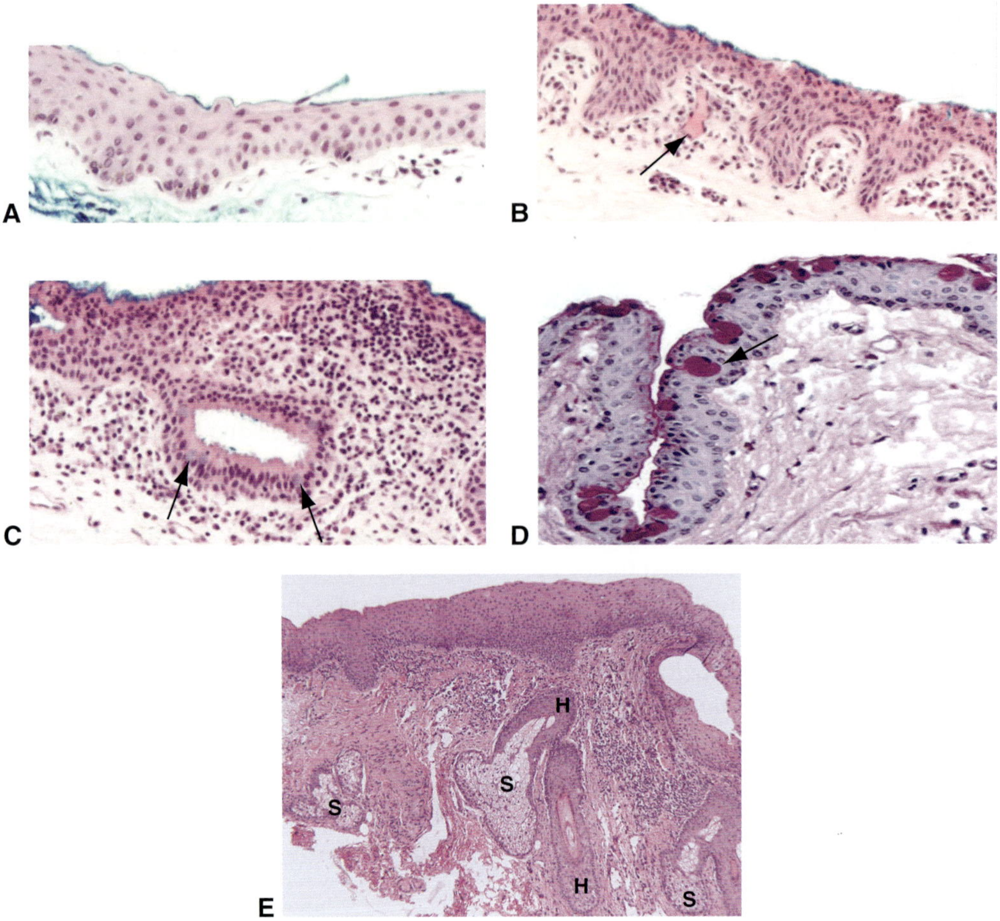

Figure 5-1 **A,** Bulbar conjunctiva with regular, nonkeratinized stratified squamous epithelium. **B,** Palpebral conjunctiva with epithelial ridges. The stroma *(arrow)* contains vessels and inflammatory cells. **C,** Conjunctiva at the fornix may contain pseudoglands of Henle (infoldings of conjunctival epithelium with abundant goblet cells *[arrows]*). **D,** Periodic acid–Schiff (PAS) stain highlights the mucin in goblet cells *(arrow)*. **E,** Caruncular conjunctiva, containing sebaceous glands (S) and hair follicles (H). *(Parts A–D courtesy of Patricia Chévez-Barrios, MD; part E courtesy of George J. Harocopos, MD.)*

the orbit. Lipodermoids are composed of a significant amount of mature adipose tissue, which makes them softer and yellower than dermoids. Dermal adnexal structures may or may not be present (Fig 5-2D). Lipodermoids, like dermoids, may be associated with Goldenhar syndrome or linear nevus sebaceous syndrome.

Osseous choristomas contain bone. *Complex choristomas* possess features of multiple types of choristomas, for example, dermoid or lipodermoid and osseous choristoma (Fig 5-2E). Clinically, complex choristomas are often indistinguishable from dermoids or lipodermoids. They may be associated with linear nevus sebaceous syndrome. See also BCSC Section 6, *Pediatric Ophthalmology and Strabismus.*

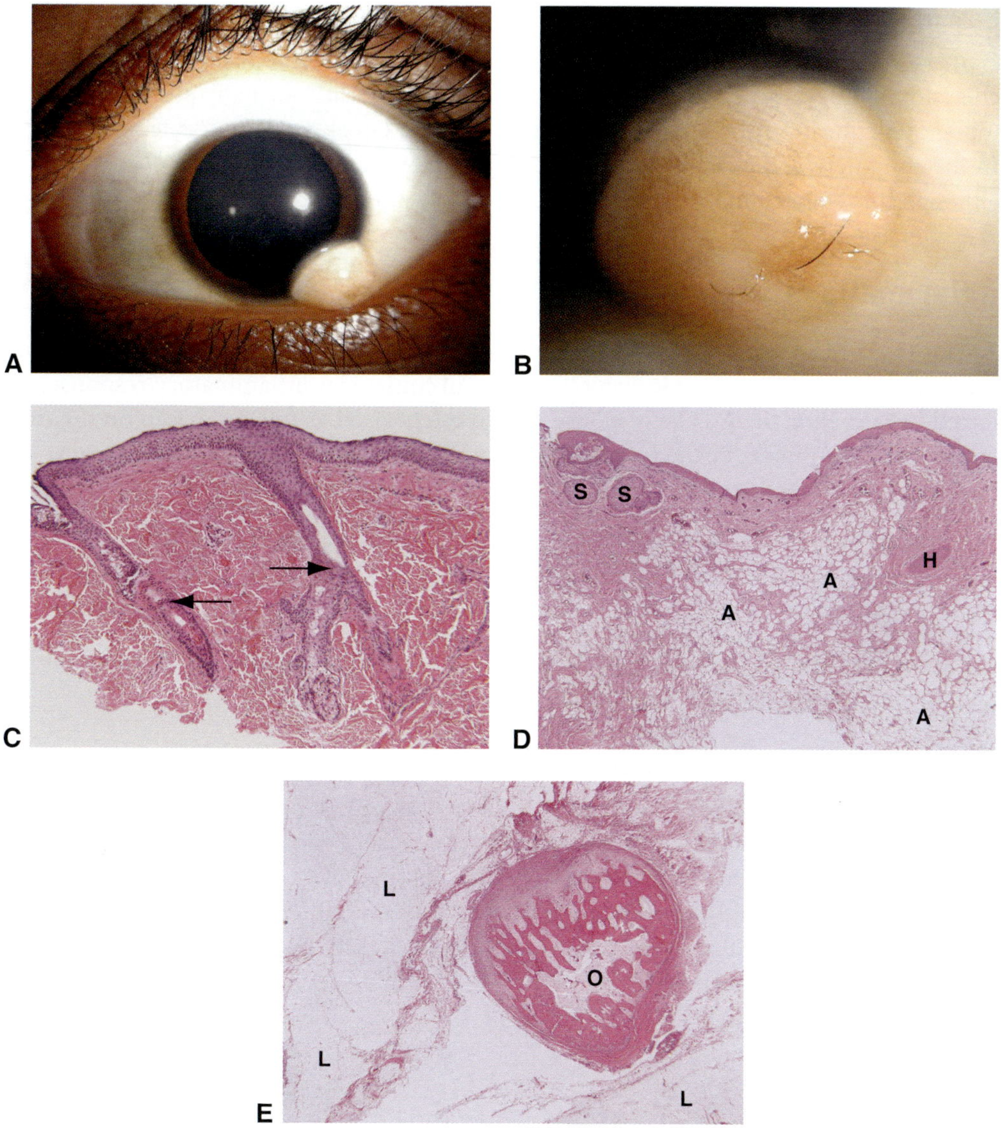

Figure 5-2 Ocular surface choristomas. **A,** Limbal dermoid, clinical appearance. **B,** Higher magnification shows hairs emanating from the dermoid. **C,** Histology shows keratinized epithelium, dense stroma, and sebaceous glands with hair follicles *(arrows)*. **D,** A lipodermoid differs from a dermoid in that it contains a significant amount of mature adipose tissue (A). This lipodermoid also contains dermal adnexal structures, including sebaceous glands (S) and hair follicles (H). **E,** Complex choristomas combine features of multiple types of choristomas, in this case osseous (O) and lipodermoid (L) choristomas. *(Parts A and B courtesy of Morton E. Smith, MD; parts C–E courtesy of George J. Harocopos, MD.)*

Hamartomas

Hamartomas, like choristomas, are benign congenital proliferations; but in contrast to choristomas, they are abnormal overgrowths of mature tissue normally present at a given topographic location (hence the derivation from the Greek word for "defect or error"). In the conjunctiva, the most common variety of hamartoma is a *capillary hemangioma,* although this hamartoma most often involves the eyelid (see Chapter 13).

Inflammations

Because part of the conjunctiva is an exposed surface, it can be affected by a variety of organisms, allergens, and toxic agents, which can initiate an inflammatory response, referred to as *conjunctivitis.* The response can be categorized as follows, based on the time frame, the constituents of the inflammatory infiltrate, macroscopic and microscopic appearance of the conjunctiva, or etiology

- acute or chronic
- papillary, follicular, or granulomatous
- infectious or noninfectious

See BCSC Section 6, *Pediatric Ophthalmology and Strabismus,* and Section 8, *External Disease and Cornea,* for additional discussion.

Papillary Versus Follicular Conjunctivitis

Most cases of conjunctivitis may be categorized as either papillary or follicular, according to the macroscopic and microscopic appearance of the conjunctiva (Fig 5-3). Neither type is pathognomonic for a particular disease entity. Clinically, *papillary conjunctivitis* shows a cobblestone arrangement of flattened nodules with central vascular cores (Fig 5-4A). Histologically, papillae appear as closely packed, flat-topped projections, with numerous inflammatory cells in the stroma surrounding a central vascular channel (Fig 5-4B).

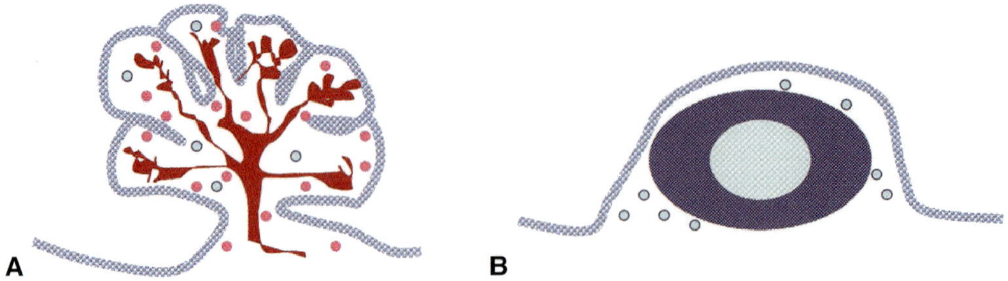

Figure 5-3 Schematic representation of papillary and follicular conjunctivitis. **A,** In papillary conjunctivitis, the conjunctival epithelium *(checkered blue)* covers fibrovascular cores with blood vessels *(red),* and the stroma contains eosinophils *(pink circles),* lymphocytes, and plasma cells *(blue circles).* **B,** In follicular conjunctivitis, the conjunctival epithelium covers lymphoid follicles, which have a paler germinal center surrounded by a darker corona *(central pale blue surrounded by purple),* and the surrounding stroma contains lymphocytes and plasma cells *(small blue circles).* *(Courtesy of Patricia Chévez-Barrios, MD.)*

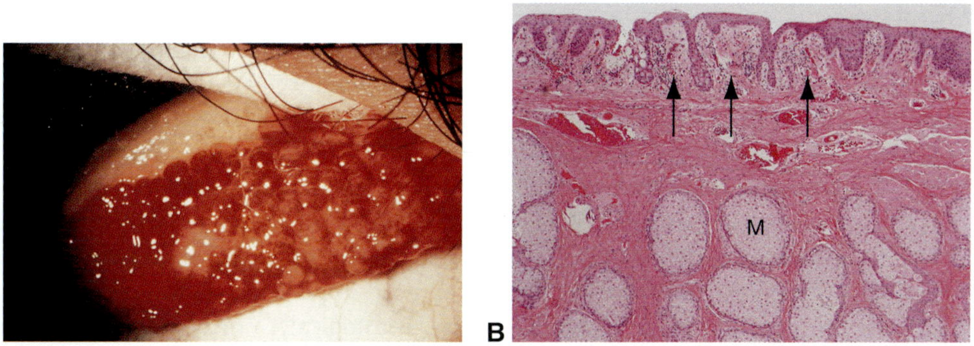

Figure 5-4 Papillary conjunctivitis. **A,** Clinical appearance. Papillae efface the normal palpebral conjunctival surface and form a confluent cobblestone pattern. **B,** Low-magnification photomicrograph shows the characteristic closely packed, flat-topped papillae with central fibrovascular cores *(arrows)*. The normal meibomian glands (M) of the tarsus are also shown. *(Part A courtesy of Harry H. Brown, MD; part B courtesy of George J. Harocopos, MD.)*

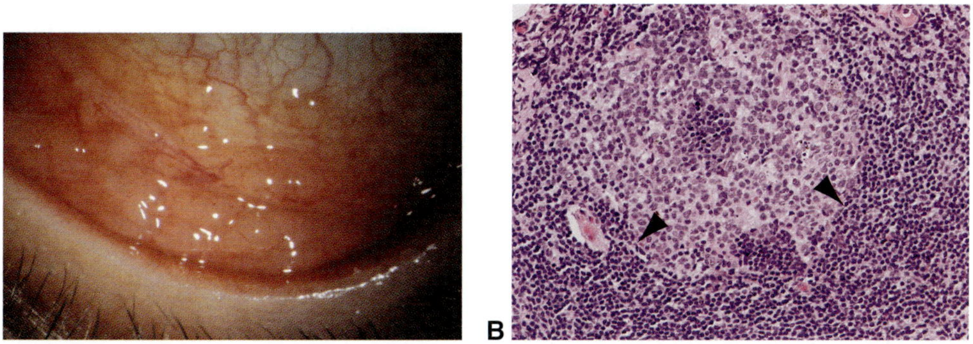

Figure 5-5 Follicular conjunctivitis. **A,** Clinical photograph showing follicles. **B,** High-magnification photomicrograph shows a lymphoid follicle and the boundary between the germinal center and the mantle zone *(arrowheads)*. Note the paler, relatively larger, immature lymphocytes in the germinal center, as compared with the darker, small, mature lymphocytes in the corona. *(Part A courtesy of Anthony J. Lubniewski, MD; part B courtesy of George J. Harocopos, MD.)*

Follicular conjunctivitis is characterized by the presence of follicles (Fig 5-5A): small, pale, dome-shaped nodules without a prominent central vessel. Histologically, a lymphoid follicle appears as a stromal, nodular aggregate of lymphocytes, occasionally arranged in a germinal center with a surrounding mantle zone (Fig 5-5B).

Granulomatous Conjunctivitis

Granulomatous conjunctivitis is less common than papillary conjunctivitis and follicular conjunctivitis and has both infectious and noninfectious causes. Clinically, the nodular elevations of granulomatous conjunctivitis may be difficult to distinguish from follicles, but the clinical history and systemic symptoms may point to the diagnosis. Granulomatous conjunctivitis occurring in association with preauricular lymphadenopathy is known as *Parinaud oculoglandular syndrome*. Bacteria such as *Bartonella henselae* (cat-scratch disease) and *Francisella tularensis* (tularemia), mycobacteria (eg, *Mycobacterium tuberculosis*), treponemes (eg, syphilis), and fungi (eg, sporotrichosis) are possible causes.

Microorganisms may be demonstrated with Gram, acid-fast, or silver stains, depending on the organism. The diagnosis can be made based on the culture results, serologic testing, PCR analysis, or a combination of these. If conjunctival biopsy is performed, the granulomas in infectious granulomatous conjunctivitis will typically demonstrate central necrosis.

One, presumably noninfectious cause of granulomatous conjunctivitis is *sarcoidosis,* a systemic disease that may involve all ocular tissues, including the conjunctiva. It manifests as small tan nodules without overt inflammatory signs, primarily within the forniceal conjunctiva (Fig 5-6A). Conjunctival biopsy can be a simple, expedient way of providing diagnostic confirmation of this systemic disease. Histologically, noncaseating granulomatous "tubercles" (round to oval aggregates of epithelioid histiocytes with or without multinucleated giant cells) are present within the conjunctival stroma, typically with a minimal cuff of lymphocytes and plasma cells (Fig 5-6B). Central necrosis is not characteristic and, if present, should suggest infectious etiologies. The diagnosis of sarcoidosis is tenable only when supported by clinical findings and after infectious causes of granulomatous inflammation have been excluded by histochemical stains and/or by culture results. As an exposed surface, the conjunctiva is vulnerable to contact with foreign bodies. Some may be transient and/or inert, whereas others may become embedded and incite a foreign-body reaction, identifiable histologically as a granuloma surrounding the foreign object. Multinucleated giant cells are common. Viewing the tissue section under polarized light may be helpful in identifying the offending foreign material (Fig 5-7). See Chapter 12 in this volume and BCSC Section 9, *Intraocular Inflammation and Uveitis,* for additional discussion.

Infectious Conjunctivitis

A wide variety of pathogens may infect the conjunctiva, including viruses, bacteria, atypical bacteria (eg, chlamydiae), fungi, and parasites. The most common offending agents in children are bacteria *(Haemophilus influenzae, Streptococcus pneumoniae)* and, in adults, viruses (adenovirus and the herpesviruses [simplex and zoster]). Specific diagnosis of infectious conjunctivitis may be made based on clinical history and examination findings (typically sufficient for viral disease), or it may require special stains for microorganisms

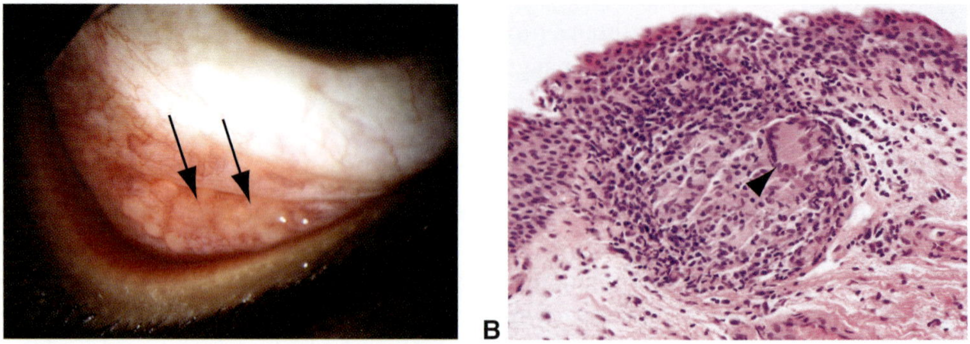

A B

Figure 5-6 Sarcoidosis. **A,** Clinical appearance of sarcoid granulomas *(arrows)* of the conjunctiva. **B,** Histology shows a noncaseating granuloma, with pale-staining histioctyes, including a multinucleated giant cell *(arrowhead).* Note the minimal cuff of lymphocytes and plasma cells. *(Courtesy of George J. Harocopos, MD.)*

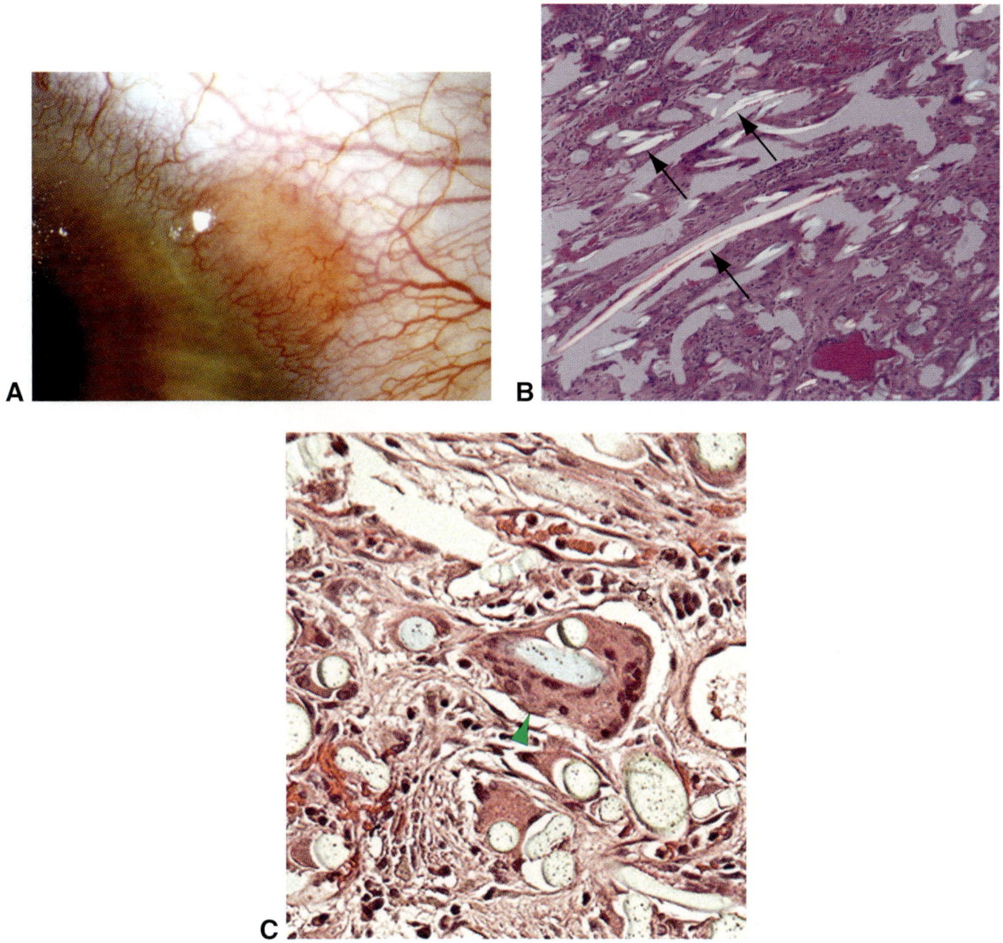

Figure 5-7 Conjunctival foreign-body granuloma. **A,** Clinical appearance on the bulbar conjunctiva. **B,** Histologic analysis of the specimen (from a different patient) under polarized light shows multiple foreign fibers *(arrows).* **C,** Hematoxylin-eosin (H&E) stain demonstrates fibers with surrounding foreign-body granulomatous reaction, including multiple giant cells *(arrowhead).* *(Part A courtesy of Anthony J. Lubniewski, MD; part B courtesy of George J. Harocopos, MD; part C courtesy of Tatyana Milman, MD.)*

(eg, Gram, Giemsa), culture, PCR analysis, or serology, depending on the organism. In cases of diagnostic uncertainty or cases unresponsive to initial treatment, cytologic evaluation of ocular surface epithelium (Fig 5-8) or tissue biopsy may be helpful in establishing a definitive diagnosis.

Noninfectious Conjunctivitis

Toxic follicular conjunctivitis, most etiologies of papillary conjunctivitis, and some forms of granulomatous conjunctivitis are noninfectious.

Mucous membrane pemphigoid (MMP; also known as ocular cicatricial pemphigoid) is a form of cicatrizing conjunctivitis that is of autoimmune etiology. Typically, it involves not only the conjunctiva, but other mucous membranes as well; in approximately

25% of patients, MMP involves the skin. When this diagnosis is suspected clinically, conjunctival biopsy is performed to establish the diagnosis. Half of the specimen should be submitted in formalin for routine histologic examination and half submitted in a special medium (Michel or Zeus) or saline for direct immunofluorescence analysis. Histologic findings are generally nonspecific but typically show a subepithelial, bandlike, mixed inflammatory cell infiltrate rich in plasma cells. The overlying epithelium may demonstrate squamous metaplasia with loss of goblet cells. Bullae are occasionally present (Fig 5-9).

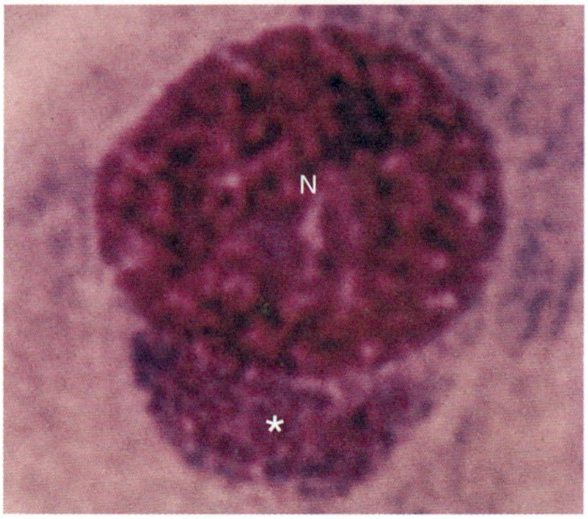

Figure 5-8 *Chlamydia,* conjunctival scraping, Giemsa stain. The cytoplasmic inclusion body *(asterisk),* composed of chlamydial organisms, can be seen capping the nucleus (N). A distinct space separates the inclusion body from the nuclear chromatin.

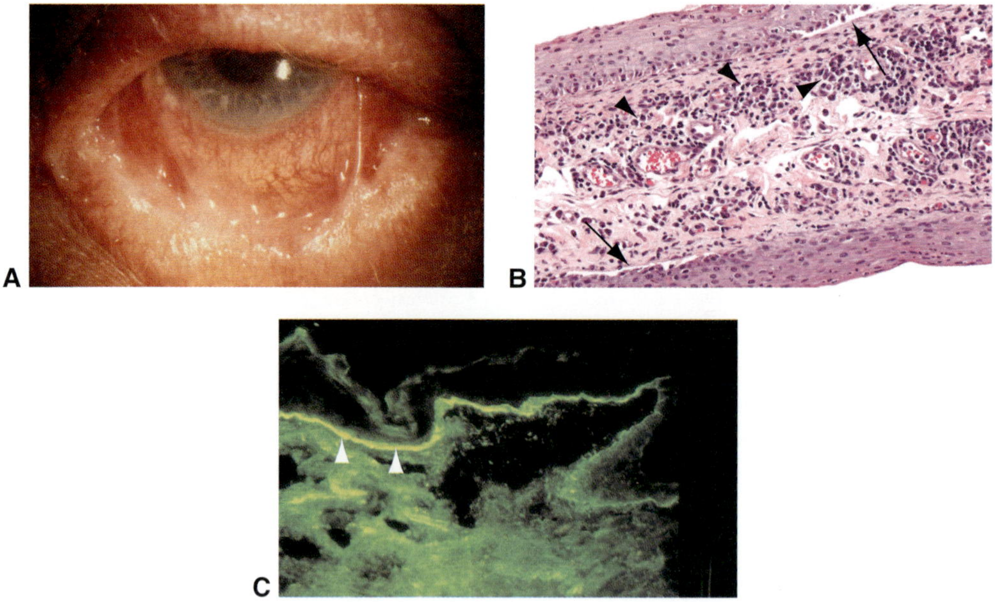

Figure 5-9 Mucous membrane pemphigoid (MMP). **A,** Clinical appearance. Note the conjunctival injection, symblepharon formation, shortening of inferior fornix, and conjunctival/eyelid cicatrization. **B,** Histology shows epithelial bullae *(arrows)* and dense chronic inflammatory cell infiltrate in the stroma *(arrowheads).* **C,** Direct immunofluorescence staining of the epithelial basement membrane *(arrowheads)* in MMP. *(Part A courtesy of Andrew J.W. Huang, MD; part B courtesy of George J. Harocopos, MD.)*

Immunofluorescence is the gold standard for diagnosis and demonstrates a linear deposition of immunoglobulins (IgG, IgM, and/or IgA) and/or complement (C3) in the epithelial basement membrane zone. The clinician must bear in mind that the sensitivity of immunofluorescence may be as low as 50% (particularly in long-standing cases with severe cicatrization). Thus, a negative result does not rule out the possibility of MMP.

Pyogenic Granuloma (Exuberant Granulation Tissue)

Pyogenic granuloma appears as a fleshy, pedunculated, nodular elevation on the ocular surface, typically occurring in association with a chalazion (on the palpebral conjunctiva) or at a site of prior accidental or surgical trauma. The name of this condition is a misnomer because the lesion is not pus-producing and is not a true granuloma. Rather, pyogenic granuloma is exuberant granulation tissue composed of a mixture of acute and chronic inflammatory cells with proliferating capillaries that classically form a radiating or "spoke-wheel" pattern (Fig 5-10).

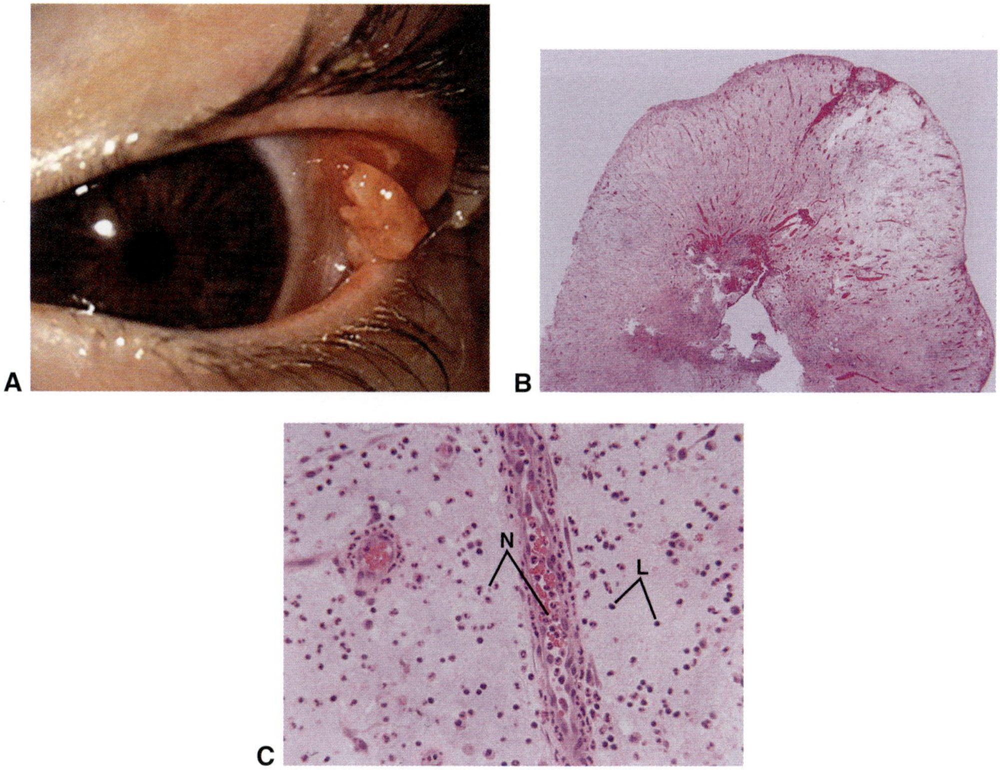

Figure 5-10 Pyogenic granuloma. **A,** Clinical appearance, at a site of prior strabismus surgery. **B,** Histology; this low-magnification photograph shows a pedunculated mass of granulation tissue, with a "spoke-wheel" vascular pattern. **C,** High magnification shows a mixture of acute and chronic inflammatory cells. Note neutrophils (N), both within the lumen of blood vessels and also infiltrating the tissue. Chronic inflammatory cells are also present, predominantly lymphocytes (L) in this field. *(Part A courtesy of Gregg T. Lueder, MD; parts B and C courtesy of George J. Harocopos, MD.)*

Degenerations

Pinguecula and Pterygium

A *pinguecula* is a small, yellowish nodule, often bilateral and typically located at the nasal and/or temporal limbus (Fig 5-11A). A manifestation of actinic damage (exposure to sunlight) or other environmental trauma, such as dust and wind, this growth is more common with advancing years. On histologic examination, the stromal collagen shows fragmentation and basophilic degeneration, referred to as *elastotic degeneration* because the degenerated collagen stains positively with histochemical stains for elastic fibers such as the Verhoeff–van Gieson stain (Fig 5-11B, C).

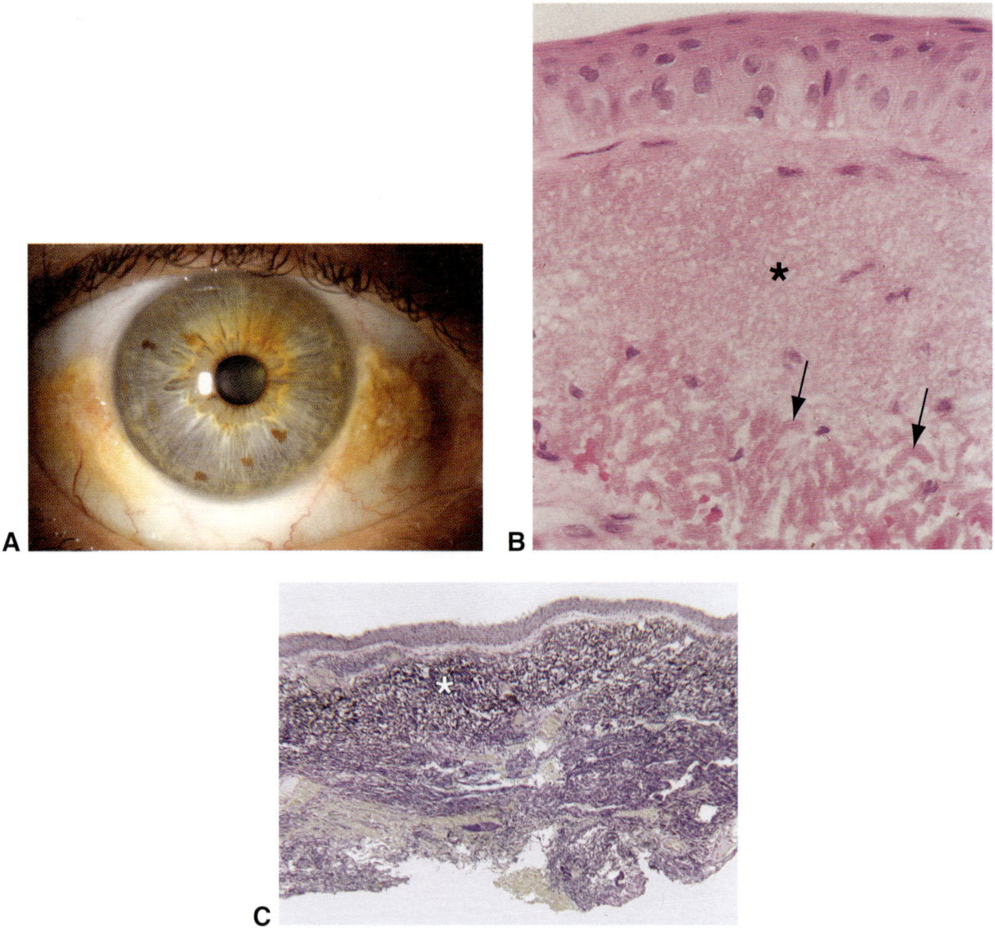

Figure 5-11 Pinguecula. **A,** Clinical appearance adjacent to the nasal and temporal limbus. **B,** Histologic examination demonstrates the acellular, amorphous, slightly basophilic material in the stroma *(asterisk)* and thick, curly fibers *(arrows)* indicative of elastotic degeneration. **C,** With Verhoeff–van Gieson stain for elastin, the basophilic material stains black *(asterisk)*. *(Parts A and C courtesy of George J. Harocopos, MD; part B courtesy of Hans E. Grossniklaus, MD.)*

A *pterygium* is similar to a pinguecula in its etiology and location but differs from the latter in its invasion of the superficial cornea as a vascular, wing-shaped growth (Fig 5-12A). Histologic examination typically shows elastotic degeneration, as in a pinguecula; prominent blood vessels correlating with the vascularity seen clinically (Fig 5-12B, C); and variable degrees of chronic inflammation. So-called *recurrent pterygia* may completely lack the histologic feature of elastotic degeneration and are thus more accurately classified as an exuberant fibroconnective tissue response.

In pingueculae and pterygia, the overlying epithelium may exhibit mild squamous metaplasia, for example, loss of goblet cells and surface keratinization. Some studies have demonstrated that there is abnormal expression of Ki-67 (a proliferation marker); dysregulation of tumor suppressor genes, such as *p53* and *p63,* and other genes associated with DNA repair; cell proliferation, migration, and angiogenesis; loss of heterozygosity; and microsatellite instability. Thus, as with actinic damage to the skin, there is the potential for future malignant transformation, although this occurs only in rare

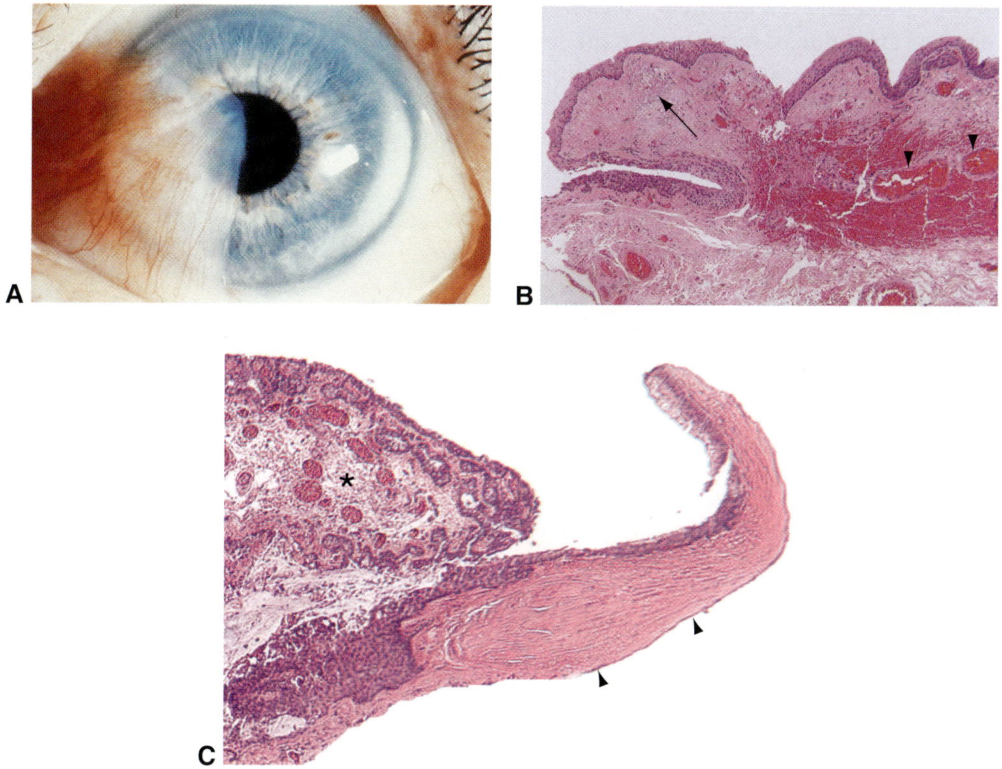

Figure 5-12 Pterygium. **A,** Clinical appearance. **B,** Histologically, a focus of elastotic degeneration is present *(arrow),* as well as prominent blood vessels *(arrowheads),* with surgically induced hemorrhage. **C,** In this case, the conjunctival and corneal portions of the pterygium are evident. Note the prominent blood vessels in the conjunctival portion *(asterisk)* and destruction of Bowman layer by ingrowth of fibroconnective tissue *(arrowheads)* in the corneal portion. *(Part A courtesy of Hans E. Grossniklaus, MD; parts B and C courtesy of George J. Harocopos, MD.)*

cases in association with pingueculae and pterygia. When conjunctival squamous neoplasia arises, it often occurs overlying an area of preexisting elastotic degeneration. If features such as epithelial hyperplasia, nuclear hyperchromasia and pleomorphism, and excessive mitotic figures are identified in an excised pinguecula or pterygium, a diagnosis of ocular surface squamous neoplasia should be assigned (see the section "Ocular surface squamous neoplasia," later in this chapter). See also BCSC Section 8, *External Disease and Cornea.*

Liu T, Liu Y, Xie L, He X, Bai J. Progress in the pathogenesis of pterygium. *Curr Eye Res.* 2013; 38(12):1191–1197.

Amyloid Deposits

Amyloid deposition in the conjunctiva is most commonly an idiopathic (primary) localized process seen in healthy young and middle-aged adults. The deposits are typically composed of monoclonal immunoglobulin (AL amyloid), secreted by local clonal plasma cells. Less often, conjunctival amyloidosis is induced by long-standing inflammation, such as with trachoma (ie, secondary localized amyloidosis, AA amyloid). Occasionally, conjunctival amyloidosis may occur in the setting of primary conjunctival lymphoma or plasmacytoma or secondary to systemic lymphoma or plasma cell myeloma.

Clinically, conjunctival amyloidosis typically presents as a salmon-colored nodular elevation, which can be associated with hemorrhage (Fig 5-13A). Histologically, amyloid

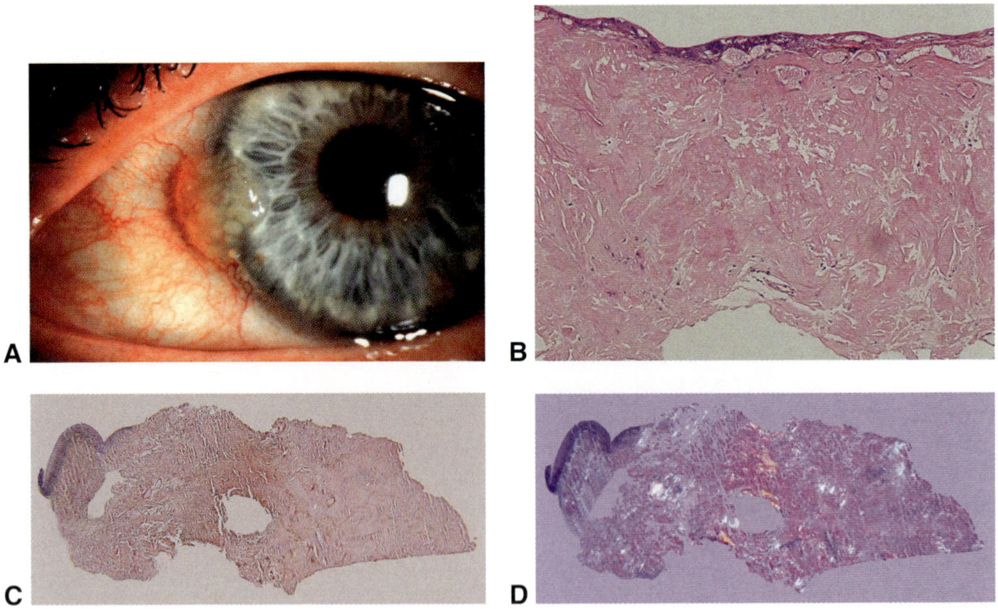

Figure 5-13 Conjunctival amyloidosis. **A,** Clinical appearance at the limbus and adjacent bulbar conjunctiva. **B,** Histologic examination reveals the diffuse, amorphous extracellular eosinophilic material throughout the stroma. **C,** Congo red stain, under standard light, highlights the amyloid orange. **D,** On Congo red stain under polarization, amyloid exhibits birefringence with dichroism (orange and apple-green colors). *(Parts A, C, and D courtesy of George J. Harocopos, MD; part B courtesy of Shu-Hong Chang, MD.)*

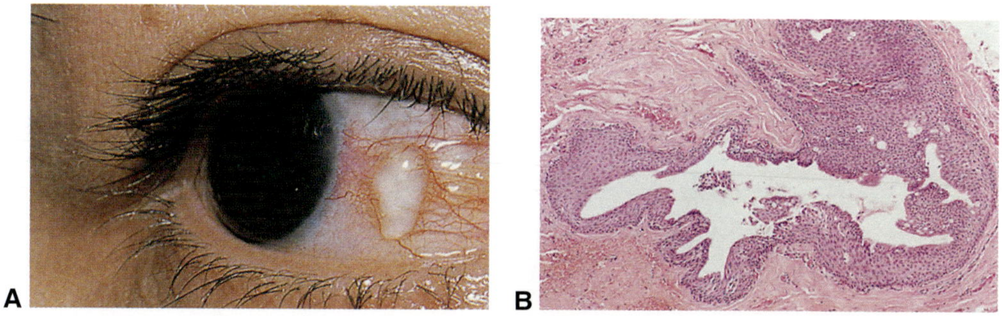

Figure 5-14 Epithelial inclusion cyst. **A,** Clinical appearance. **B,** Histologically, the cyst is lined by nonkeratinized stratified squamous epithelium with goblet cells, characteristic of conjunctiva.

appears as eosinophilic extracellular deposits within the stroma, sometimes in a perivascular distribution. On Congo red stain, under standard light, amyloid deposits appear orange. When viewed with polarized light and a rotating polarization filter, they exhibit birefringence with dichroism; that is, they change from orange to apple green as the filter is rotated (Fig 5-13B–D). Other useful staining methods include crystal violet and the fluorescent stain thioflavin T. Electron microscopy shows characteristic fibrils (see Chapter 6, Fig 6-19D). Immunohistochemical methods, sequencing, and mass spectrometry–based proteomic analysis are some of the techniques that are used in amyloid subtyping. See also BCSC Section 8, *External Disease and Cornea.*

Picken MM. Amyloidosis—where are we now and where are we heading? *Arch Pathol Lab Med.* 2010;134(4):545–551.

Epithelial Inclusion Cyst

A conjunctival epithelial inclusion cyst may form at a site of prior accidental or surgical trauma (eg, after strabismus surgery, retinal surgery, or enucleation). Clinically, the lesion appears as a transparent, cystic elevation on the ocular surface. There may be associated injection (Fig 5-14). Histologic examination shows a cystic space lined by conjunctival epithelium, located in the stroma. The lumen may be empty or may contain inspissated proteinaceous material and cellular debris.

Neoplasia

Squamous Lesions

Squamous papillomas

The most common ocular surface neoplasms are those of the squamous family. Squamous papillomas may be divided clinically into pedunculated and sessile subtypes.

Pedunculated papillomas are exophytic, pink-red, strawberry-like papillary growths frequently localized to the caruncle (Fig 5-15A), plica semilunaris, or forniceal conjunctiva. They occur more commonly in children than adults, with multiple lesions often present in affected patients. Pedunculated papillomas are associated with human papillomavirus

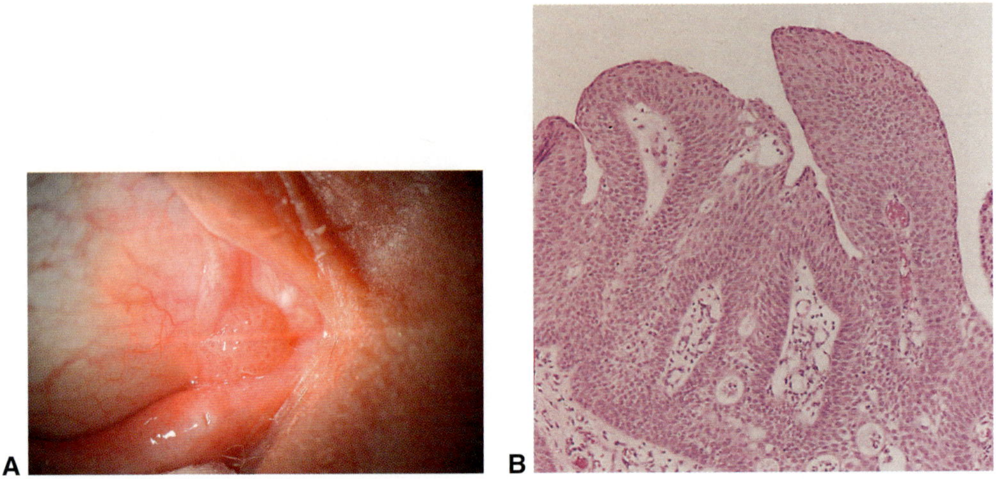

Figure 5-15 Squamous papilloma. **A,** Clinical appearance at the caruncle. **B,** The epithelium is hyperplastic and draped over fibrovascular cores. *(Part A courtesy of George J. Harocopos, MD.)*

(HPV) infection, subtypes 6 and 11. Histologic examination of a pedunculated papilloma demonstrates papillary fibrovascular cores covered by hyperplastic squamous epithelium (Fig 5-15B). Goblet cells may be present as in normal conjunctival epithelium. If there is overlying tear film disruption resulting in exposure, the number of goblet cells may be reduced and the surface keratinized. Neutrophils may be seen within the epithelium, and a chronic inflammatory infiltrate is frequently present in the stroma. Pedunculated papillomas typically exhibit benign behavior.

Sessile papillomas typically arise on the bulbar conjunctiva, especially adjacent to the limbus, and occur more commonly in adults. These papillomas are associated with HPV infection, subtypes 16 and 18—the same subtypes associated with squamous neoplasia. Clinical features worrisome for malignant transformation include leukoplakia (white patch indicative of keratinization), inflammation, atypical vascularity, and corneal involvement. Histologically, a sessile papilloma exhibits a broad base and lacks the prominent fingerlike projections seen in a pedunculated papilloma. The epithelium is hyperplastic but lacks prominent atypia. Evidence of nuclear hyperchromasia and pleomorphism, altered cell polarity, and abundant mitotic figures suggest a diagnosis of ocular surface squamous neoplasia.

Ocular surface squamous neoplasia

Ocular surface squamous neoplasia (OSSN) comprises a wide spectrum of dysplastic changes of the ocular surface epithelium, including corneal and conjunctival intraepithelial neoplasia (CIN) and squamous cell carcinoma (SCC). OSSN typically arises in the interpalpebral limbal area. The prevalence of OSSN is higher in equatorial regions of the world. UV-light exposure, especially in individuals with light skin pigmentation, is a known risk factor for OSSN. Mutations associated with UV light occur in tumor suppressor genes such as *p53* and have been demonstrated in OSSN. A hereditary deficiency of DNA repair (as occurs in xeroderma pigmentosum) increases the risk of OSSN formation.

OSSN is also associated with HPV infection (subtypes 16 and 18) and with human immunodeficiency virus (HIV) infection. HIV-associated OSSN may demonstrate rapid growth and aggressive behavior; HIV should be suspected in any OSSN patient younger than 50 years. Non–HIV-related immunosuppression is also a risk factor for OSSN. Other risk factors include older age and smoking.

The clinical appearance of OSSN is characterized by epithelial thickening, with the ocular surface appearing gelatinous or leukoplakic; the lesion may extend onto the peripheral cornea. There may be a prominent "corkscrew" vascular pattern with feeder vessels leading to the lesion (Fig 5-16). Histologically, the epithelium exhibits hyperplasia, loss of goblet cells, loss of cell polarity, nuclear hyperchromasia and pleomorphism, and mitotic figures. Frequently, there is surface keratinization, which correlates with the leukoplakia observed clinically. A chronic inflammatory response and increased vascularity are often present in the stroma.

The most important assessment to be made histologically in OSSN is whether the neoplasia is contained by the basement membrane (ie, intraepithelial or in situ) or whether neoplastic cells have traversed the epithelial basement membrane and invaded the stroma. For lesions contained by the basement membrane, the term *conjunctival intraepithelial neoplasia (CIN)* is used. The neoplasia may be graded as mild, moderate, or severe according to the degree of cellular atypia. In cases with the most severe atypia, there is full-thickness involvement of the epithelium, often with squamous eddies or keratin whorls or pearls. For these more advanced lesions, the term *squamous carcinoma in situ* is used. Invasion of the stroma by neoplastic cells is diagnostic of *squamous cell carcinoma* (Fig 5-17; see also Fig 5-16D). Invasion through the sclera or cornea with intraocular spread is an uncommon complication of invasive squamous cell carcinoma, typically occurring at the site of a previous surgical procedure or in the setting of immunosuppression. In addition, rare variants of conjunctival carcinoma, *mucoepidermoid carcinoma* and *spindle cell carcinoma,* may demonstrate aggressive behavior, with higher rates of recurrence, intraocular spread, and orbital invasion. Although regional lymph node metastasis is not as common in OSSN with conjunctival squamous cell carcinoma as it is with squamous carcinomas of the skin or other sites, dissemination and death can occur.

Edge S, Byrd DR, Compton CC, Fritz AG, Greene FL, Trotti A, eds. Ophthalmic Sites: Carcinoma of the conjunctiva. In: *AJCC Cancer Staging Manual.* 7th ed. New York: Springer; 2010:part X, pp 531–537.

Mittal R, Rath S, Vemuganti GK. Ocular surface squamous neoplasia. Review of etiopathogenesis and an update on clinico-pathological diagnosis. *Saudi J Ophthalmol.* 2013; 27(3):177–186.

Melanocytic Lesions

Table 5-1 summarizes key clinical features of the main types of ocular surface melanocytic lesions.

Melanocytic nevi

As with hemangiomas, *melanocytic nevi* are classified by some authors as hamartomas and by others as neoplasms, with this distinction resting upon whether the lesion is congenital

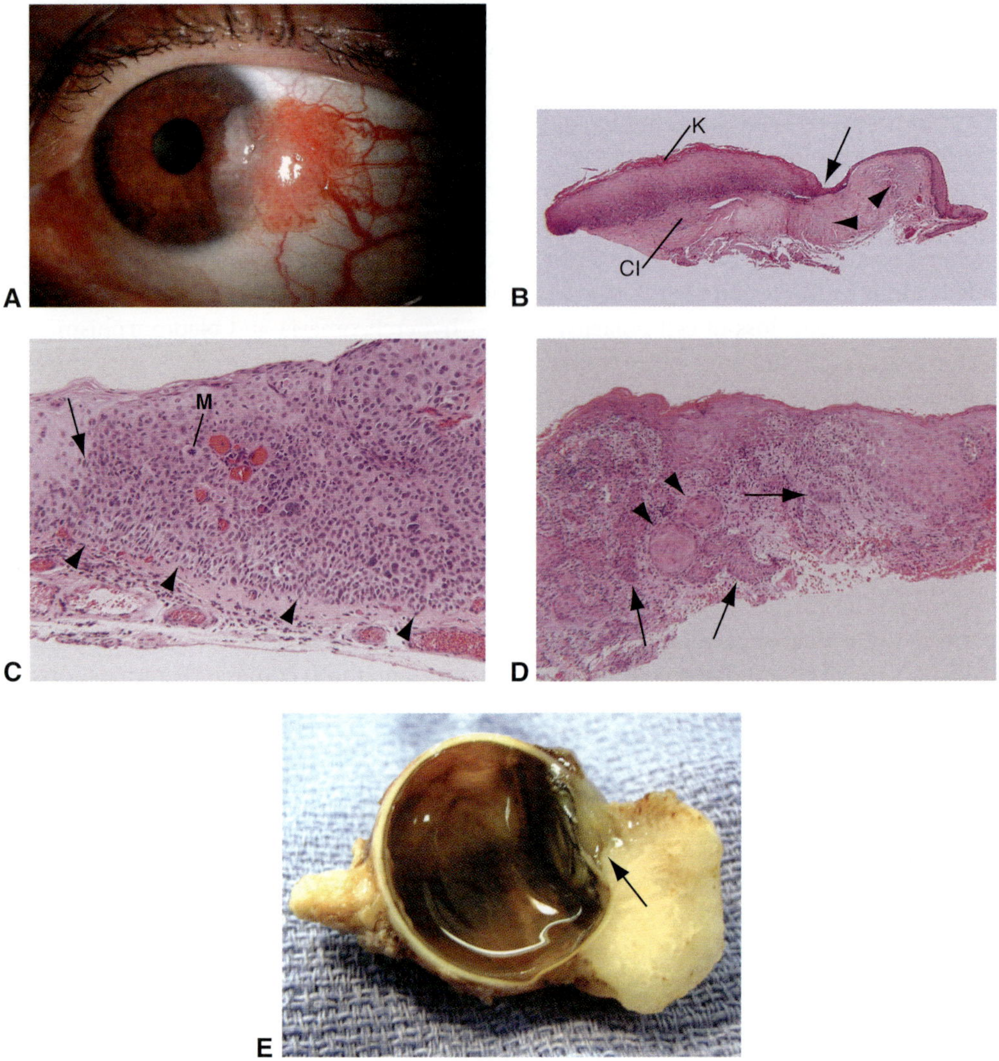

Figure 5-16 Ocular surface squamous neoplasia (OSSN). **A,** Clinical appearance. Note the "corkscrew" vascular pattern of the conjunctival portion and gelatinous appearance with focal leukoplakia of the corneal portion. Also note feeder vessels. **B,** Histologic examination shows the sharp demarcation *(arrow)* between normal and abnormal epithelium in OSSN. The epithelium is hyperplastic, with surface keratinization (K). As the basement membrane is intact, a diagnosis of conjunctival intraepithelial neoplasia (CIN) is made. There is a chronic inflammatory response in the stroma (CI). Also note areas of elastotic degeneration in the stroma *(arrowheads),* indicating that the lesion arose over a pinguecula. **C,** High magnification (different patient) shows the transition zone where neoplasia begins *(arrow).* To the right of the arrow, the epithelium exhibits mild keratinization, hyperplasia, nuclear hyperchromasia and pleomorphism, goblet cell loss, altered cell polarity, full-thickness involvement, and mitotic figures (M). The basement membrane is intact *(arrowheads).* **D,** In squamous cell carcinoma, tongues of epithelium violate the basement membrane and invade the stroma *(arrows),* with squamous eddies *(arrowheads).* **E,** Gross photograph of squamous carcinoma that has invaded the limbus and anterior chamber angle through a previous surgical incision *(arrow). (Part A courtesy of Vahid Feiz, MD; parts B–E courtesy of George J. Harocopos, MD.)*

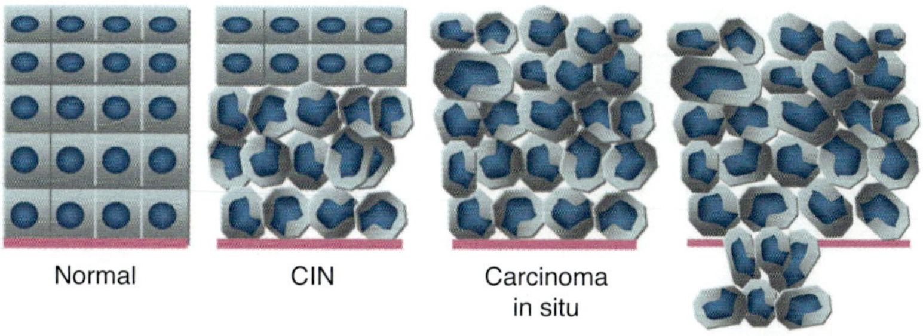

Figure 5-17 Schematic representation of the progression of OSSN. The first panel represents normal epithelium with basement membrane *(pink line).* In CIN, a portion of the epithelium is replaced with dysplastic cells. Carcinoma in situ is the complete replacement of epithelium by dysplastic cells, with the basement membrane still intact. In invasive squamous cell carcinoma, note the invasion through the basement membrane into the stroma. *(Courtesy of Patricia Chévez-Barrios, MD.)*

Table 5-1 Clinical Comparison of Ocular Surface Melanocytic Lesions

Lesion (Alternative terminology)	Onset	Characteristics	Location	Malignant Potential
Conjunctival nevus	Childhood or youth	Small, usually unilateral, cysts	Conjunctiva, mainly bulbar Caruncle	Yes, but low (conjunctival melanoma)
Ocular and oculodermal melanocytosis	Congenital	Patchy or diffuse; blue-gray; usually unilateral	Episclera/sclera (under conjunctiva)	Yes (uveal melanoma)
Complexion-associated melanosis (Primary conjunctival melanosis, hypermelanosis)	Young adulthood	Bilateral flat patches	Conjunctiva, typically bulbar and limbal	None to low
Primary acquired melanosis (PAM) Conjunctival melanocytic intraepithelial neoplasia (C-MIN)	Middle age	Diffuse; usually unilateral	Conjunctiva, mainly bulbar	Yes (conjunctival melanoma) Risk varies with degree of atypia

or acquired. Conjunctival melanocytic nevi usually arise in childhood, appearing on the bulbar conjunctiva as circumscribed pigmented lesions, frequently incorporating small, clear epithelial inclusion cysts (Fig 5-18A). Nevi also occur fairly commonly in the caruncle. Conjunctival nevi may be nonpigmented *(amelanotic),* in which case they have a pinkish appearance and the clinical diagnosis may be more challenging. The pigmentation and size of a nevus may increase during puberty, at which point the lesion may first be noticed. Melanocytic nevi occur only rarely in the palpebral conjunctiva; pigmented lesions in this area are more likely to represent intraepithelial melanosis or melanoma.

Like cutaneous melanocytic nevi, nevocellular conjunctival nevi undergo evolutionary changes. In the initial junctional phase, nevus cells are arranged in nests *(theques)* at

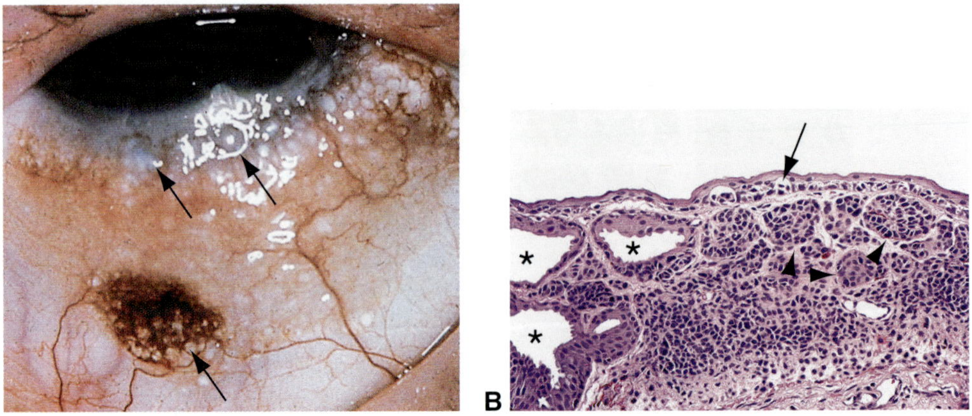

Figure 5-18 Conjunctival melanocytic nevus. **A,** Clinical appearance, with characteristic cystic areas *(arrows).* **B,** Histologically, the melanocytes are round, oval, or pear-shaped cells, mostly arranged in nests *(arrowheads).* Melanocytes are present at the epithelial–stromal junction *(arrow);* hence, this is a compound nevus. Note the epithelial inclusion cysts *(asterisks)* within the lesion, correlating with the clinical appearance. *(Part B courtesy of George J. Harocopos, MD.)*

the interface (junction) between the epithelium and the stroma. As the nevus evolves, the nests descend into the stroma and may lose connection with the epithelium. Nevus cells residing exclusively at the epithelial–stromal junction are called *junctional nevi,* whereas nevi located exclusively in the stroma are termed *subepithelial* or *stromal nevi;* nevi with both junctional and subepithelial components are designated *compound nevi.* Epithelial inclusion cysts are often encountered within compound nevi. The presence of these cysts, in conjunction with melanocytes exhibiting a nested pattern, is a histologic feature of a benign lesion (Fig 5-18B).

Nevi can be further categorized, for example, into Spitz nevus, halo nevus, and blue nevus. A blue nevus is a dark blue-gray to blue-black nevus in which the melanocytes are located in the deep stroma and have spindly morphology, similar to that of nevus cells seen in the uveal tract. Ocular, dermal, and oculodermal melanocytosis are forms of blue nevi typically seen unilaterally in darkly pigmented individuals (eg, African, Hispanic, and Asian persons). In *ocular melanocytosis,* the nevus is located in the deep episclera and sclera, giving the ocular surface a slate-gray appearance (Fig 5-19), and also in the uveal tract, often resulting in iris heterochromia; the conjunctiva (epithelium and stroma) is uninvolved. In *dermal melanocytosis,* the nevus is located in the periocular skin. Dermal melanocytosis may also occur in conjunction with orbital melanocytosis, that is, *dermal orbital melanocytosis. Oculodermal melanocytosis,* also known as *nevus of Ota,* combines the features of ocular and dermal melanocytosis. Although these conditions are rare in lightly pigmented persons, the risk of malignant transformation is increased in these individuals. When transformation into melanoma occurs, it is generally seen in the uveal tract; cutaneous, orbital, and meningeal melanomas are rare. Recent studies have shown that nevi of Ota manifest the same mutation in the G protein α-subunit genes *(GNAQ* and *GNA11)* that primary ciliochoroidal and central nervous system melanomas do. See also Chapter 17 in this volume and BCSC Section 8, *External Disease and Cornea.*

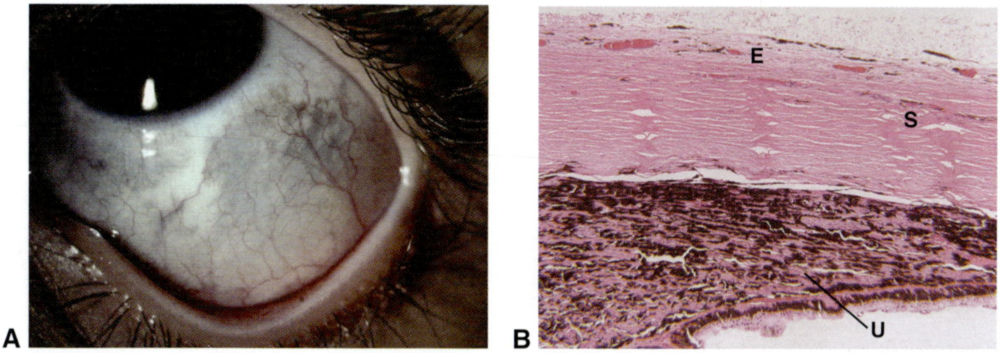

Figure 5-19 Ocular melanocytosis. **A,** Clinical appearance. **B,** Histologic examination shows an abnormally increased population of intensely pigmented spindle and dendritic melanocytes in the deep episclera (E), sclera (S), and uveal tract (U). *(Part A courtesy of Gabriela M. Espinoza, MD; part B courtesy of George J. Harocopos, MD.)*

Intraepithelial melanosis

Classification of non-nevoid conjunctival melanocytic proliferations is unique to this anatomical location and has been a subject of ongoing debate and critique. Traditionally, the acquired conjunctival pigmentation has been referred to as melanosis. Melanosis is divided into *primary acquired melanosis (PAM),* which occurs without predisposing conditions; *secondary acquired melanosis,* which occurs in a setting of systemic disease (eg, Addison disease) or secondary to another conjunctival lesion (eg, squamous papilloma or carcinoma); and *complexion-associated melanosis,* which occurs in individuals with darker complexions. PAM is further divided into *PAM without atypia* and *PAM with atypia.* The concept of PAM with atypia is controversial, as it denotes a spectrum of lesions—from those showing only mild cytologic atypia to severely atypical lesions frequently associated with invasive melanoma—and the precise definition of melanoma in situ is lacking. In an effort to distinguish between conjunctival hyperpigmentation and melanocytic proliferation and to standardize the grading of intraepithelial melanocytic proliferations, a new classification scheme has been proposed, one that divides conjunctival melanosis into *hypermelanosis, conjunctival melanocytic intraepithelial neoplasia (C-MIN),* and *melanoma in situ.* In the absence of universal terminology, both classification schemes are incorporated into the following discussion.

Complexion-associated melanosis appears as bilateral flat patches of brown pigmentation with irregular margins, typically involving the bulbar and limbal conjunctiva, in individuals with dark skin pigmentation (Fig 5-20A). Streaks and whorls of melanotic pigmentation may extend onto the peripheral cornea, a condition called *striate melanokeratosis.* The caruncle and palpebral conjunctiva may also be involved. Histologically, there is increased pigmentation, localized primarily to the epithelial cells; the basal epithelial melanocytes are normal in number and cytomorphology (hence the proposed new term, hypermelanosis) (Fig 5-20B).

Secondary acquired melanosis is similarly characterized by increased pigmentation in the absence of melanocytic atypia. The number of melanocytes may be mildly increased, however; this increase is triggered by the underlying conjunctival inflammatory

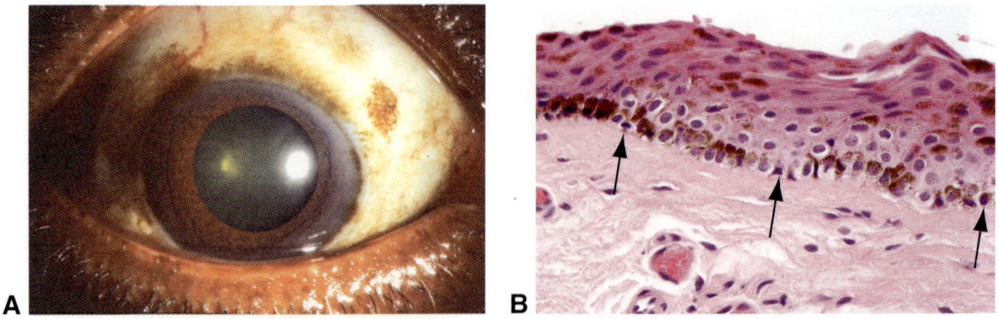

Figure 5-20 Complexion-associated melanosis (acquired hypermelanosis). **A,** Clinical appearance. **B,** Histologic examination shows a normal density of small, morphologically unremarkable melanocytes confined mainly to the basal layer of the epithelium *(arrows)* with variable extension of pigment into more superficial epithelial layers. *(Part A courtesy of George J. Harocopos, MD; part B courtesy of Tatyana Milman, MD.)*

or neoplastic process. Both complexion-associated melanosis and secondary acquired melanosis have no significant risk of progression to melanoma.

In contrast, PAM characteristically presents as a unilateral melanotic macule or patch in middle-aged light-skinned individuals. The lesion may remain stable or grow slowly over a period of 10 or more years. It may be difficult to predict clinically in any given patient whether PAM is likely to progress to melanoma; thus, the recommendations regarding when to observe versus when to perform biopsy are controversial. Retrospective data suggest that the number of clock-hours of conjunctival involvement (3 clock-hours or more) and caruncular, forniceal, or palpebral conjunctival locations are associated with a worse prognosis (Fig 5-21). Histologic criteria have been developed to identify patients at high risk for malignancy.

PAM without atypia is characterized by a normal or mildly increased number of cytologically unremarkable melanocytes along the basal epithelial layer, with the pigment, when present, being localized mainly to the epithelial cells (see Fig 5-21B). Thus, without the clinical history, the pathologist may not be able to distinguish PAM without atypia from complexion-associated melanosis or secondary acquired melanosis, as the histologic findings for these conditions may be identical. According to the proposed classification scheme, lesions lacking melanocytic hyperplasia or atypia are classified as *primary conjunctival hypermelanosis* (see Fig 5-20B), whereas those composed of a lentiginous proliferation of basal melanocytes (which are occasionally mildly enlarged) lacking cytologic atypia are termed *C-MIN without atypia* (see Fig 5-21B).

In PAM with atypia *(C-MIN with atypia),* melanocytes are cytologically atypical; they form nests, demonstrate discohesiveness, and migrate into the more superficial epithelium *(pagetoid spread).* The cells often exhibit epithelioid morphology, with large hyperchromatic nuclei, prominent nucleoli, and moderate to abundant cytoplasm. Mitotic figures may be present. A chronic inflammatory response is frequently seen in the stroma. The atypia may be graded as mild, moderate, or severe, although there is poor interobserver and intraobserver reproducibility of such grading. Typically, basilar lentiginous, mildly atypical dendritic melanocytic proliferations are graded as *PAM with mild atypia,* whereas those demonstrating pagetoid spread and epithelioid cytomorphology are categorized as

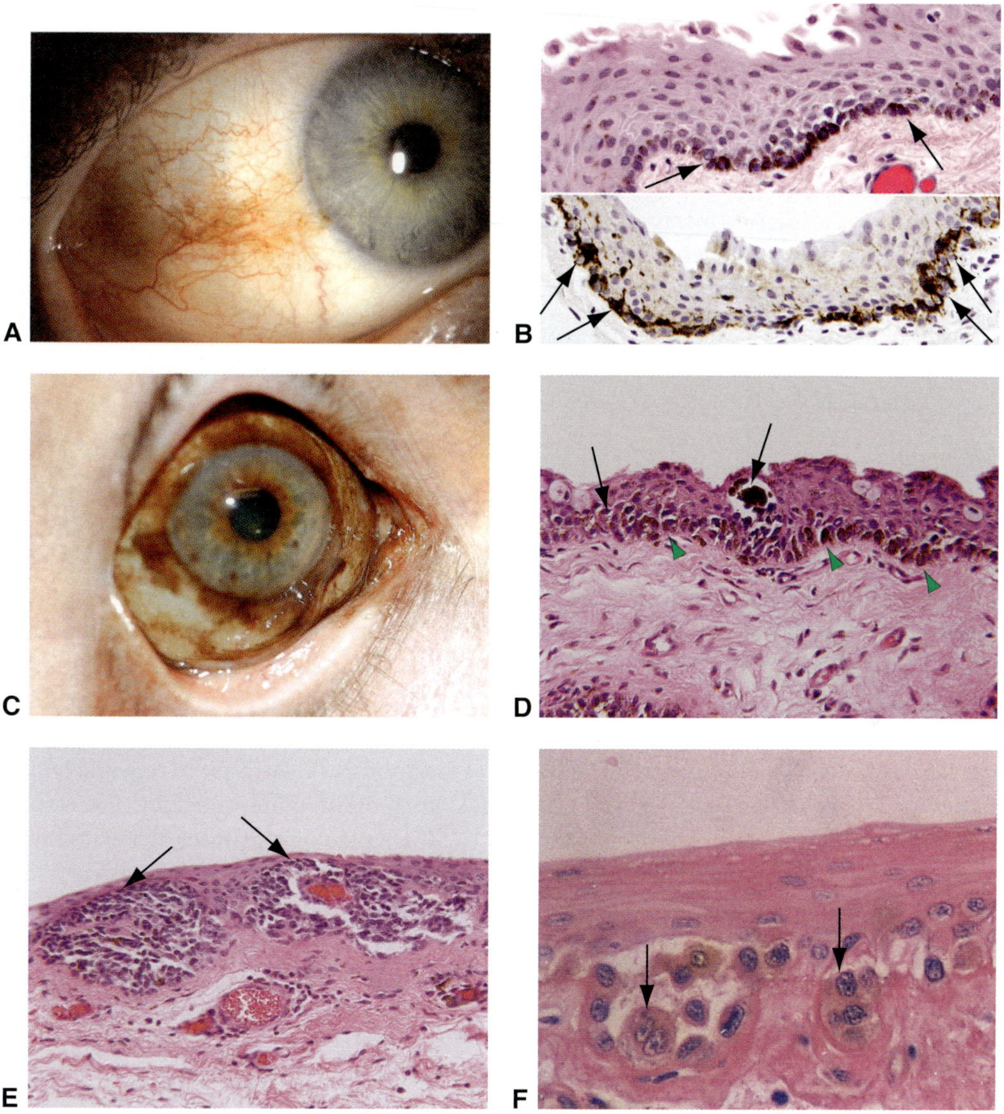

Figure 5-21 Primary acquired melanosis (PAM)/conjunctival melanocytic intraepithelial neoplasia (C-MIN). **A,** Mild PAM, involving 1 clock-hour of conjunctiva; unlikely to harbor atypia and may be observed. **B,** Histology of PAM (C-MIN) without atypia. H&E stain *(top)* shows melanocytic proliferation, confined to the basal layer of the epithelium *(between the 2 arrows)*, with no cellular atypia. Melan-A (MART-1) immunohistochemical stain *(bottom)* highlights the increased number of small dendritic melanocytes, arranged linearly in the region of the basal epithelium *(arrows)*. **C,** Extensive PAM, involving much of the ocular surface, including the caruncle, palpebral conjunctiva, and eyelid margin; likely harbors atypia and warrants biopsy. **D,** Histology of PAM (C-MIN) with mild to moderate atypia, mostly in the basal epithelial layer *(arrowheads)*; the melanocytes are small, without prominent nucleoli. Some melanocytes are seen in the superficial epithelium, singly and in nests *(arrows)*. There is a moderate risk of transformation to melanoma. **E,** Histology of PAM with severe atypia (melanoma in situ). The minimally pigmented melanocytic proliferation *(arrows)* involves most of the epithelial thickness. Some atypical melanocytes have epithelioid morphology. **F,** PAM with severe atypia (different patient). Higher magnification shows epithelioid melanocytes *(arrows)* within the epithelium. These latter two lesions are at significant risk for progression to melanoma. *(Parts A, D, and E courtesy of George J. Harocopos, MD; part B courtesy of Tatyana Milman, MD; part C courtesy of Vahid Feiz, MD.)*

PAM with moderate to severe atypia. According to the seventh edition of the American Joint Committee on Cancer (AJCC) staging system, involvement of greater than 75% of the conjunctival epithelium by atypical epithelioid melanocytes and/or presence of pagetoid spread are defining features of *conjunctival melanoma in situ* (see Fig 5-21E–F). PAM with mild atypia carries minimal, if any, risk of malignant transformation. In contrast, PAM with moderate or severe atypia carries a substantial risk of progression to melanoma.

See also BCSC Section 8, *External Disease and Cornea.*

Shields JA, Shields CL, Mashayekhi A, et al. Primary acquired melanosis of the conjunctiva: risks for progression to melanoma in 311 eyes. The 2006 Lorenz E. Zimmerman lecture. *Ophthalmology.* 2008;115(3):511–519.

Melanoma

Approximately 50%–70% of cases of *conjunctival melanoma* arise from PAM with atypia (Fig 5-22); the remainder develop from either a nevus or de novo. Melanomas are usually nodular growths with vascularity that may involve any portion of the conjunctiva. The nodule may be pigmented or amelanotic. Histologically, the cellular morphology in melanomas ranges from spindle to epithelioid (see Fig 5-22B). These cytologic features do not have the same prognostic significance that they have in uveal melanoma. In more aggressive lesions, mitotic figures may present. Immunohistochemical stains for melanocytes such as Melan-A (MART-1) and HMB-45, ideally complexed with red chromogen, may be of help in diagnostically challenging cases. Conjunctival melanomas metastasize to regional lymph nodes in 25% of patients, as well as to the lungs, liver, brain, bone, and skin. The overall mortality rate in these cases ranges from 15% to 30%. Histologic features associated with a worse prognosis include nonbulbar conjunctival location (ie, plica semilunaris/caruncle, forniceal or palpebral conjunctiva, palpebral conjunctiva) and greater tumor thickness.

Occasionally, extrascleral extension of an anterior uveal melanoma presents as an episcleral/conjunctival mass. This diagnosis should be considered, particularly for a nonmobile pigmented or amelanotic episcleral nodule overlying the ciliary body that is associated with sentinel vessels and without surrounding PAM (Fig 5-23). A complete

A
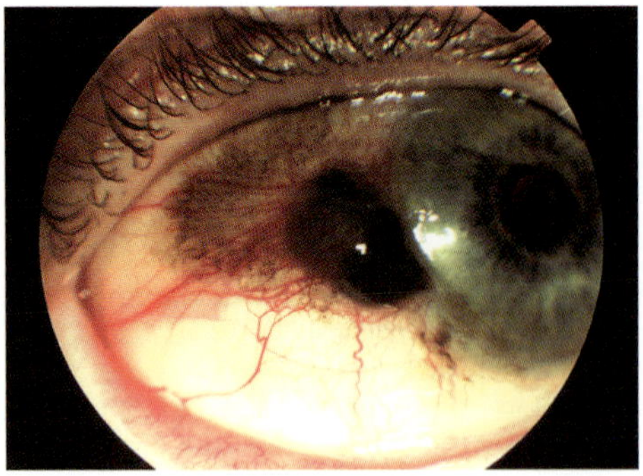
B
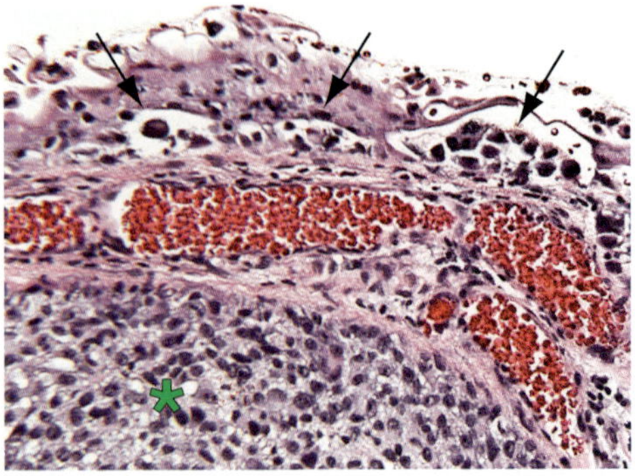

Figure 5-22 Melanoma arising from PAM with atypia. **A,** Clinical appearance. Note the elevated melanoma nodule, adjacent to the limbus, arising from a background of PAM (diffuse, flat, brown pigmentation). Also note the prominent vascularity. **B,** Histologic examination shows melanoma *(asterisk)* arising from PAM *(arrows)*. *(Part A courtesy of Morton E. Smith, MD; part B courtesy of Tatyana Milman, MD.)*

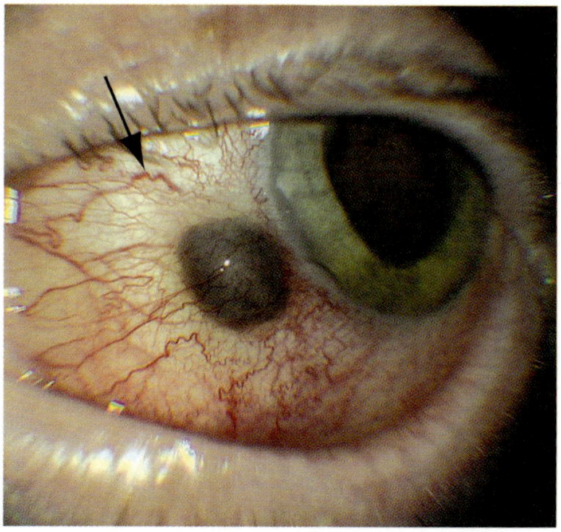

Figure 5-23 Melanoma of the ciliary body with extrascleral extension, presenting as an ocular surface mass. Note that there is no PAM surrounding the nodule, a clue that the lesion might have an intraocular origin. Also note that the lesion is associated with deep episcleral/scleral vessels (sentinel vessels, *arrow*) and does not obscure the overlying conjunctival vessels. This indicates that the lesion is deep to the conjunctiva. *(Courtesy of J. William Harbour, MD.)*

eye examination, including gonioscopy and dilated ophthalmoscopy, should always be performed in any patient with a conjunctival mass. In individuals with darker complexions, conjunctival squamous cell carcinoma may occasionally be associated with reactive pigmentation, masquerading as melanoma. See also BCSC Section 8, *External Disease and Cornea.*

Damato B, Coupland SE. Conjunctival melanoma and melanosis: a reappraisal of terminology, classification and staging. *Clin Experiment Ophthalmol.* 2008;36(8): 786–795.

Edge S, Byrd DR, Compton CC, Fritz AG, Greene FL, Trotti A, eds. Ophthalmic Sites: Malignant melanoma of the conjunctiva. In: *AJCC Cancer Staging Manual.* 7th ed. New York: Springer; 2010:part X, pp 538–546.

Shields JA, Shields CL, Mashayekhi A, et al. Primary acquired melanosis of the conjunctiva: risks for progression to melanoma in 311 eyes. The 2006 Lorenz E. Zimmerman lecture. *Ophthalmology.* 2008;115(3):511–519.

Zembowicz A, Mandal RV, Choopong P. Melanocytic lesions of the conjunctiva. *Arch Pathol Lab Med.* 2010;134(12):1785–1792.

Lymphoid Lesions

The normal conjunctiva contains MALT, and a few small follicles are often visible clinically in the normal inferior fornix. As described previously, the reactive lymphoid follicle consists of a germinal center and surrounding corona (see Fig 5-5). The corona is divided into marginal and mantle zones, although these zones are not well delineated histologically without the use of immunohistochemical stains.

Lymphoid tissue may proliferate in the conjunctiva abnormally, often in the absence of inflammation, and this lymphoid hyperplasia may be benign (reactive) or malignant. Clinically, both benign and malignant lymphoproliferative conjunctival lesions appear as soft, mobile, salmon-pink masses with a smooth-surface, characteristically localized to the forniceal and the bulbar conjunctiva (Fig 5-24A, B). The condition may be unilateral or bilateral, and an orbital component may be present. Incisional biopsy is generally required to make a precise diagnosis.

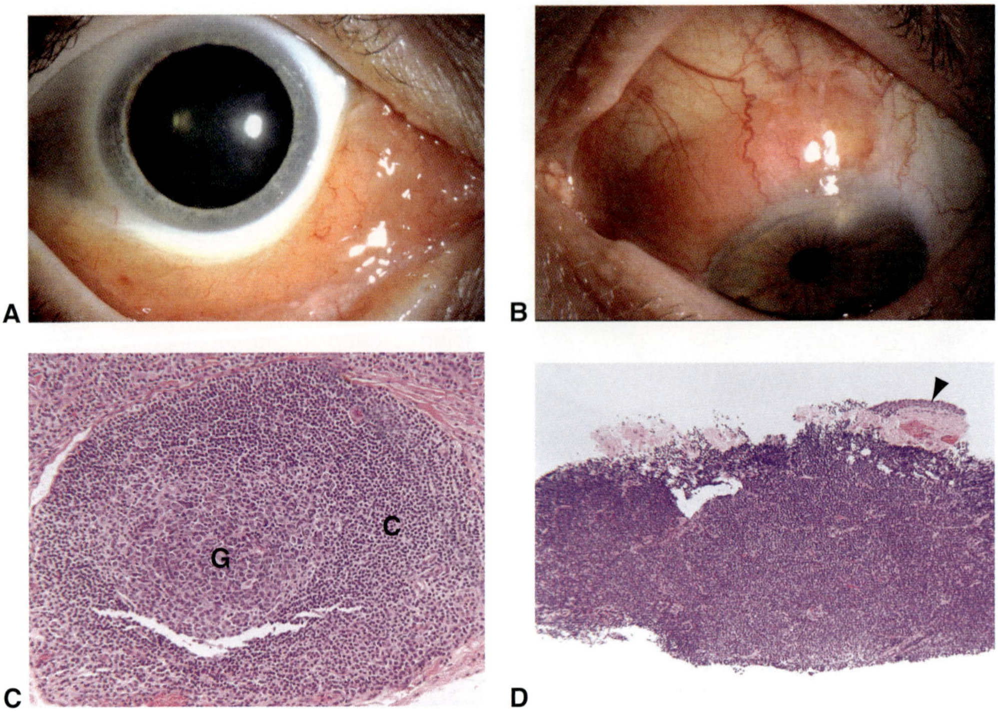

Figure 5-24 Lymphoid lesions of the conjunctiva. Clinical appearance ("salmon patch") in the inferior fornix **(A)** and in the bulbar conjunctiva **(B). C,** Histologic examination of benign lymphoid hyperplasia, showing normal follicular architecture, with a well-defined germinal center (G) and corona (C). **D,** Histologic examination of lymphoma shows a sheet of lymphocytes infiltrating the stroma, without well-defined follicles. Note the conjunctival epithelium *(arrowhead). (Part A courtesy of Anthony J. Lubniewski, MD; part B courtesy of Anjali K. Pathak, MD; parts C and D courtesy of George J. Harocopos, MD.)*

Evaluation of conjunctival lymphoid lesions is limited by the size of the biopsy specimen. Thus, communication with the pathologist regarding recommendations for optimal specimen submission is essential. Histologic examination and immunohistochemistry are routinely used in the workup. When the submitted tissue is sufficient for additional studies, flow cytometry and molecular genetic studies can also be performed (see Chapters 3 and 4).

On routine hematoxylin-eosin sections, histologic features favoring a diagnosis of *benign lymphoid hyperplasia* include the presence of normal-appearing lymphoid follicles with distinct germinal centers and with small, mature coronal lymphocytes (Fig 5-24C). In contrast, *lymphoma* frequently demonstrates a diffuse or vaguely nodular proliferation of monomorphic lymphocytes in the stroma, without well-defined follicles (Fig 5-24D). As is true for most ocular adnexal lymphomas, conjunctival lymphoma is often a low-grade small B-cell lymphoma, classified as extranodal marginal zone B-cell lymphoma of MALT type (MALT lymphoma) (Fig 5-25).

Of all ocular adnexal lymphomas, conjunctival lymphoma has the best prognosis, as approximately 80% of conjunctival lymphomas are localized to the conjunctiva and not associated with systemic disease. See BCSC Section 8, *External Disease and Cornea,* and Section 7, *Orbit, Eyelids, and Lacrimal System,* for additional discussion.

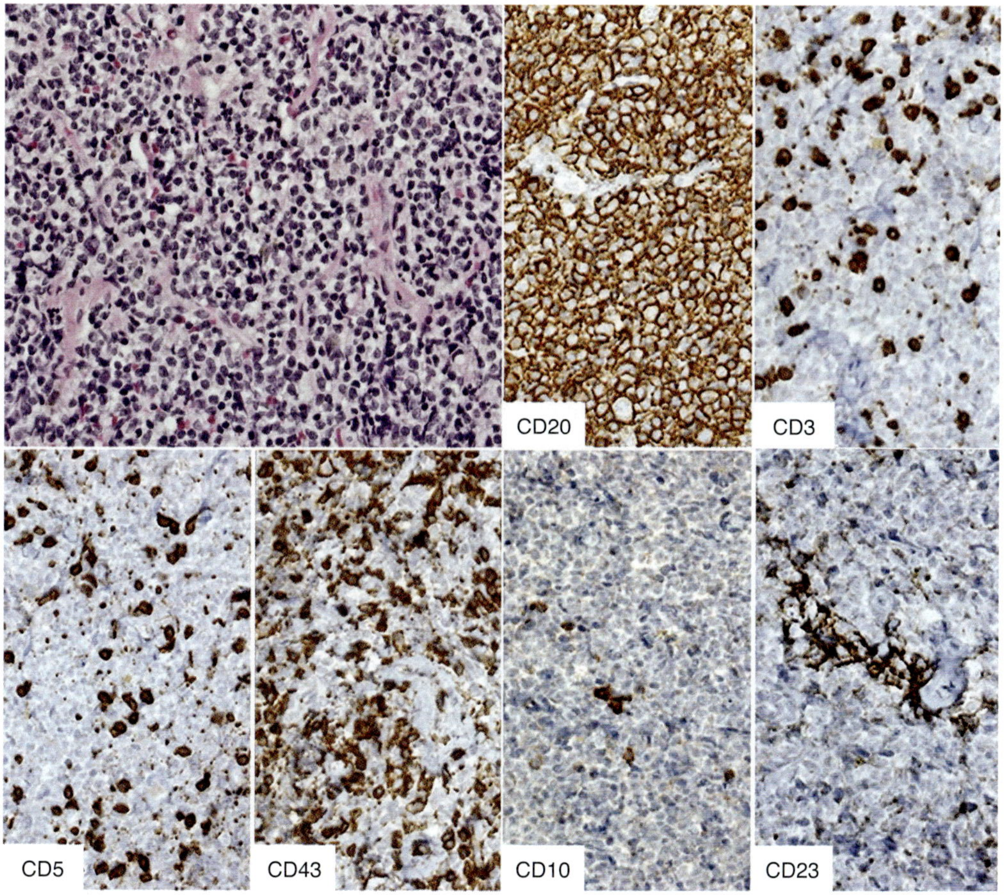

Figure 5-25 Histology of conjunctival extranodal marginal zone B-cell lymphoma of mucosa-associated lymphoid tissue (MALT lymphoma) type. H&E-stained preparation demonstrates a diffuse proliferation of small lymphocytes with mildly irregular nuclear contours, inconspicuous nucleoli, and scant cytoplasm. Immunohistochemical staining shows that the atypical lymphocytes are CD20+ B cells, which coexpress CD43 and are negative for CD5, CD10, and CD23. Rare reactive T cells are CD3+, CD5+, and CD43+. The disrupted follicular dendritic meshworks of the residual germinal center are highlighted with CD23 immunostain. Rare germinal center B cells are CD10+. *(Courtesy of Tatyana Milman, MD.)*

Edge S, Byrd DR, Compton CC, Fritz AG, Greene FL, Trotti A, eds. Ophthalmic Sites: Ocular adnexal lymphoma. In: *AJCC Cancer Staging Manual.* 7th ed. New York: Springer; 2010: part X, pp 583–589.

Shields CL, Shields JA, Carvalho C, et al. Conjunctival lymphoid tumors: clinical analysis of 117 cases and relationship to systemic lymphoma. *Ophthalmology.* 2001;108(5):979–984.

Swerdlow SH, Campo E, Harris NL, et al. *WHO Classification of Tumours of Haematopoietic and Lymphoid Tissues.* 4th ed. Lyon, France: IARC; 2008.

Glandular Lesions

Oncocytoma is a benign proliferation of apocrine or accessory lacrimal gland epithelium, that is, an adenoma. It typically arises in the caruncle, but it may occasionally be located

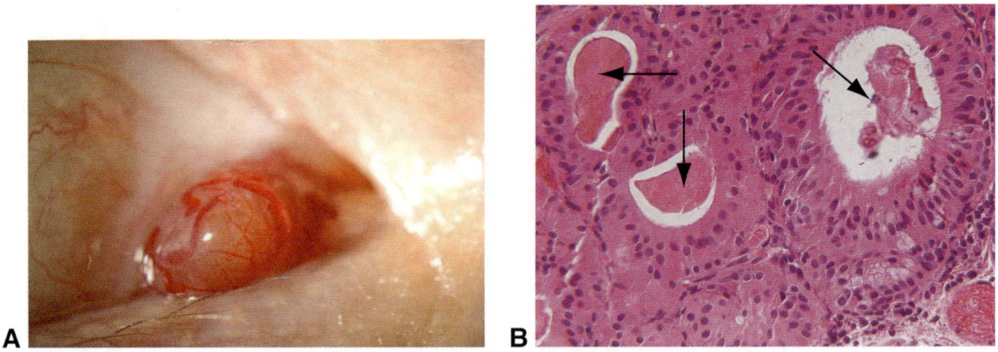

Figure 5-26 Oncocytoma. **A,** Clinical appearance at the caruncle. **B,** Histology shows cystadenomatous proliferation of columnar epithelial cells, with deeply eosinophilic cytoplasm. Some of the cells surround protein-filled lumina *(arrows)*. *(Part A courtesy of Mark J. Mannis, MD; part B courtesy of George J. Harocopos, MD.)*

elsewhere on the conjunctiva. Oncocytoma most commonly occurs in elderly women. Clinically, it appears as a tan to reddish, vascularized nodule (Fig 5-26). Histologically, the lesion is composed of a cystadenomatous proliferation of columnar epithelium with abundant, intensely eosinophilic cytoplasm (reflecting the presence of numerous mitochondria) and granular eosinophilic material in the lumen.

Other Neoplasms

Virtually any neoplasm that can occur in the orbit and eyelid skin can occur, though less frequently, in the conjunctiva, including sebaceous, neural, muscular, vascular, and fibrocytic tumors. Metastatic lesions to the conjunctiva are rare. Orbital neoplasms are discussed in Chapter 14. See also BCSC Section 8, *External Disease and Cornea,* and Section 7, *Orbit, Eyelids, and Lacrimal System.*

CHAPTER 6

Cornea

Topography

The normal cornea is avascular and is composed of 5 layers: epithelium, Bowman layer, stroma, Descemet membrane, and endothelium (Fig 6-1).

The corneal *epithelium* is nonkeratinized stratified squamous epithelium without goblet cells; it ranges from 5 to 7 cell layers in thickness. The epithelial basement membrane is thin and is best seen with periodic acid–Schiff (PAS) stain.

Bowman layer, which is located immediately beneath the epithelial basement membrane, is an acellular, modified region of the anterior stroma that is composed of irregularly arranged collagen fibrils.

The corneal *stroma* makes up 90% of the total corneal thickness. It consists of collagen-producing keratocytes (corneal stromal fibrocytes), collagenous lamellae, and proteoglycan ground substance. The lamellar collagen fibrils are uniform in size and periodicity, contributing to corneal transparency. The posteriormost stroma forms a thin, acellular layer that strongly adheres to the underlying Descemet membrane (pre–Descemet layer).

Descemet membrane is a PAS-positive true basement membrane that is elaborated by the corneal endothelium.

The corneal *endothelium* is composed of a single layer of cells. The cells appear mostly hexagonal *en face,* such as on confocal microscopy. In a histologic cross section of the cornea, the endothelial cells have a cuboidal appearance. See BCSC Section 2, *Fundamentals and Principles of Ophthalmology,* and Section 8, *External Disease and Cornea,* for a discussion of the embryology, structure, and physiology of the cornea.

Dua HS, Faraj LA, Said DG, Gray T, Lowe J. Human corneal anatomy redefined: a novel pre-Descemet's layer (Dua's layer). *Ophthalmology.* 2013;120(9):1778–1785.

Fine BS, Yanoff M. *Ocular Histology: A Text and Atlas.* 2nd ed. Hagerstown, MD: Harper and Row; 1979:176–177.

Congenital Anomalies

Dermoid

Dermoid, a type of choristoma that may involve the cornea, is discussed in Chapter 5 (see Fig 5-2). See also BCSC Section 6, *Pediatric Ophthalmology and Strabismus.*

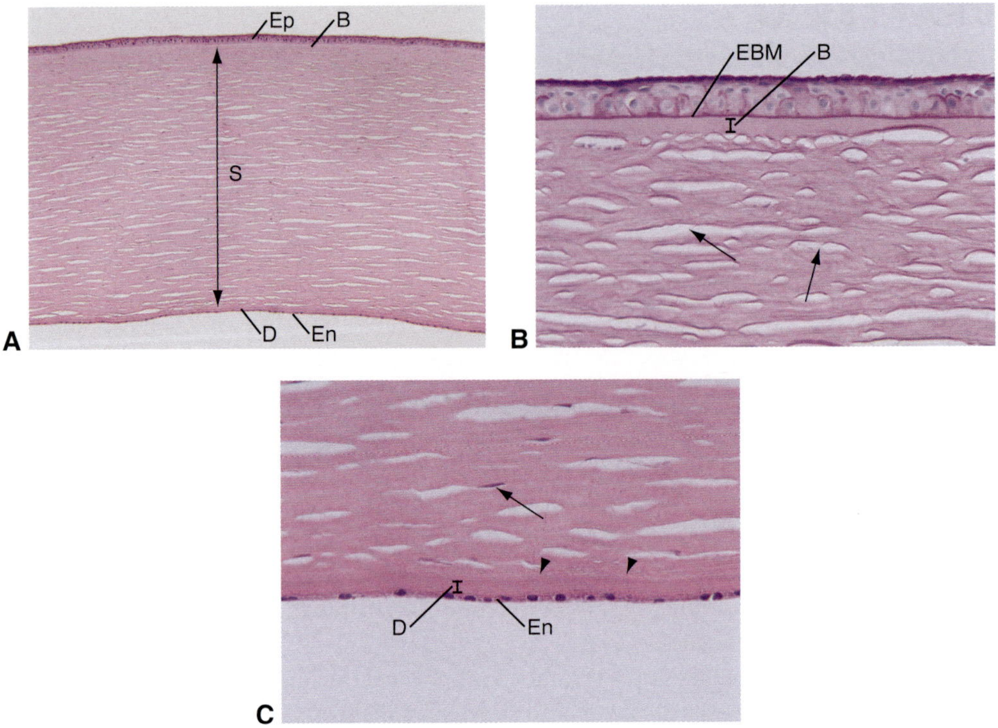

Figure 6-1 Normal cornea. **A,** The cornea is composed of epithelium (Ep), Bowman layer (B), stroma (S), Descemet membrane (D), and endothelium (En). **B,** On higher magnification, periodic acid–Schiff (PAS) stain highlights the epithelial basement membrane (EBM), distinguishing it from Bowman layer (B). Because of dehydration of the tissue during processing for paraffin embedding, multiple areas of separation (clefts) of the stromal lamellae are evident *(arrows).* If the stromal clefts are absent, corneal edema or fibrosis is suspected (the former if the cornea is thick, and the latter if thin). This is an example of a meaningful artifact. **C,** Higher magnification (hematoxylin-eosin [H&E] stain) also delineates Descemet membrane (D), endothelium (En), and a thin, acellular stromal pre–Descemet membrane layer *(arrowheads).* The keratocyte nuclei *(arrow)* are apparent. (Note that PAS stain also highlights Descemet membrane.) *(Courtesy of George J. Harocopos, MD.)*

Peters Anomaly

Peters anomaly represents the severe end of the spectrum of anterior segment dysgenesis syndromes, in which the neural crest does not properly migrate, disrupting anterior segment development and cleavage of the lens from the corneal endothelium. This condition is typically bilateral and sporadic, but autosomal dominant and recessive modes of inheritance have also been reported. In this anomaly, a localized defect, known as *internal ulcer of von Hippel,* appears in the central or paracentral portion of Descemet membrane; at the edges of the defect, iris strands are typically adherent to the posterior corneal surface. In the most severe form of Peters anomaly, the lens also adheres to the posterior corneal surface. The anterior chamber angle may be malformed, predisposing patients to congenital glaucoma. Associated findings include *sclerocornea,* which is characterized by peripheral corneal stromal opacification and vascularization, and *cornea plana,* in which the curvature of the cornea is flattened (Fig 6-2).

See also BCSC Section 8, *External Disease and Cornea,* and Section 6, *Pediatric Ophthalmology and Strabismus.*

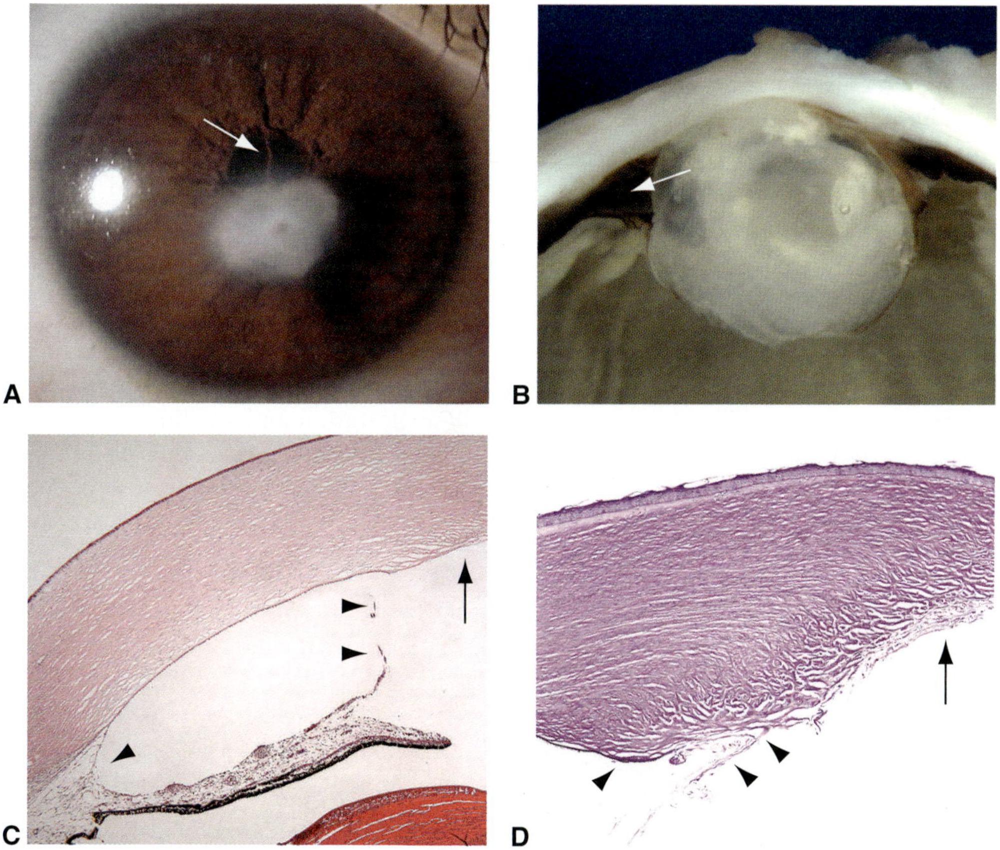

Figure 6-2 Peters anomaly. **A,** Clinical appearance. Note the central corneal opacity (leukoma) with attached iris strands *(arrow).* The lens is uninvolved. **B,** Gross photograph of a more severe form of Peters anomaly demonstrates attachment of a cataractous lens to the opacified cornea (adherent leukoma). Note the accompanying peripheral flattening of the corneal curvature and opacification (cornea plana and sclerocornea, respectively). The iris and anterior chamber angle structures are malformed *(arrow).* **C,** Low-magnification photomicrograph demonstrates internal ulcer of von Hippel *(arrow)* with attached iris strands *(double arrowhead).* Incomplete cleavage of the anterior chamber angle structures (fetal angle deformity) is also present *(single arrowhead).* **D,** PAS stain highlights peripheral Descemet membrane *(single arrowhead).* The central cornea is fibrotic and demonstrates absence of posterior stroma and Descemet membrane *(arrow).* A fibrotic iris strand *(double arrowhead)* is attached to the edge of the corneal defect. *(Courtesy of Tatyana Milman, MD.)*

Inflammations

Infectious Keratitis

Infectious processes caused by a number of microbial agents may affect the cornea. Severe inflammation can lead to corneal necrosis, ulceration, and perforation. See also BCSC Section 8, *External Disease and Cornea.*

Bacterial infections

Corneal infections caused by bacterial agents often follow a disruption in the corneal epithelial integrity resulting from contact lens wear, trauma, alteration in immunologic defenses (eg, use of topical or systemic immunosuppressive agents), antecedent corneal disease (eg, dry eye disease, exposure keratopathy), ocular medication toxicity, or contamination of ocular medications. Bacterial organisms commonly involved in corneal infections include *Pseudomonas aeruginosa, Staphylococcus aureus, Streptococcus pneumoniae,* and Enterobacteriaceae.

Scrapings from infected corneas show collections of neutrophils admixed with necrotic debris. Gram stain may demonstrate the presence of organisms (Fig 6-3). A culture is helpful for accurate identification of specific organisms and for assessment of antibiotic sensitivities.

Herpes simplex virus keratitis

Usually a self-limited corneal epithelial disease, herpes simplex virus keratitis is characterized by a linear arborizing pattern of shallow ulceration and swelling of epithelial cells called a *dendrite* (Fig 6-4A). Corneal scrapings obtained from a dendrite and prepared using Giemsa or hematoxylin-eosin stain reveal intranuclear viral inclusions. Viral

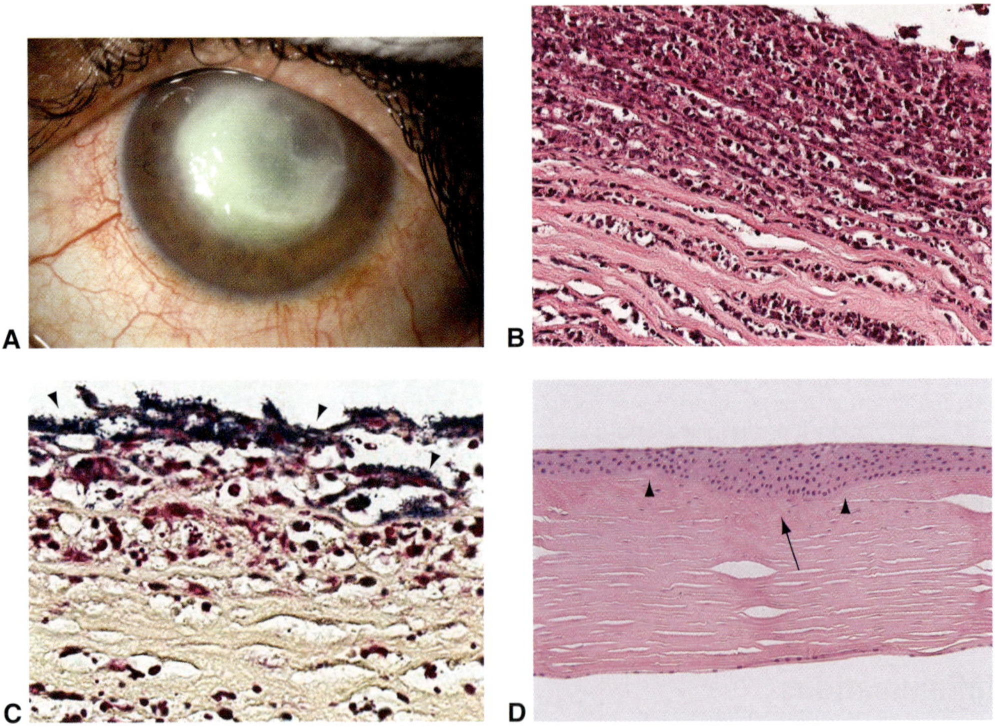

Figure 6-3 Bacterial ulcer. **A,** Clinical appearance. **B,** H&E stain demonstrates acute necrotizing ulcerative keratitis, with numerous neutrophils infiltrating corneal stromal lamellae and necrotic cellular debris. **C,** Gram stain shows numerous gram-positive cocci *(arrowheads).* **D,** Keratoplasty specimen (different patient) showing a scar from healed keratitis. Note loss of Bowman layer *(between arrowheads)* and stromal thinning with fibrosis *(arrow)* and compensatory epithelial thickening. *(Part A courtesy of Andrew J.W. Huang, MD; parts B and C courtesy of Tatyana Milman, MD; part D courtesy of George J. Harocopos, MD.)*

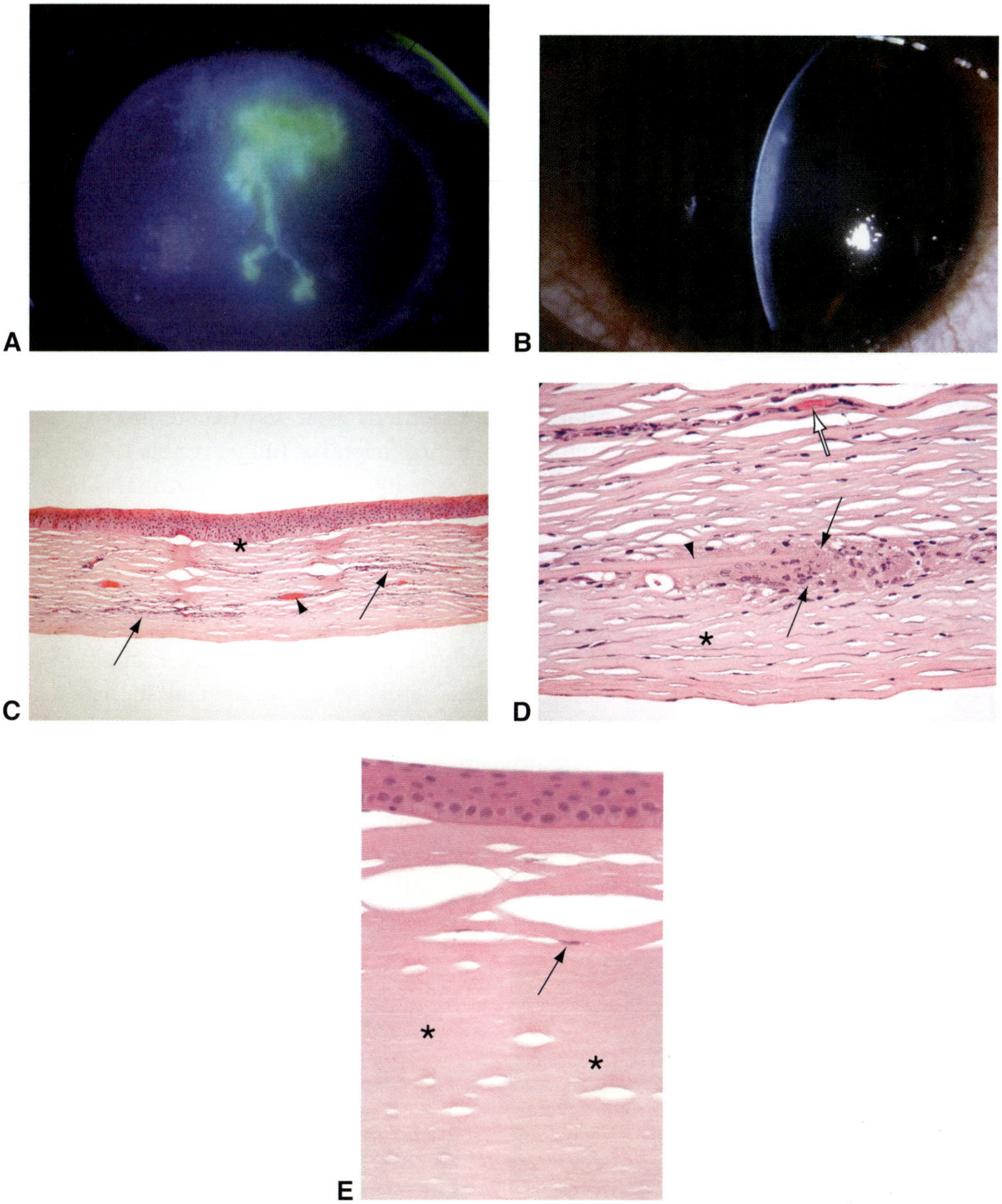

Figure 6-4 Herpes simplex virus keratitis. Clinical photographs depicting dendritic **(A)** and stromal (disciform) **(B)** keratitis. Note the central stromal haze and thickening in **B. C,** Histology of corneal button shows stromal keratitis with loss of Bowman layer *(asterisk)*, stromal scarring and vascularization *(arrowhead)*, and scattered chronic inflammatory cells *(arrows)*. **D,** Higher-magnification photomicrograph shows granulomatous reaction *(between arrows)* in the region of Descemet membrane *(arrowhead)*. Note the fibrous retrocorneal membrane *(asterisk)*, scattered chronic inflammatory cells, and blood vessel *(open arrow)*. **E,** Postherpetic neurotrophic keratopathy. Photomicrograph shows featureless corneal stroma *(asterisks)* with only rare keratocytes *(arrow)*. *(Parts A and B courtesy of Anthony J. Lubniewski, MD; parts C and D courtesy of Tatyana Milman, MD; part E courtesy of Robert H. Rosa, Jr, MD.)*

culture, antigen detection, or polymerase chain reaction (PCR) techniques may be helpful in atypical cases. Stromal and/or *disciform keratitis* (Fig 6-4B) may accompany or follow epithelial infection, leading to stromal scarring and possibly vascularization. Histologically, chronic inflammatory cells and blood vessels may be seen tracking between stromal lamellae, a phenomenon called *interstitial keratitis* (Fig 6-4C) (discussed later). Endotheliitis may also occur, with a granulomatous reaction at the level of Descemet membrane (Fig 6-4D). Postherpetic neurotrophic keratopathy may result from corneal hypoesthesia or anesthesia; it is characterized histologically by a corneal stroma that is essentially devoid of keratocytes (Fig 6-4E).

Fungal keratitis

Mycotic keratitis is often a complication of trauma, especially trauma involving plant or vegetable matter, or microtrauma related to contact lens wear. Corticosteroid use, especially topical, is another major risk factor. Unlike most bacteria, fungi are able to penetrate the cornea and extend through Descemet membrane into the anterior chamber. The most common organisms are the septated, filamentous fungi *Aspergillus* and *Fusarium* and the yeast *Candida; Mucor* (nonseptated, filamentous) is less common. Cultures, particularly on Sabouraud agar, are helpful for accurate identification of specific organisms and for assessment of antifungal sensitivities. When the culture is negative and organism identity remains elusive, corneal biopsy may be considered, for both histologic evaluation and PCR. Many fungi can be seen in tissue sections with the use of special stains such as Grocott-Gomori methenamine–silver nitrate (GMS) or PAS (Fig 6-5). Fungi (eg, *Mucor*) are sometimes apparent on routine hematoxylin-eosin sections.

Acanthamoeba *keratitis*

Acanthamoeba protozoa most commonly cause infection in soft contact lens wearers who do not take appropriate precautions in cleaning and disinfecting their lenses or whose

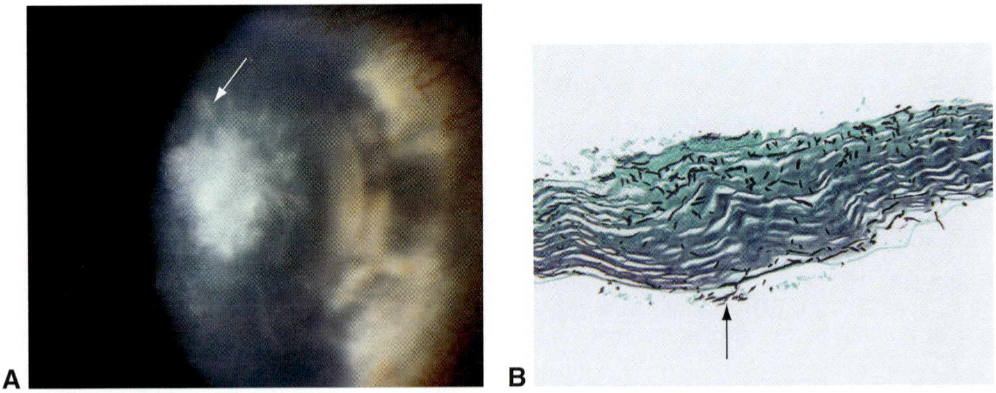

Figure 6-5 *Fusarium* keratitis. **A,** Clinical photograph shows gray-white, dry-appearing stromal infiltrate with feathery margins and satellite lesions *(arrow).* **B,** Grocott-Gomori methenamine–silver nitrate (GMS) stain of corneal button demonstrates fungal hyphae *(black).* Note that fungal hyphae have penetrated through Descemet membrane *(arrow).* *(Part A courtesy of Andrew J.W. Huang, MD; part B courtesy of George J. Harocopos, MD.)*

lenses come into contact with contaminated stagnant water (eg, as found in hot tubs and ponds). Patients presenting with *Acanthamoeba* keratitis usually have severe eye pain caused by radial keratoneuritis. In late stages, a ring infiltrate may be present (Fig 6-6A). Special culture techniques and media, including nonnutrient blood agar layered with *Escherichia coli,* are required to grow *Acanthamoeba.* In later stages of disease, the organisms penetrate into deeper layers of the stroma and may be difficult to isolate from a superficial scraping. Because of these challenges, PCR-based methods for diagnosis of *Acanthamoeba* keratitis have become more widely used. Histologically, corneal scrapings, biopsy specimens, or corneal buttons may show cysts and trophozoites (Fig 6-6B). The organisms are generally easily visualized with routine hematoxylin-eosin sections but may also be highlighted with PAS and GMS stains. Calcofluor white or acridine orange stain may also be used.

Infectious pseudocrystalline keratopathy

Infectious pseudocrystalline keratopathy typically occurs in patients on long-term topical corticosteroid therapy—for example, following penetrating keratoplasty. The infection typically arises along a suture track or a surgical wound. The most common etiologic microorganism is viridans (α-hemolytic) streptococci, but other organisms have been reported, including bacteria, mycobacteria, and fungi. Chronic immunosuppression, when combined with properties of the organism's glycocalyx that sequester the organism from the immune system, may promote growth of the organism in this condition. No true crystals are involved; rather, this condition derives its name from the crystalloid clinical appearance of the opacity (Fig 6-7A). In many cases, the diagnosis is missed clinically and

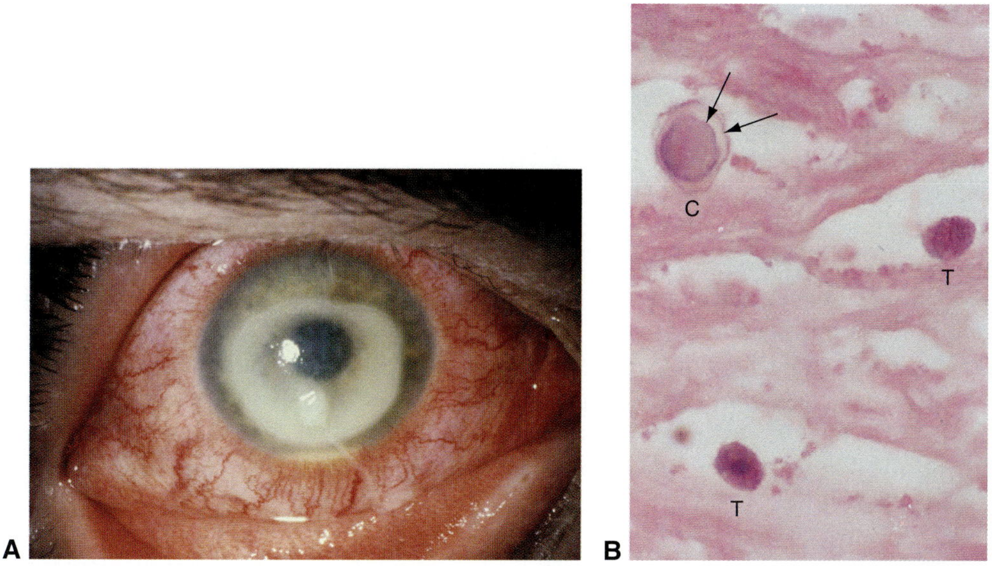

Figure 6-6 *Acanthamoeba* keratitis. **A,** Clinical photograph depicting ring infiltrate and small hypopyon. **B,** Note the cyst (C) and trophozoite (T) forms. The cyst has a double wall, that is, endocyst and exocyst *(arrows)*. *(Part A courtesy of Sander Dubovy, MD.)*

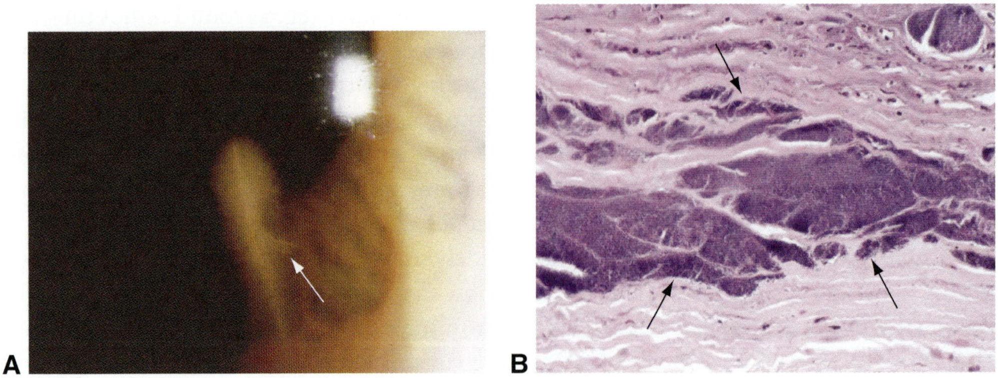

Figure 6-7 Infectious pseudocrystalline keratopathy. **A,** Clinical photograph depicting crystalloid-appearing (or "fernlike") stromal infiltrate *(arrow),* with intact overlying epithelium. The infection arose along a suture track following repair of a corneal laceration. **B,** Gram stain demonstrates colonies of gram-positive cocci interposed between stromal collagen lamellae *(arrows)* without appreciable inflammatory response. *(Part A courtesy of Anthony J. Lubniewski, MD; part B courtesy of Morton E. Smith, MD.)*

is made histologically after failure of a corneal graft. Histologically, colonies of organisms are present within the interlamellar spaces of the stroma. The inflammatory cell infiltrate is typically insignificant. The organisms are sometimes apparent on hematoxylin-eosin stain but may also be highlighted by Gram, PAS, GMS, or acid-fast stain, depending on the etiologic agent (Fig 6-7B).

Interstitial keratitis

In interstitial keratitis (IK), nonsuppurative inflammatory cells infiltrate the interlamellar spaces of the corneal stroma, often with vascularization; typically, the overlying epithelium remains intact. The changes observed in IK are thought to result from an immunologic response to infectious microorganisms or their antigens. Transplacental infection of the fetus by *Treponema pallidum* (congenital syphilis) may cause IK (Fig 6-8A). Histologically, chronic syphilis-related (luetic) IK is characterized by the presence of stromal ghost vessels devoid of erythrocytes with surrounding stromal fibrosis and a variable degree of chronic inflammation. Bowman layer and Descemet membrane are characteristically intact. In addition, Descemet membrane may demonstrate focal multilaminated excrescences (Fig 6-8B), reminiscent of *guttae,* drop-like excrescences of Descemet membrane (Latin for *drop*), seen in Fuchs endothelial corneal dystrophy (discussed later in this chapter).

Although congenital syphilis represents the "classic" cause of IK, the most common etiologic agent of IK is the herpes virus (see Fig 6-4). Other organisms that can cause IK include *Mycobacterium tuberculosis, Mycobacterium leprae, Borrelia burgdorferi,* and Epstein-Barr virus.

Noninfectious Keratitis

Corneal inflammation can also be caused by noninfectious agents. For example, autoimmune diseases, especially rheumatoid arthritis and graft-vs-host disease, may be associated with sterile corneal ulceration. Topical medication toxicity (eg, overuse of topical

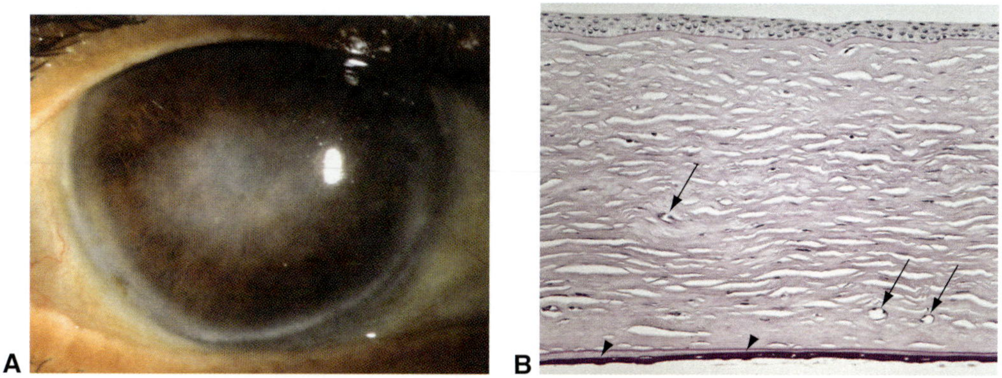

Figure 6-8 Interstitial keratitis of congenital syphilis. **A,** Clinical photograph depicting stromal opacity, with intact overlying epithelium. **B,** PAS stain shows ghost vessels *(arrows)* in the midstroma and deep stroma, with surrounding fibrosis and sparse chronic inflammatory cell infiltrate. Descemet membrane is multilaminated and demonstrates nodular excrescences *(arrowheads).* Note the intact epithelium and Bowman layer. Corneal thickness measured less than 400 µm, indicative of visually significant stromal fibrosis. *(Part A courtesy of Anthony J. Lubniewski, MD; part B courtesy of Tatyana Milman, MD.)*

anesthetics, nonsteroidal anti-inflammatory drugs [NSAIDs], or antivirals) may also result in corneal melting. Histology varies, depending on the etiology, but the unifying feature is absence of organisms. See also BCSC Section 8, *External Disease and Cornea.*

Degenerations and Dystrophies

Degenerations

Corneal degenerations are secondary changes that occur in previously normal tissue. They are often associated with aging, are not inherited, and are not necessarily bilateral. See also BCSC Section 8, *External Disease and Cornea.*

Salzmann nodular degeneration

Salzmann nodular degeneration may occur secondary to long-standing keratitis or may be idiopathic. It may be bilateral and is more commonly seen in female patients who are middle-aged and older, often in association with blepharitis. Lesions that are gray-white or bluish and flat or raised appear where the eyelid margin contacts the cornea in primary gaze and/or in the central and paracentral cornea (Fig 6-9A). Histologic examination reveals variably thick epithelium and replacement of Bowman layer with disorganized collagenous tissue (Fig 6-9B).

Clinical and histologic findings of Salzmann nodular degeneration overlap with those of the recently characterized peripheral hypertrophic subepithelial corneal degeneration, which also demonstrates components resembling pterygia.

Calcific band keratopathy

Seen clinically as a band-shaped calcific plaque in the interpalpebral zone and typically sparing the most peripheral clear cornea, calcific band keratopathy is characterized by the

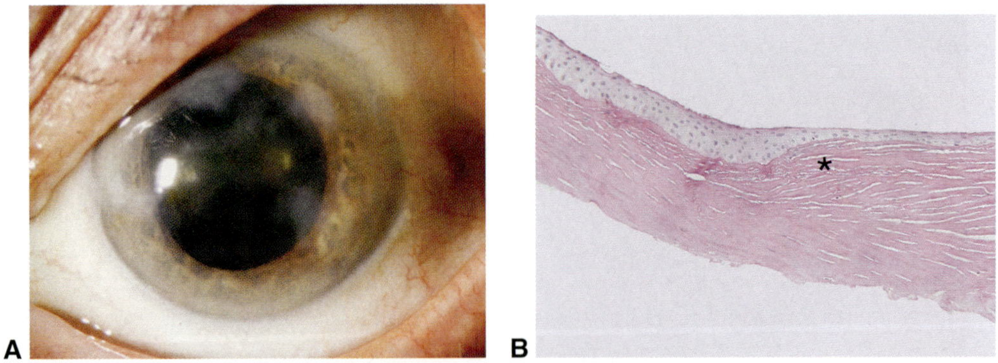

Figure 6-9 Salzmann nodular degeneration. **A,** Clinical appearance. Note the gray-white corneal opacities. **B,** Histology of superficial keratectomy specimen (PAS stain) shows irregular epithelial thickness and diffuse loss of Bowman layer, as well as replacement of the latter with disorganized collagenous tissue *(asterisk)*. *(Courtesy of George J. Harocopos, MD.)*

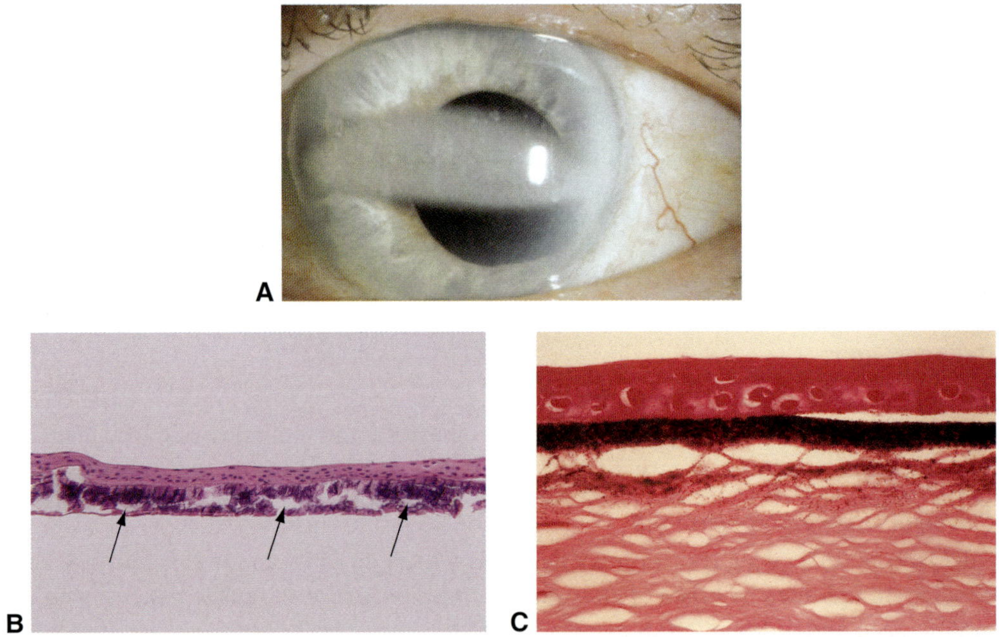

Figure 6-10 Calcific band keratopathy. **A,** Clinical appearance. **B,** Calcific band keratopathy may be treated with epithelial scraping and chelation with ethylenediaminetetraacetic acid (EDTA "scrub"). The calcium is deposited at the level of Bowman layer *(arrows)*, appearing deeply basophilic (purple) on H&E stain. **C,** Calcium deposits appear black on von Kossa stain. *(Part A courtesy of Anthony J. Lubniewski, MD; part B courtesy of George J. Harocopos, MD; part C courtesy of Hans E. Grossniklaus, MD.)*

deposition of calcium at the level of Bowman layer and the anterior stroma. The calcium deposits appear as basophilic granules in hematoxylin-eosin sections; the presence of calcium can be further confirmed with the use of special stains such as alizarin red or von Kossa stain (Fig 6-10). Band keratopathy may develop in chronically inflamed and/or traumatized eyes, following therapy (eg, intravitreal silicone oil), and, less commonly, in association with systemic hypercalcemic states.

Actinic keratopathy

Also known as *spheroidal degeneration, Labrador keratopathy,* or *climatic droplet keratopathy,* actinic keratopathy is characterized by aggregates of translucent, golden-brown spheroidal deposits in the interpalpebral superficial cornea (Fig 6-11A). The condition is generally bilateral and is more common in males. It is frequently associated with calcific band keratopathy. In addition, smaller spheroidal deposits may mimic calcific band keratopathy; this phenomenon has been described as "actinic" band keratopathy. The etiology is controversial, but the cumulative evidence suggests that the deposits develop from ultraviolet (UV) radiation–induced alteration of preexisting structural connective tissue components or from the synthesis of abnormal extracellular material in limbal conjunctiva. This abnormal material progressively diffuses into the superficial cornea, precipitates over a prolonged period of time, and may be further modified by UV light. Histologic examination reveals basophilic globules beneath the epithelium in the region of Bowman layer and the anterior stroma (Fig 6-11B). Analogous to the actinic degeneration of collagen in pingueculae and pterygia, the deposits stain black with special stains for elastin, such as Verhoeff–van Gieson stain.

Pannus

Pannus, the growth of fibrovascular or fibrous tissue between the epithelium and Bowman layer (Fig 6-12), is frequently seen in cases of chronic corneal edema or following prolonged corneal inflammation. Bowman layer may be disrupted.

Bullous keratopathy

Bullous keratopathy can occur after cataract surgery (*pseudophakic* or *aphakic bullous keratopathy*) or after other forms of intraocular surgery, such as penetrating keratoplasty, glaucoma procedures, or retinal detachment repair. Bullous keratopathy is induced by extensive endothelial cell loss. This leads to corneal decompensation, characterized by the initial development of stromal edema and Descemet membrane folds, followed by

A B
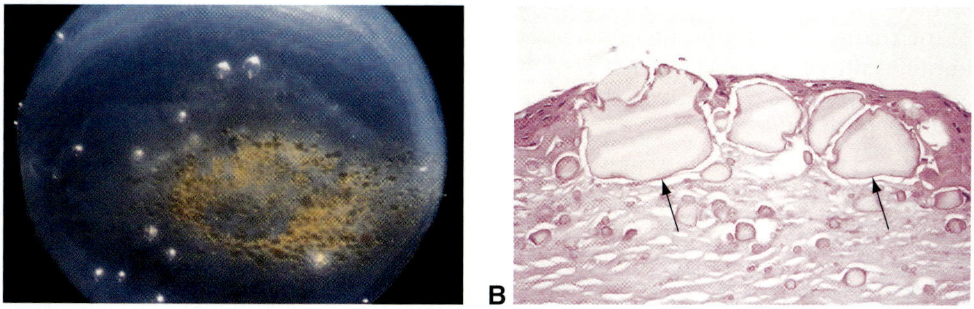

Figure 6-11 Actinic keratopathy (also called *spheroidal degeneration* or *climatic droplet keratopathy*). **A,** Gross appearance of corneal button. The air bubbles are artifacts. **B,** Histology shows lightly staining basophilic globules *(arrows)* in the epithelium and superficial stroma. *(Courtesy of Hans E. Grossniklaus, MD.)*

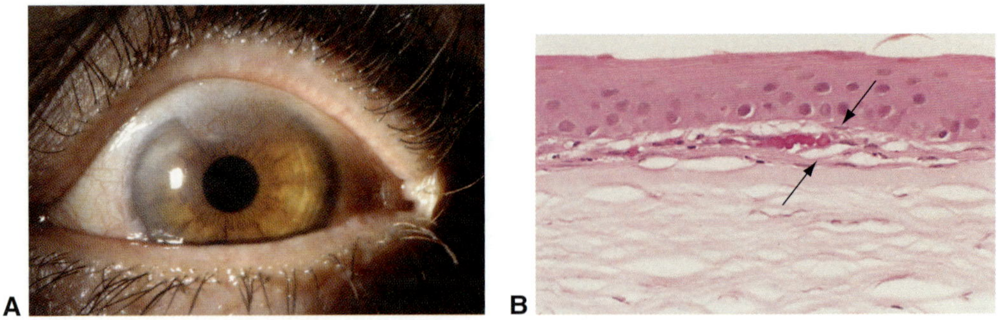

Figure 6-12 Pannus. **A,** Clinical appearance in the superior cornea. **B,** Fibrovascular pannus *(between arrows)* is interposed between the epithelium and Bowman layer. *(Part A courtesy of George J. Harocopos, MD.)*

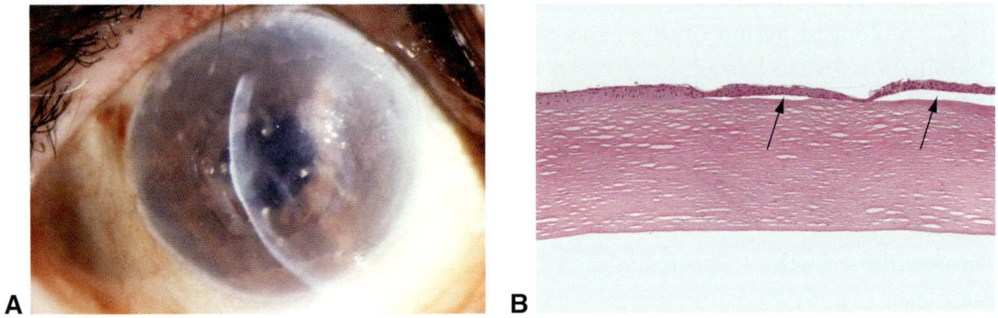

Figure 6-13 Pseudophakic bullous keratopathy. **A,** Clinical appearance of severe bullous keratopathy associated with an iris clip anterior chamber lens implant. **B,** Corneal button from penetrating keratoplasty. Note the subepithelial bullae *(arrows).* Also note stromal edema, characterized by focal absence of interlamellar spaces, and diffuse endothelial cell loss without thickening of Descemet membrane or guttae. *(Part A courtesy of Andrew J.W. Huang, MD; part B courtesy of George J. Harocopos, MD.)*

intracellular epithelial edema and, ultimately, separation of the epithelium from Bowman layer. Small separations called *microcysts* may coalesce to form large separations, known as *bullae.* In advanced cases of bullous keratopathy, secondary epithelial basement membrane changes and fibrous pannus may develop. Descemet membrane may be thickened but typically lacks guttae (Fig 6-13).

Corneal graft failure

Failure of an existing corneal graft is one of the most common indications for penetrating keratoplasty (PK) or lamellar keratoplasty. In PK or endothelial keratoplasty, graft failure may develop gradually over time or follow an acute rejection episode. The final common pathway is endothelial cell loss. When endothelial failure occurs, associated bullous keratopathy often develops. A delicate, fibrous retrocorneal membrane is frequently seen (Fig 6-14A, B). Wound-related complications, such as *fibrous* or *epithelial ingrowth* or *downgrowth,* can also contribute to graft failure; they are more common in PK grafts. In various lamellar keratoplasty procedures, additional important etiologies of graft failure are suboptimal trephination and abnormal lenticule positioning (Fig 6-14C–E).

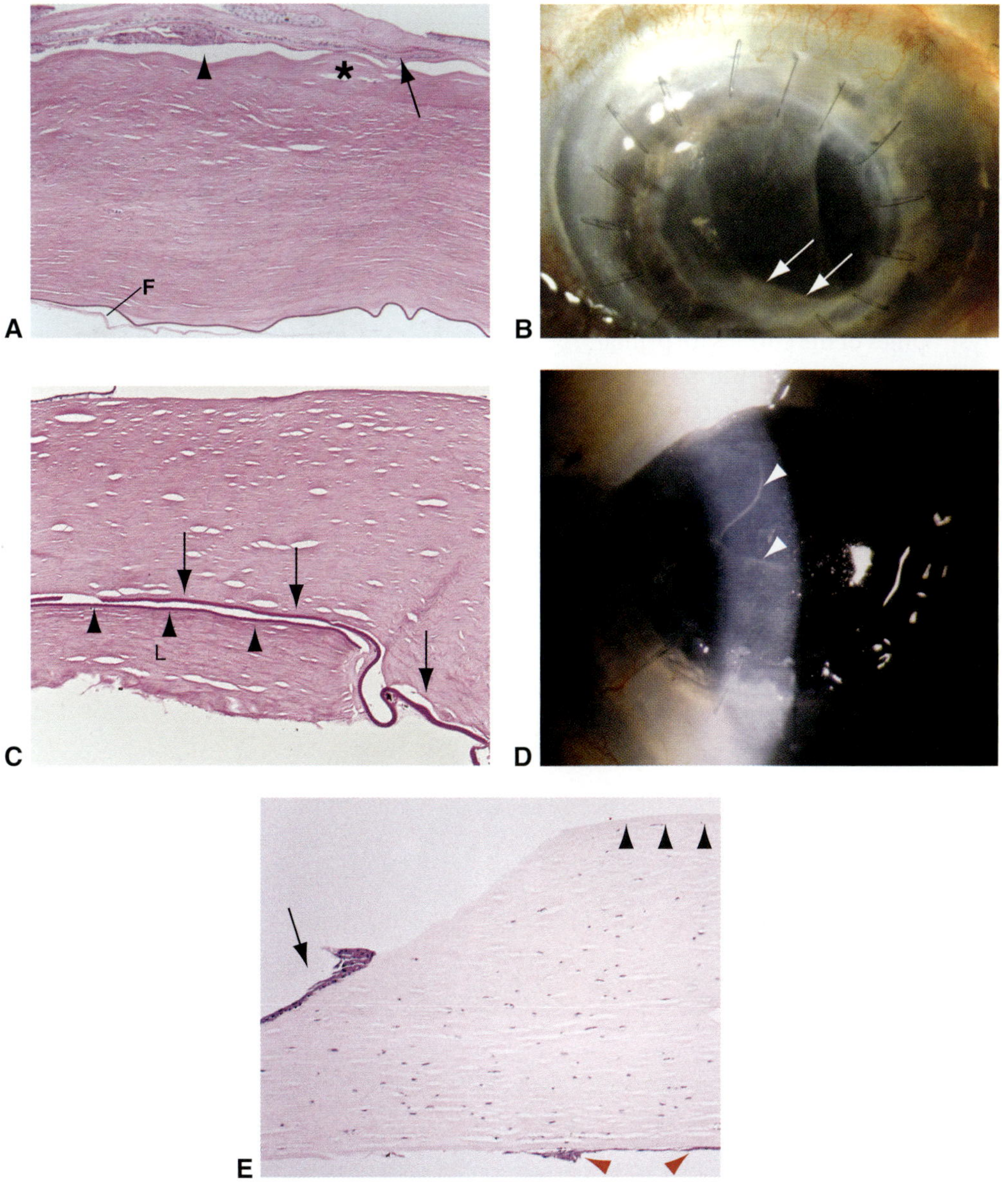

Figure 6-14 Corneal graft failure. **A,** PAS stain of failed penetrating keratoplasty (PK) graft with diffuse endothelial cell loss, fibrous retrocorneal membrane (F), secondary stromal edema with bullous keratopathy *(arrowhead)*, epithelial basement membrane thickening *(arrow)*, and thick fibrous pannus *(asterisk)*. **B,** Clinical appearance of fibrous downgrowth *(arrows)*. **C,** PAS stain of a failed graft following Descemet-stripping automated endothelial keratoplasty (DSAEK). The abnormally positioned donor lenticule (L) with donor Descemet membrane *(arrowheads)* faces the recipient's Descemet membrane *(arrows)*. Note the endothelial attenuation and marked stromal edema. **D,** Clinical appearance of epithelial downgrowth in a PK graft *(arrowheads)*. **E,** Histology of an explanted donor lenticule from a failed DSAEK graft (different patient) shows full-thickness cornea with Bowman layer *(arrowheads)* on the right and partial-thickness cornea on the left. Retention of donor epithelium led to the epithelial ingrowth *(red arrowheads)*. *(Part A courtesy of George J. Harocopos, MD; parts B and D courtesy of Anthony J. Lubniewski, MD; parts C and E courtesy of Tatyana Milman, MD.)*

Pigment deposits

Blood staining of the cornea may complicate hyphema when intraocular pressure (IOP) is very high for a long duration; however, if the endothelium is compromised, blood staining can occur even at normal or low IOP (Fig 6-15A). Histologically, red blood cells and their breakdown products (mostly hemoglobin and also small amounts of hemosiderin) are seen in the corneal stroma. The hemosiderin is located in the cytoplasm of keratocytes and may be demonstrated with iron stains, such as Prussian blue (Fig 6-15B, C).

Dystrophies

Dystrophies of the cornea are primary, generally inherited, bilateral disorders, categorized by the layer of the cornea most involved (ie, epithelial, stromal, or endothelial) and by the identified genetic alterations. Although traditional pathologic methods continue to play an important role in the diagnosis of corneal dystrophies, clinicians are increasingly relying on ancillary clinical diagnostic modalities, such as confocal microscopy and optical coherence tomography (OCT), and on molecular genetic studies, particularly in the evaluation of dystrophies induced by a mutation in the *transforming growth factor beta-induced gene (TGFBI).* These studies, which are commercially available, can be performed on peripheral blood. Only the most common corneal dystrophies are discussed in this chapter. See also BCSC Section 8, *External Disease and Cornea.*

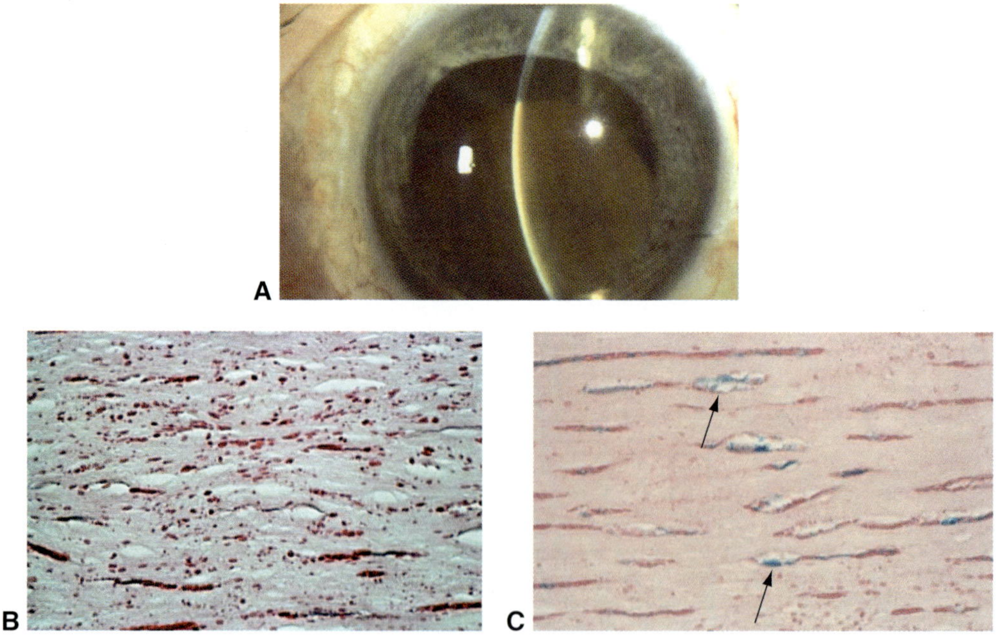

Figure 6-15 Corneal blood staining. **A,** Clinical appearance. Note the tan coloration of the central cornea. **B,** Masson trichrome stain. The red particles represent erythrocytic debris and hemoglobin in the corneal stroma. **C,** An iron stain demonstrates hemosiderin *(arrows)* within stromal keratocytes. *(Part A courtesy of Anthony J. Lubniewski, MD; parts B and C courtesy of Hans E. Grossniklaus, MD.)*

Epithelial and subepithelial dystrophies

Epithelial basement membrane dystrophy Also called *map-dot-fingerprint dystrophy,* epithelial basement membrane dystrophy (EBMD) is characterized by clinically observed patterns resembling maps, dots, and fingerprints. Regional thickening of epithelial basement membrane with deposition of intraepithelial basal laminar material results in lines resembling a geographic map. Intraepithelial pseudocysts containing degenerated epithelial debris resemble dots. Riblike intraepithelial extensions of basal laminar material result in patterns resembling fingerprints (Fig 6-16). Many patients with presumed EBMD have an underlying degenerative process, such as recurrent corneal erosions or bullous keratopathy.

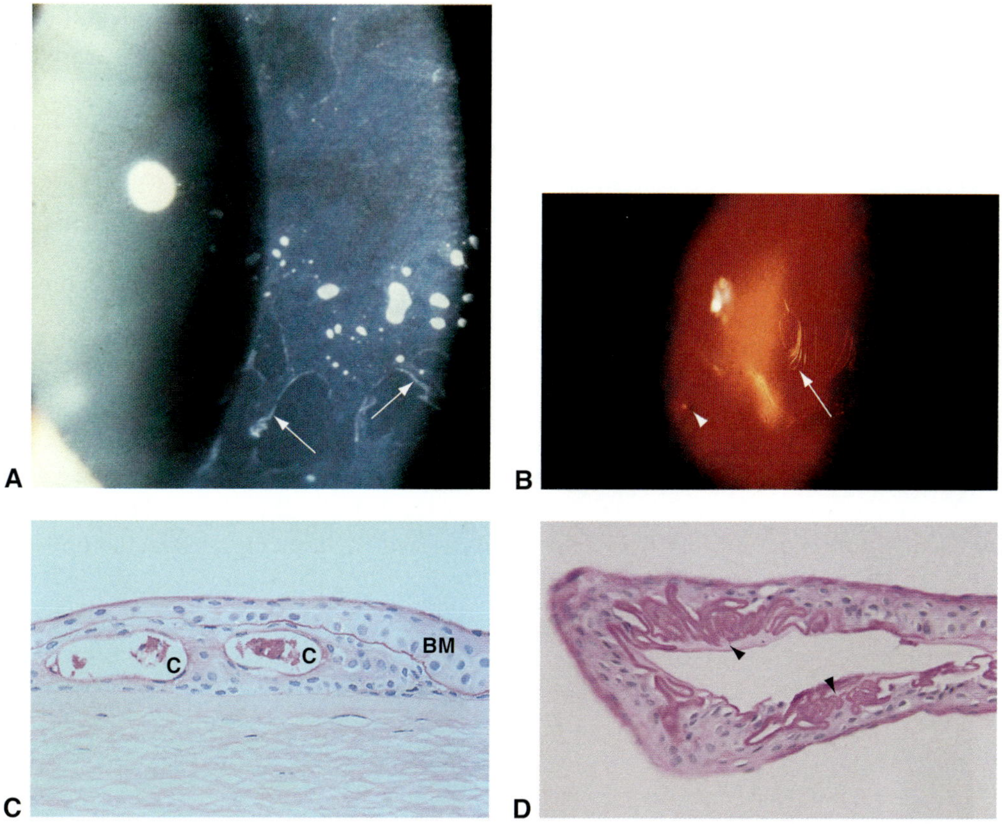

Figure 6-16 Epithelial basement membrane dystrophy (EBMD, also called *map-dot-fingerprint dystrophy*). **A,** Clinical appearance, showing fine, lacy opacities *(arrows).* **B,** Retroillumination demonstrating wavy lines *(arrow)* and dotlike lesions *(arrowhead).* **C,** The changes in primary EBMD are essentially identical to those seen in cases of chronic corneal edema secondary to endothelial decompensation. Note the intraepithelial basement membrane (BM) highlighted with PAS stain and the degenerating epithelial cells trapped within cystoid spaces (C). **D,** When surgical treatment is required for EBMD, removal of abnormal epithelium (superficial keratectomy) may be performed, as in this case. PAS stain highlights folding and thickening *(arrowheads)* of the epithelial basement membrane. *(Part A courtesy of Andrew J.W. Huang, MD; part D courtesy of George J. Harocopos, MD.)*

Epithelial–stromal TGFBI *dystrophies*

A mutation in the *TGFBI* gene on chromosome 5q31 results in the most common dystrophies chiefly involving epithelium and stroma. This gene encodes *keratoepithelin,* a protein elaborated predominantly by the corneal epithelium. Thus, contrary to the current anatomical terminology, these dystrophies are primarily epithelial in origin.

Reis-Bücklers corneal dystrophy Formerly known as corneal dystrophy of Bowman layer type I, Reis-Bücklers corneal dystrophy (RBCD) is an autosomal dominant disorder characterized by confluent, irregular, and coarse geographic-like opacities with varying densities at the level of Bowman layer and superficial stroma (Fig 6-17A). OCT demonstrates a homogenous, confluent layer of hyperreflective deposits, which often has a serrated anterior border, at the level of Bowman layer and anterior stroma. Histologically, Bowman layer is replaced by a sheetlike layer of granular deposits, which stain intensely red with Masson trichrome stain and immunoreact with anti-*TGFBI* antibodies. The overlying epithelium is irregular in thickness (Fig 6-17B).

Thiel-Behnke corneal dystrophy Formerly known as corneal dystrophy of Bowman layer type II, Thiel-Behnke corneal dystrophy (TBCD) clinically manifests as solitary flecks or irregularly shaped, scattered opacities at the level of Bowman layer that progress to symmetrical subepithelial honeycomb opacities. OCT demonstrates prominent hyperreflective material at the level of Bowman layer that extends into the epithelium in a characteristic "saw-toothed" pattern. Histologic evaluation shows diffuse replacement of Bowman layer by fibrous pannus and the "saw-toothed" pattern observed with OCT (Fig 6-18). Ultrastructurally, TBCD can be distinguished from RBCD by the presence of curly collagen fibers that are about 10 nm in diameter.

Lattice corneal dystrophy, *TGFBI* Type: Classic lattice corneal dystrophy and variants Classic lattice corneal dystrophy (LCD), or lattice corneal dystrophy type 1 (LCD1), is an autosomal dominant stromal dystrophy characterized by branching, refractile lines in

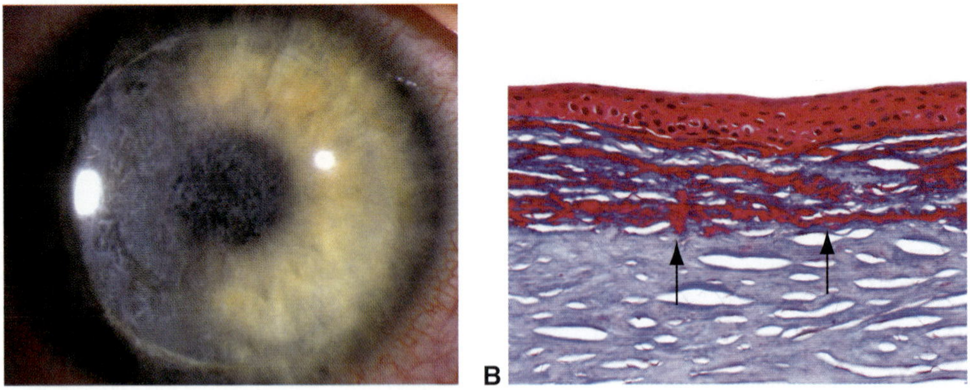
A B

Figure 6-17 Reis-Bücklers corneal dystrophy. **A,** Clinical photograph demonstrates coarse opacities resembling a geographic map in the superficial cornea. Note the circumferential linear scar in the peripheral cornea associated with a lamellar graft in this recurrent corneal dystrophy. **B,** Masson trichrome stain demonstrates diffuse loss of Bowman layer, superficial stromal fibrosis, and numerous red deposits *(arrows)*. *(Part A courtesy of Brandon Ayres, MD; part B courtesy of Tatyana Milman, MD.)*

the central corneal stroma, as well as intervening stromal haze in the later stages of disease (Fig 6-19A). Histologic examination reveals poorly demarcated, fusiform amyloid deposits, most conspicuously in the anterior stroma and Bowman layer. These deposits stain orange with Congo red on standard light microscopy and exhibit birefringence with dichroism (orange and apple green coloration) under polarized light (Fig 6-19B–D).

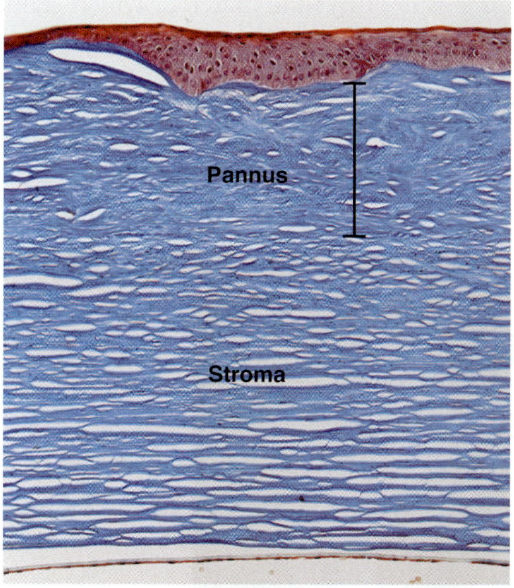

Figure 6-18 Thiel-Behnke corneal dystrophy. Masson trichrome stain demonstrates diffuse replacement of Bowman layer by a thick fibrous pannus (bracket). The overlying epithelium exhibits a "saw-toothed" configuration. The underlying stroma appears to be uninvolved. *(Courtesy of Tero Kivelä, MD.)*

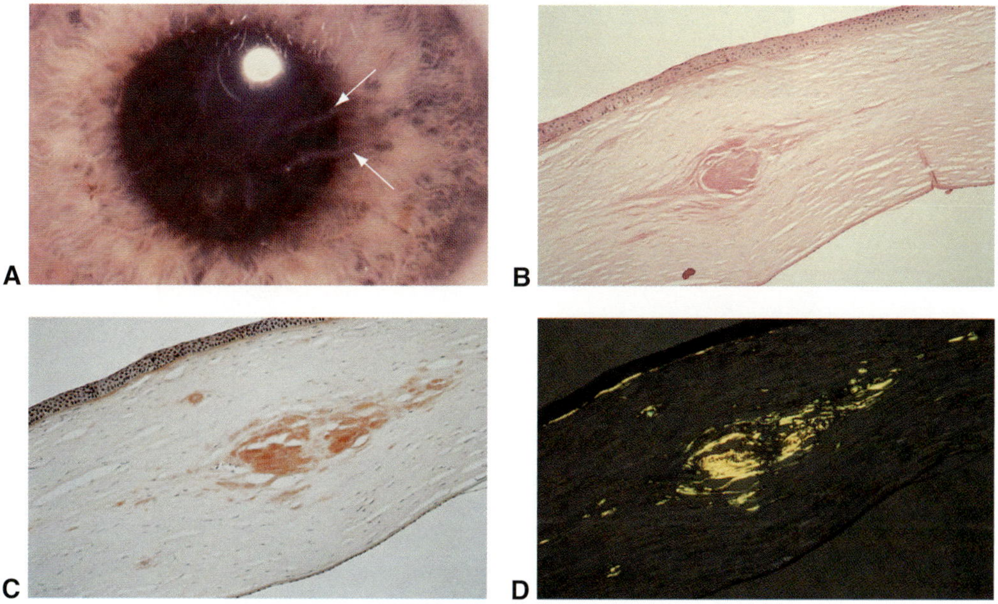

Figure 6-19 Lattice corneal dystrophy *TGFBI* type. **A,** Clinical appearance. Note the lattice lines *(arrows)*. **B,** H&E stain shows scattered fusiform, eosinophilic material deposited in the anterior and mid-stroma. **C,** Congo red stain (orange) demonstrates that the fusiform deposits are amyloid. **D,** With Congo red stain, under polarized light, amyloid deposits exhibit dichroism (orange and apple green). *(Parts B–D courtesy of Hans E. Grossniklaus, MD.)*

Amyloid demonstrates metachromasia with crystal violet stain. The fluorescent stain thioflavin T may also be used to demonstrate amyloid.

Granular corneal dystrophy type 1 Granular corneal dystrophy type 1 (GCD1) is an autosomal dominant disorder characterized by sharply demarcated (granular) central corneal stromal deposits separated by clear intervening stroma (Fig 6-20A). Histologically, irregularly shaped, well-circumscribed, "crumblike" deposits of hyaline material, which stain bright red with Masson trichrome stain, are visible in the stroma (Fig 6-20B, C).

Granular corneal dystrophy type 2 Formerly known as *Avellino dystrophy,* granular corneal dystrophy type 2 (GCD2) demonstrates clinical, histologic, and ultrastructural features of both granular and lattice dystrophy (Fig 6-21). See Table 6-1 for a histologic comparison of macular corneal dystrophy, GCD1, LCD1, and GCD2.

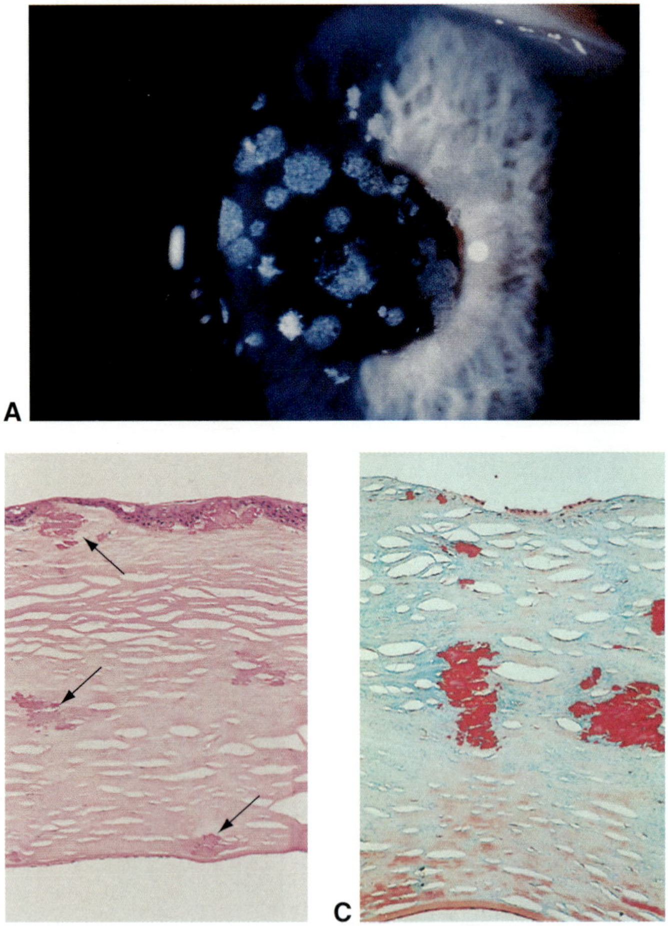

Figure 6-20 Granular corneal dystrophy type 1. **A,** Clinical appearance. Note the well-demarcated stromal opacities with clear intervening stroma. **B,** H&E stain. Note the eosinophilic deposits *(arrows)* at all levels of the corneal stroma. **C,** Masson trichrome stain. The stromal collagen stains blue, and the granular deposits stain brilliant red.

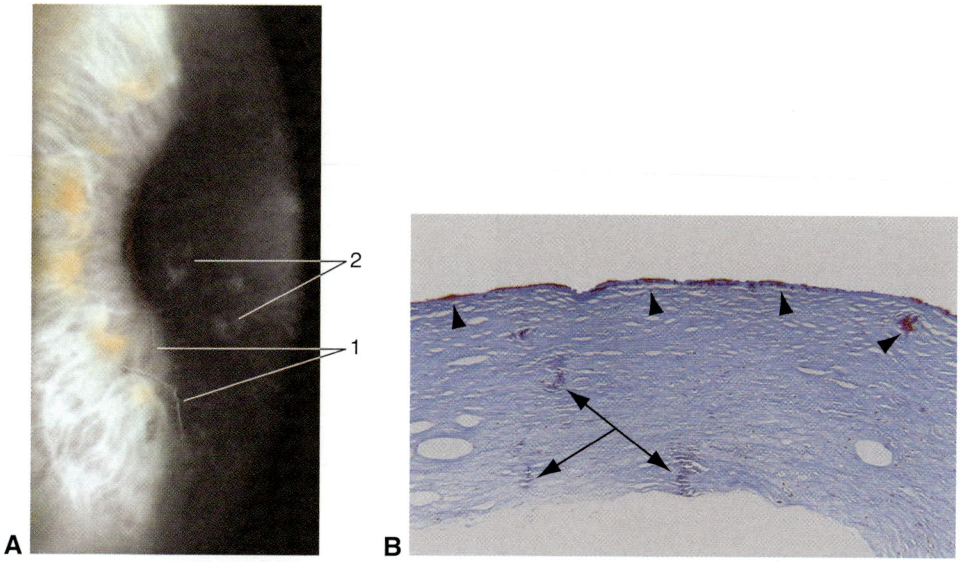

Figure 6-21 Granular corneal dystrophy type 2 (Avellino). **A,** Clinical appearance, showing both lattice lines (1) and granular deposits (2). **B,** Trichrome stain of deep anterior lamellar keratoplasty (DALK) button highlights hyaline deposits at the level of Bowman layer and anterior stroma *(arrowheads).* Other deposits at various levels of the stroma stain a darker blue than the stromal background *(triple arrow);* Congo red stain confirmed that these deposits are amyloid. The empty spaces in the posterior stroma were caused by pneumatic dissection. *(Part A modified with permission from Krachmer JH, Palay DA.* Cornea Atlas. *2nd ed. Philadelphia: Mosby-Elsevier; 2006:163. Part B courtesy of George J. Harocopos, MD.)*

Table 6-1 Histologic Differentiation of Corneal Dystrophies

Dystrophy	Trichrome	Alcian Blue	Congo Red	Periodic Acid–Schiff
Granular, type 1	+ (strong)	–	–	–
Granular, type 2 (Avellino)	+ (strong)	–	+ (dichroism)	+ (amyloid)
Lattice, type 1	–	–	+ (dichroism)	+ (amyloid)
Macular	–	+	–	+
Reis-Bücklers	+ (strong)	–	–	–
Thiel-Behnke	–/+ (weak)	–	–	–

Stromal dystrophies

Macular corneal dystrophy Macular corneal dystrophy (MCD), an autosomal recessive corneal stromal dystrophy, caused by mutations in the *carbohydrate sulfotransferase 6* gene on chromosome 16q22. This dystrophy is characterized by diffuse stromal haze that extends limbus to limbus and is associated with poorly demarcated focal opacities (macules) (Fig 6-22A). Alcian blue and colloidal iron stains highlight nonsulfated glycosaminoglycan deposits, which accumulate intracellularly in the stromal keratocytes and endothelium and extracellularly in the stroma. Pathologic changes in the endothelium are frequently accompanied by guttae (Fig 6-22B–D).

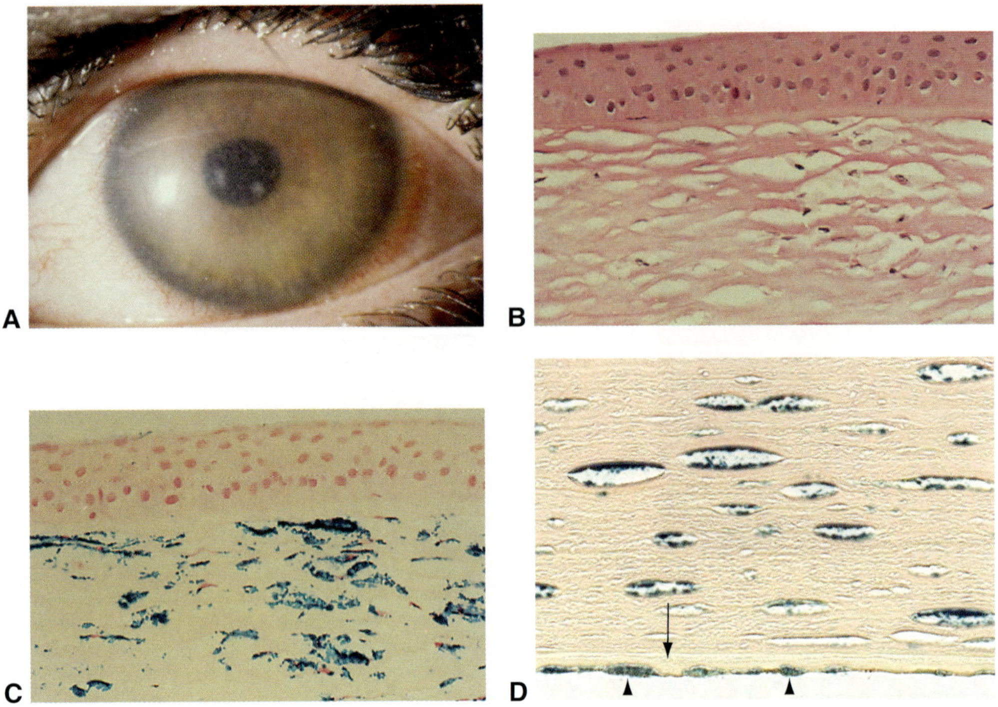

Figure 6-22 Macular corneal dystrophy. **A,** Clinical appearance, showing diffusely hazy cornea with focal opacities. **B,** H&E stain. Note the pale-gray fluffy material within keratocytes and extracellularly in the stroma. **C,** Colloidal iron stains mucopolysaccharides (nonsulfated glycosaminoglycans) in the keratocytes and stroma. **D,** Colloidal iron stain also highlights mucopolysaccharides in the corneal endothelium *(arrowheads).* Note Descemet membrane excrescences, or *guttae (arrow). (Part A courtesy of Sander Dubovy, MD; part D courtesy of Tatyana Milman, MD.)*

Descemet membrane and endothelial dystrophies

Fuchs endothelial corneal dystrophy Although Fuchs endothelial corneal dystrophy can be inherited in an autosomal dominant fashion, most cases are sporadic. It is one of the leading causes of bullous keratopathy (previously discussed), characterized in its early stage by the presence of guttae. In some cases, progressive endothelial cell loss occurs over time, ultimately resulting in visually significant corneal edema and bullous keratopathy, typically in middle-aged to older individuals. Histologically, Descemet membrane is thickened and studded with anvil-shaped or drop-like guttae, which may protrude into the anterior chamber or may be buried within a new layer of Descemet membrane (Fig 6-23A, B). The epithelium demonstrates changes identical to those of bullous keratopathy from degenerative causes and to the findings seen in epithelial basement membrane dystrophy. In cases of endothelial decompensation without extensive subepithelial fibrosis, endothelial keratoplasty may be a surgical alternative to PK (Fig 6-23C).

Congenital hereditary endothelial dystrophy Traditionally, there have been 2 recognized forms of congenital hereditary endothelial dystrophy (CHED): autosomal dominant

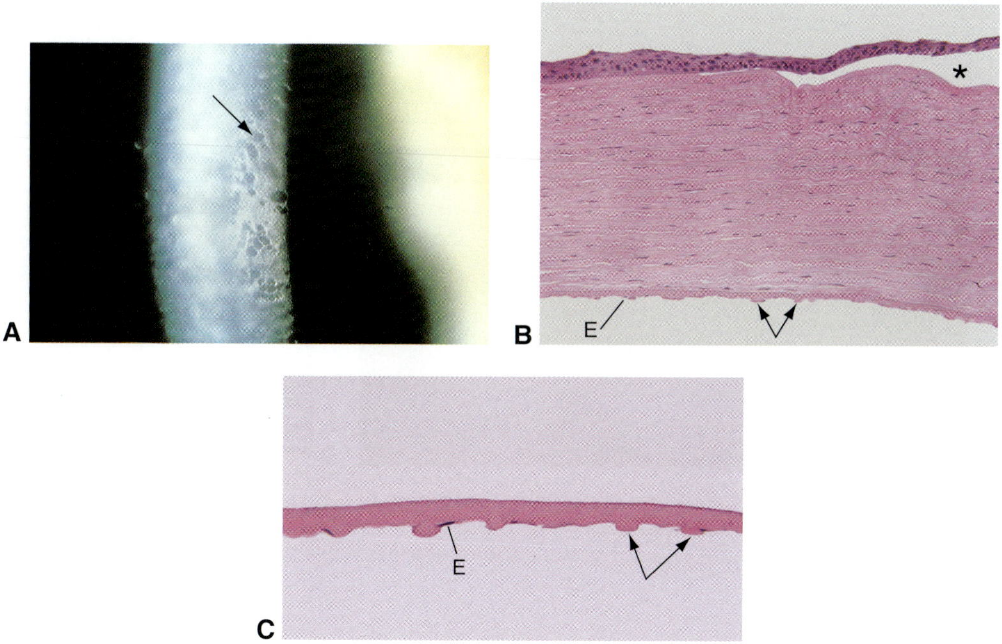

Figure 6-23 Fuchs endothelial corneal dystrophy. **A,** Slit-lamp illumination of the cornea shows "beaten bronze" appearance of Descemet membrane *(arrow).* **B,** Corneal button from PK shows endothelial cell loss, with few surviving endothelial cells (E). Numerous guttae are seen in Descemet membrane *(arrows).* The result of endothelial decompensation is diffuse stromal edema (note loss of interlamellar clefts) and epithelial bulla *(asterisk).* **C,** Specimen from Descemet membrane–stripping endothelial keratoplasty (DSEK) shows few endothelial cells (E) and numerous guttae *(arrows).* *(Part A reproduced from* External Disease and Cornea: A Multimedia Collection. *San Francisco: American Academy of Ophthalmology; 2000. Parts B and C courtesy of George J. Harocopos, MD.)*

and recessive. However, recent evidence suggests that the autosomal dominant variant (CHED1) is not sufficiently distinct from posterior polymorphous corneal dystrophy (discussed next) to be considered a separate dystrophy. CHED (formerly CHED2) presents early with diffuse or ground-glass, milky, and frequently asymmetric corneal clouding, associated with marked corneal thickening (Fig 6-24A). The primary abnormality in CHED is thought to be a degeneration of endothelial cells during or after the fifth month of gestation. Histologically, Descemet membrane is diffusely thickened and occasionally laminated. The corneal endothelium is markedly atrophic (Fig 6-24B).

Posterior polymorphous corneal dystrophy Posterior polymorphous corneal dystrophy (PPCD) is an autosomal dominant dystrophy that presents early, frequently with asymmetric opacities of various shapes at the level of Descemet membrane, including nodular, vesicular (blisterlike), and "railroad track"–like lesions (Fig 6-25A). The condition can be progressive and is associated with corneal edema, peripheral iridocorneal adhesions, and IOP elevation. Histologically, Descemet membrane is thickened and multilaminated with focal nodular and fusiform excrescences. Although the corneal endothelium is generally

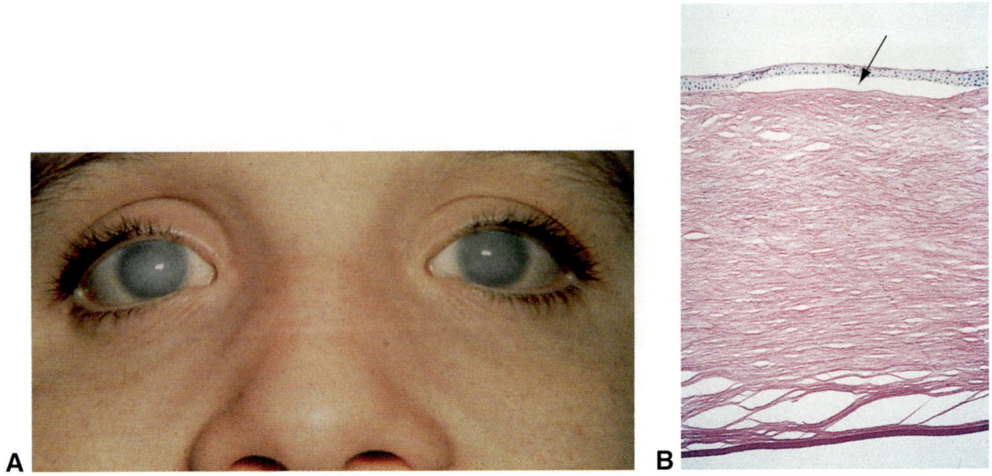

Figure 6-24 Congenital hereditary endothelial dystrophy. **A,** Clinical appearance with bilateral corneal clouding. **B,** Note diffuse edema with bullous keratopathy *(arrow).* Descemet membrane is diffusely thickened, without guttae, and endothelial cells are absent. *(Courtesy of Hans E. Grossniklaus, MD.)*

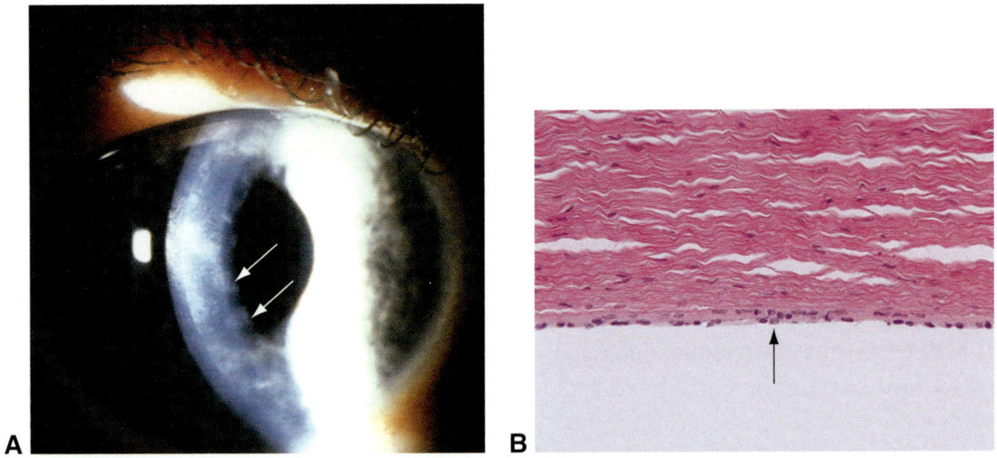

Figure 6-25 Posterior polymorphous corneal dystrophy. **A,** Clinical appearance, showing nummular opacities *(arrows)* and linear opacities on the endothelial surface. **B,** Note overlapping or multilayering of endothelial cells *(arrow).* *(Part A courtesy of Andrew J.W. Huang, MD; part B courtesy of George J. Harocopos, MD.)*

atrophic, overlapping or multilayered aggregates of endothelial cells with spindle morphology are focally present (Fig 6-25B). These transformed endothelial cells demonstrate the immunophenotypic and ultrastructural features of epithelial cells (ie, epithelialization of the endothelium).

Aldave AJ, Han J, Frausto RF. Genetics of the corneal endothelial dystrophies: an evidence-based review. *Clin Genet.* 2013;84(2):109–119.

Weiss JS, Møller HU, Aldave AJ, et al. IC3D classification of corneal dystrophies—edition 2. *Cornea.* 2015;34(2):117–159.

Ectatic Disorders

Keratoectasias (keratoconus, keratoglobus, and pellucid marginal degeneration) are noninflammatory, typically bilateral, and predominantly sporadic disorders that share a unifying feature: stromal thinning. See also BCSC Section 8, *External Disease and Cornea.*

Keratoconus

Keratoconus, which is typically diagnosed during adolescence or young adulthood, is characterized by central or inferocentral corneal stromal ectasia (Fig 6-26A). Although

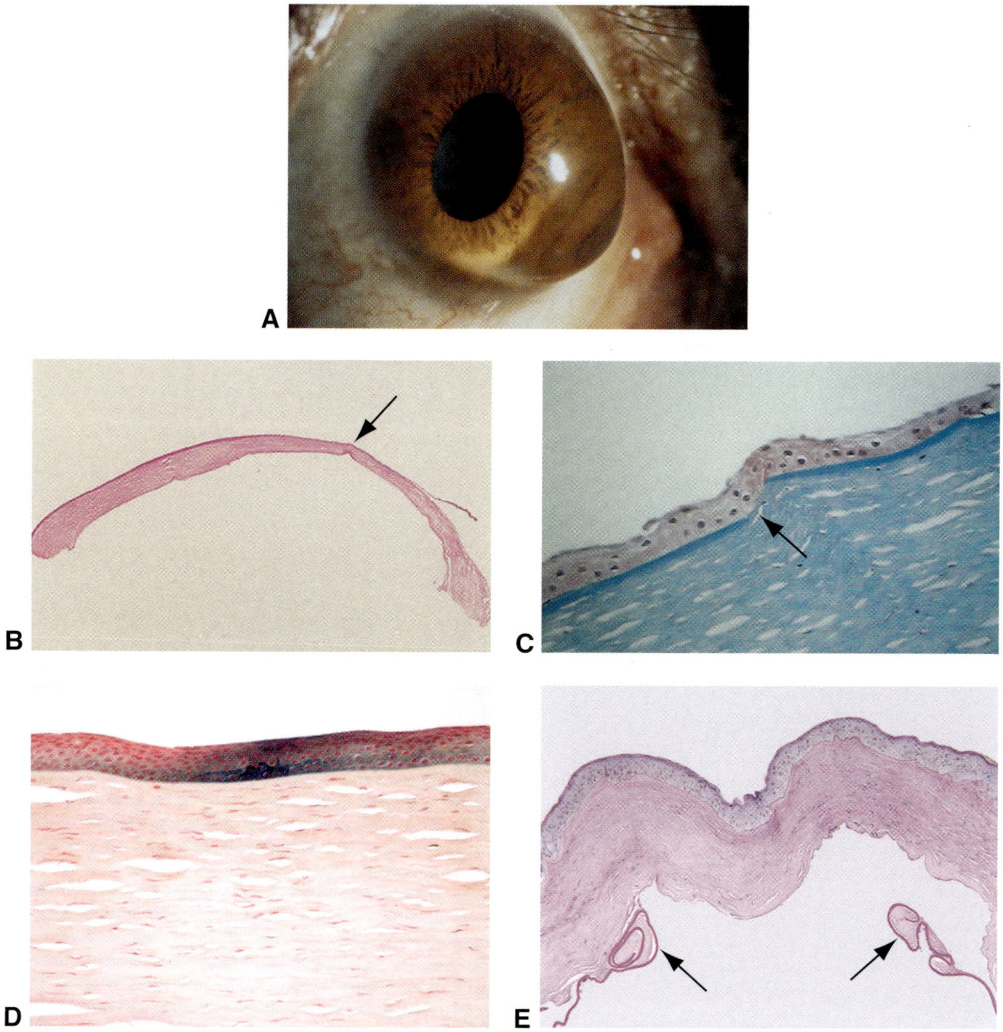

Figure 6-26 Keratoconus. **A,** Clinical appearance. **B,** Low-magnification view shows apical stromal thinning *(arrow).* **C,** Masson trichrome stain demonstrates focal disruption of Bowman layer *(arrow).* **D,** Prussian blue stain demonstrates intraepithelial iron deposition (Fleischer ring). **E,** In a patient with prior hydrops, PAS stain highlights rupture of Descemet membrane, with rolled-up edges on either side *(arrows).* *(Part A courtesy of Sander Dubovy, MD; part C courtesy of Hans E. Grossniklaus, MD; part D courtesy of Tatyana Milman, MD; part E courtesy of George J. Harocopos, MD.)*

frequently sporadic and isolated, familial inheritance and association with other ocular and systemic conditions, including atopy, Down syndrome, and Marfan syndrome, have been described. The unifying pathophysiologic change is loss of stromal structural integrity, leading to keratoectasia. The alteration in the normal corneal contour produces irregular astigmatism, occasionally requiring deep anterior lamellar keratoplasty (DALK). Advanced cases with significant apical scarring are managed with PK.

Histologic findings in keratoconus include central stromal thinning and focal discontinuities in Bowman layer. Apical anterior stromal fibrosis is often present (Fig 6-26B, C). Iron deposition in the epithelium at the base of the cone *(Fleischer ring)* can sometimes be demonstrated with Prussian blue stain (Fig 6-26D). In patients with a history of *corneal hydrops,* a break in Descemet membrane may be observed (Fig 6-26E).

Neoplasia

Primary conjunctival intraepithelial neoplasia, melanocytic processes, and sebaceous carcinoma may extend from adjacent structures and involve the corneal epithelium. This condition is described further in Chapter 5. In rare cases, intraepithelial squamous neoplasia may arise in the cornea.

CHAPTER 7

Anterior Chamber and Trabecular Meshwork

Topography

The anterior chamber is bounded anteriorly by the corneal endothelium, posteriorly by the anterior surface of the iris–ciliary body and pupillary portion of the lens, and peripherally by the trabecular meshwork (Fig 7-1). The normal depth of the anterior chamber is approximately 3.0–3.5 mm. The trabecular meshwork is derived predominantly from the neural crest. See BCSC Section 2, *Fundamentals and Principles of Ophthalmology,* for more detail.

The histologic features of the anterior chamber angle correlate with its gonioscopic landmarks (Fig 7-2). For example, the termination of Descemet membrane manifests gonioscopically as Schwalbe line. The scleral spur, a triangular extension of the sclera

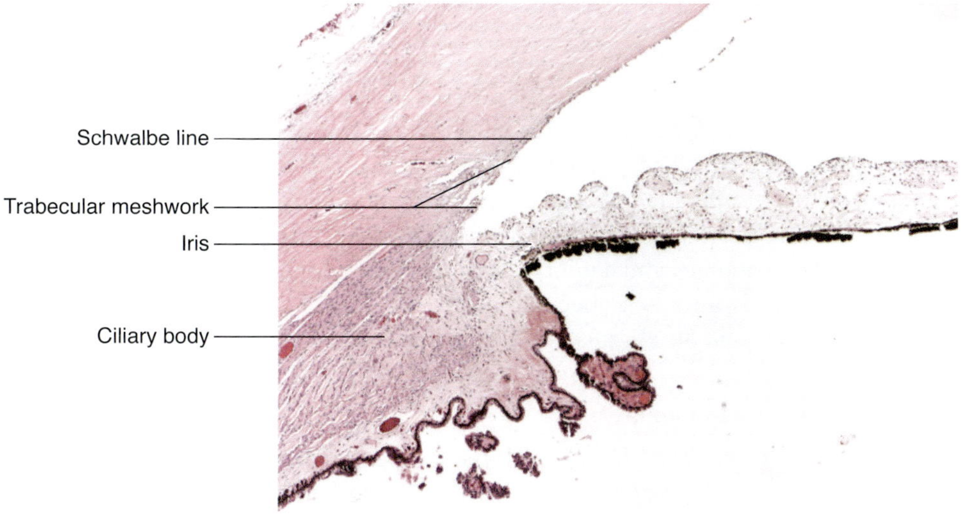

Figure 7-1 The normal anterior chamber angle, the site of drainage for the major portion of the aqueous humor flow, is defined by the anterior border of the iris, the face of the ciliary body, the internal surface of the trabecular meshwork, and the posterior surface of the cornea. *(Courtesy of Nasreen A. Syed, MD.)*

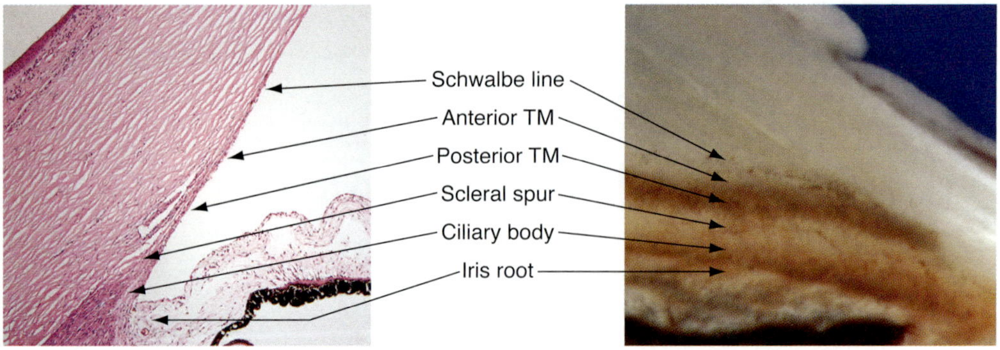

Figure 7-2 Gonioscopic landmarks of a normal anterior chamber angle with histologic correlation. TM = trabecular meshwork. *(Courtesy of Tatyana Milman, MD.)*

that appears gonioscopically as a white band, can be identified histologically by tracing the outermost longitudinal ciliary body muscle to its insertion. The groove formed by the scleral spur and corneoscleral tissue (internal scleral sulcus) accommodates the trabecular meshwork and Schlemm canal. See also Figure 2-3 in BCSC Section 10, *Glaucoma.*

Congenital Anomalies

See BCSC Section 10, *Glaucoma,* for additional discussion on the conditions described in the following sections.

Primary Congenital Glaucoma

Primary congenital glaucoma (PCG), also referred to as *congenital* or *infantile glaucoma,* can be evident at birth or become evident within the first few years of life. The pathogenesis of PCG may be related to arrested development of the anterior chamber angle structures. Histologically, the anterior chamber angle retains an "embryonic" or "fetal" conformation, characterized by anterior insertion of the iris root, mesenchymal tissue in the anterior chamber angle, and a poorly developed scleral spur in which the ciliary body muscle inserts directly into the trabecular meshwork (Fig 7-3). See BCSC Section 6, *Pediatric Ophthalmology and Strabismus,* for detailed discussion of PCG.

Anterior Segment Dysgenesis

The term *anterior segment dysgenesis* comprises a spectrum of developmental anomalies resulting from abnormalities of neural crest migration and differentiation during embryologic development (eg, Axenfeld-Rieger syndrome, Peters anomaly, posterior keratoconus, and iridoschisis). Maldevelopment of the anterior chamber angle is most prominent in *Axenfeld-Rieger syndrome,* an autosomal dominant disorder, which itself encompasses a spectrum of anomalies, ranging from isolated bilateral ocular defects to a fully manifested systemic disorder.

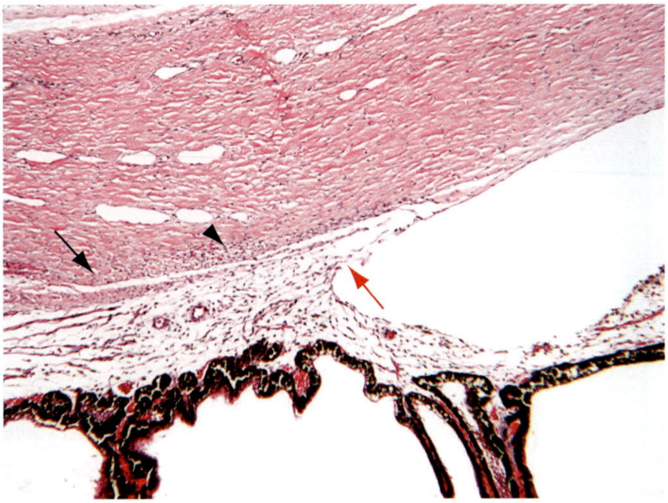

Figure 7-3 Congenital glaucoma. This micrograph of a fetal anterior chamber angle demonstrates the anterior insertion of the iris root *(red arrow)*, the anteriorly displaced ciliary processes, and a poorly developed scleral spur *(black arrow)* and trabecular meshwork *(arrowhead)*. *(Courtesy of Tatyana Milman, MD.)*

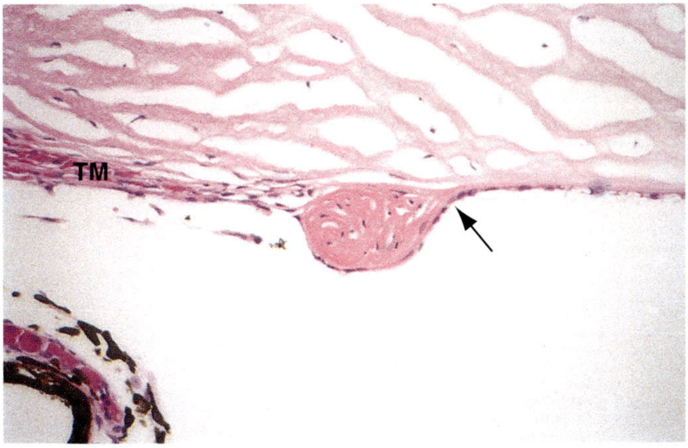

Figure 7-4 Posterior embryotoxon. Light micrograph shows a nodular prominence at the termination of Descemet membrane *(arrow)*. TM = trabecular meshwork. *(Courtesy of Hans E. Grossniklaus, MD.)*

Ocular manifestations of Axenfeld-Rieger syndrome include posterior embryotoxon (a thickened and anteriorly displaced Schwalbe line), iris strands adherent to Schwalbe line, iris hypoplasia, corectopia and polycoria, a maldeveloped or "fetal" anterior chamber angle (discussed earlier), and glaucoma in 50% of the cases occurring in late childhood or adulthood (Figs 7-4, 7-5). See also BCSC Section 8, *External Disease and Cornea.*

Chang TC, Summers CG, Schimmenti LA, Grajewski AL. Axenfeld-Rieger syndrome: new perspectives. *Br J Ophthalmol.* 2012;96(3):318–322.

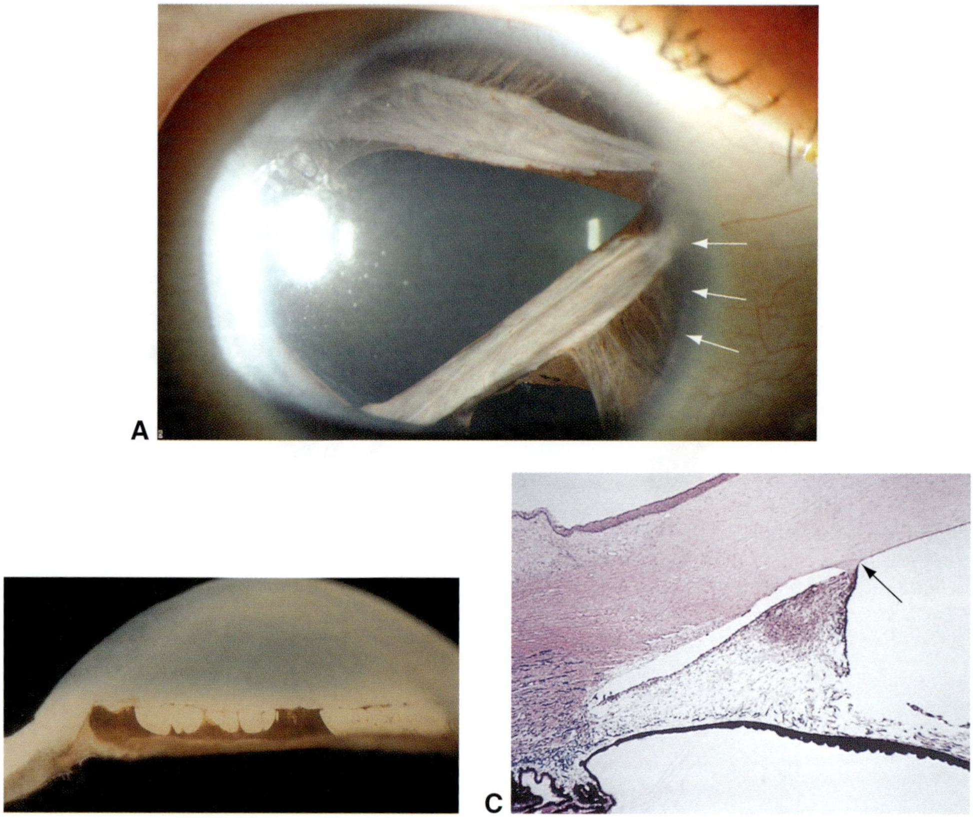

Figure 7-5 Axenfeld-Rieger syndrome. **A,** Clinical photograph of the anterior segment in a patient with Axenfeld-Rieger syndrome. Iris atrophy, polycoria, and iris strands in the periphery are present. Posterior embryotoxon can be seen laterally *(arrows).* **B,** Gross photograph shows a prominent Schwalbe line and the anterior insertion of iris strands (Axenfeld anomaly). **C,** Light micrograph shows iris strands that insert anteriorly on Schwalbe line *(arrow).* *(Part A courtesy of Wallace L.M. Alward, MD. Copyright University of Iowa. Part B courtesy of Robert Y. Foos, MD; part C modified with permission from Yanoff M, Fine BS.* Ocular Pathology: A Color Atlas. *New York: Gower; 1988.)*

Degenerations

Iridocorneal Endothelial Syndrome

Iridocorneal endothelial (ICE) syndrome, which typically affects young to middle-aged adults, is a spectrum of acquired unilateral abnormalities of the corneal endothelium, anterior chamber angle, and iris. There are 3 recognized clinical variants of ICE (when combined, the first letter of each variant also forms the mnemonic *ICE*):

- iris nevus (Cogan-Reese) syndrome
- Chandler syndrome
- essential progressive iris atrophy

All forms of ICE syndrome have the following 2 features in common: epithelial-like metaplasia and abnormal proliferation of the corneal endothelium. Abnormal endothelial cells migrate over the anterior chamber angle, leading to the formation of peripheral anterior synechiae (PAS) and subsequent secondary angle-closure glaucoma in approximately half of patients with this condition (Fig 7-6). See BCSC Section 8, *External Disease and Cornea,* and Section 10, *Glaucoma,* for further discussion.

Levy SG, Kirkness CM, Moss J, Ficker L, McCartney AC. The histopathology of the iridocorneal-endothelial syndrome. *Cornea.* 1996;15(1):46–54.

Secondary Glaucoma

Pseudoexfoliation syndrome

Pseudoexfoliation syndrome is a systemic condition that is usually identified in individuals older than 50 years. It is characterized by the production and progressive accumulation

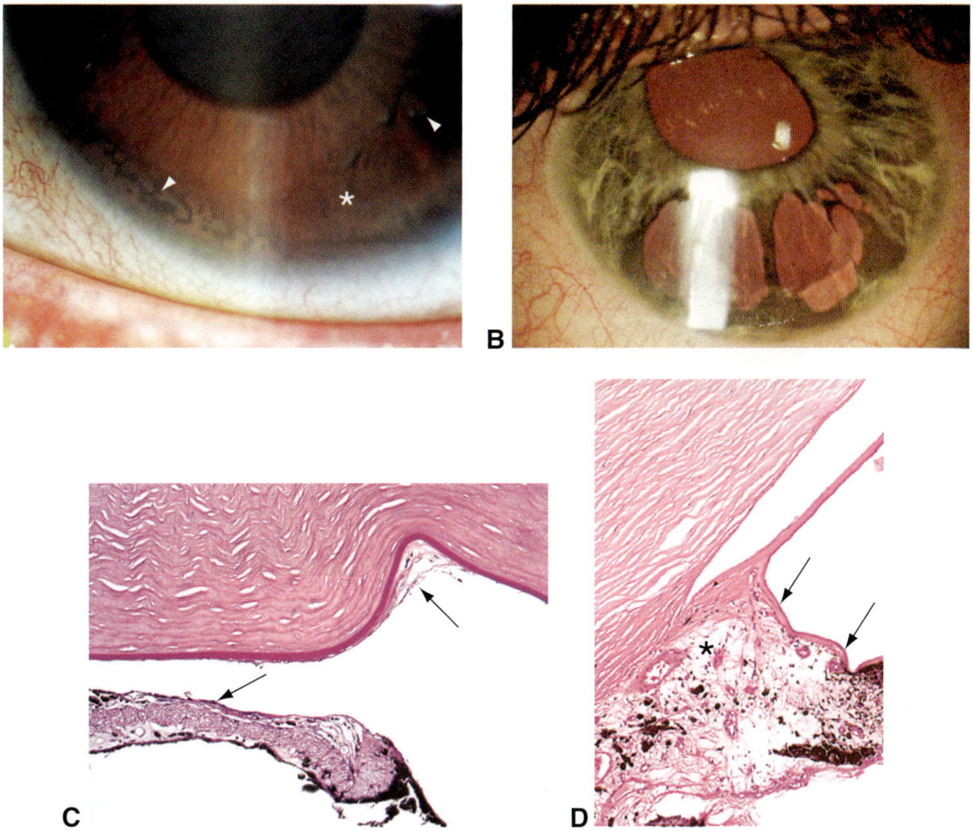
A B C D

Figure 7-6 Iridocorneal endothelial (ICE) syndrome. **A,** Iris nevus syndrome. The normal anterior iris architecture is effaced by a membrane growing on the anterior iris surface *(asterisk).* The membrane pinches off islands of normal iris stroma, resulting in a nodular, nevus-like appearance *(arrowheads).* **B,** Essential iris atrophy. Atrophic holes in the iris and a narrow anterior chamber, consistent with peripheral anterior synechiae formation. **C,** A membrane composed of spindle cells lines the posterior surface of the cornea and the anterior surface of the atrophic iris *(arrows).* Metaplastic endothelial cells deposit on the iris surface a thin basement membrane that exhibits positive periodic acid–Schiff staining and is analogous to Descemet membrane. **D,** Descemet membrane lines the anterior surface of the iris *(arrows).* The iris is apposed to the cornea (peripheral anterior synechiae, *asterisk*). *(Part A courtesy of Paul A. Sidoti, MD; parts B and C courtesy of Tatyana Milman, MD.)*

of a fibrillar material in tissues throughout the anterior segment and in the connective tissue of various visceral organs (Fig 7-7). These deposits help differentiate pseudoexfoliation syndrome from true exfoliation, in which infrared radiation induces splitting of the lens capsule.

Recent data suggest that the pathogenesis of pseudoexfoliation syndrome is a combination of excessive production and abnormal aggregation of elastic microfibril and extracellular matrix components (protein sink), as well as abnormal biomechanical properties of the elastic components of the trabecular meshwork and lamina cribrosa. Polymorphisms in the lysyl oxidase–like 1 gene, *LOXL1,* on chromosome 15 (15q24) are markers for pseudoexfoliation syndrome. Lysyl oxidase is a pivotal enzyme in extracellular matrix formation, catalyzing covalent crosslinking of collagen and elastin.

Pseudoexfoliative material is most apparent on the surface of the anterior segment structures, where it exhibits a positive periodic acid–Schiff reaction and presents as delicate, feathery or brushlike fibrils arranged perpendicular to the surfaces of the intraocular structures (Fig 7-8A). Pseudoexfoliative material also accumulates in the trabecular

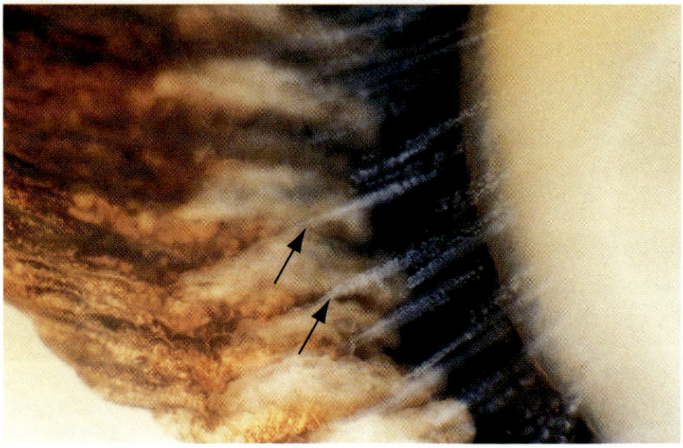

Figure 7-7 Gross photograph shows fibrillar deposits on the lens zonular fibers *(arrows)* in pseudoexfoliation syndrome. *(Courtesy of Hans E. Grossniklaus, MD.)*

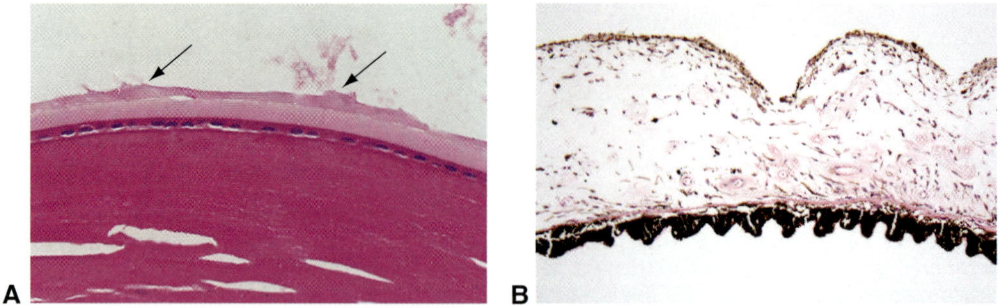

Figure 7-8 Pseudoexfoliation syndrome. **A,** Abnormal material appears on the anterior lens capsule like iron filings on the edge of a magnet *(arrows).* **B,** The iris pigment epithelium demonstrates a "saw-toothed" configuration, consistent with pseudoexfoliation. *(Part B courtesy of Tatyana Milman, MD.)*

meshwork and the wall of Schlemm canal. Associated degenerative changes in the iris pigment epithelium manifest histologically in a "saw-toothed" configuration (Fig 7-8B). These degenerative changes lead to pigment aggregation in the angle. See also BCSC Section 10, *Glaucoma,* and Section 11, *Lens and Cataract.*

Vazquez LE, Lee RK. Genomic and proteomic pathophysiology of pseudoexfoliation glaucoma. *Int Ophthalmol Clin.* 2014;54(4):1–13.

Phacolytic glaucoma

Phacolytic glaucoma develops when denatured lens protein leaks from a hypermature cataract through an intact but permeable lens capsule. The trabecular meshwork becomes occluded by both the lens protein and macrophages that are engorged with phagocytosed proteinaceous, eosinophilic lens material (Fig 7-9).

Trauma

Following an intraocular hemorrhage, blood breakdown products may accumulate in the trabecular meshwork. The rigidity and spherical shape of hemolyzed erythrocytes make it difficult for them to escape through the trabecular meshwork, leading to *ghost cell glaucoma* (Fig 7-10).

In *hemolytic glaucoma,* macrophages in the anterior chamber phagocytose erythrocytes and their breakdown products. These hemoglobin-laden and hemosiderin-laden macrophages block the trabecular outflow channels (Fig 7-11). The macrophages may be a sign of trabecular obstruction rather than the actual cause of an obstruction.

In other cases of secondary open-angle glaucoma associated with chronic intraocular hemorrhage, histologic examinations have revealed hemosiderin within the trabecular endothelium and within many ocular epithelial structures (see Fig 7-11). The presence of hemosiderin may be a sign of damage that occurred during oxidation of hemoglobin. The iron stored in the cells may be the result of an enzyme toxin that damages trabecular function in *hemosiderosis bulbi.* The Prussian blue reaction can demonstrate iron deposition in hemosiderosis bulbi.

Blunt injury to the globe may be associated with *angle recession, cyclodialysis,* and *iridodialysis.* Progressive degenerative changes in the trabecular meshwork can contribute

A
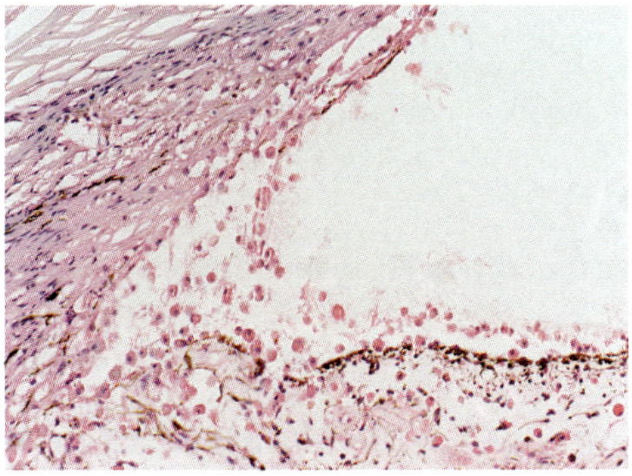
B
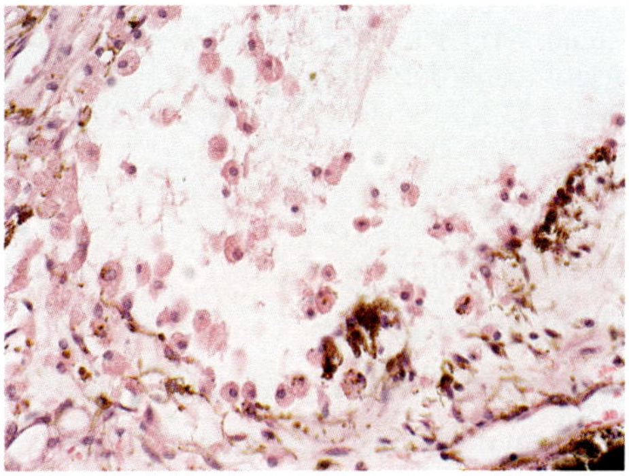

Figure 7-9 Phacolytic glaucoma. **A,** Photomicrograph of macrophages filled with degenerated lens cortical material in the angle (hematoxylin-eosin, 200×). **B,** Higher magnification (hematoxylin-eosin, 400×). *(Courtesy of Michele M. Bloomer, MD.)*

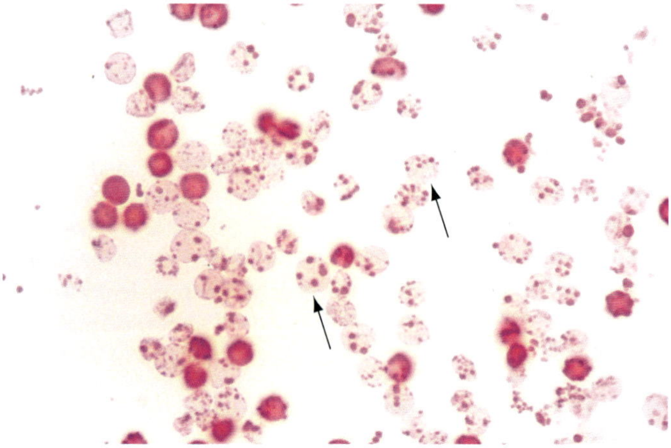

Figure 7-10 Aqueous aspirate demonstrating numerous ghost red blood cells. The degenerating hemoglobin is present as small globules known as Heinz bodies *(arrows)*. *(Courtesy of Nasreen A. Syed, MD.)*

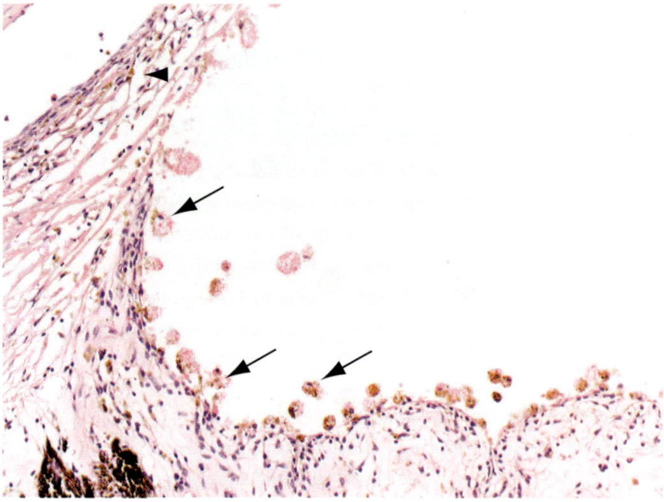

Figure 7-11 Hemolytic glaucoma. The anterior chamber angle contains macrophages with erythrocytic debris and rust-colored intracytoplasmic material, hemosiderin *(arrows)*. Hemosiderin is also observed within the trabecular meshwork endothelium *(arrowhead)*. *(Courtesy of Michele M. Bloomer, MD.)*

to the development of glaucoma after injury. See the section Histologic Sequelae of Ocular Trauma in Chapter 2.

Pigment dispersion associations

Pigment dispersion may be associated with a variety of other conditions in which pigment epithelium or uveal melanocytes are injured, such as uveitis or uveal melanoma. These conditions are characterized by the presence of pigment within the trabecular meshwork as well as in macrophages littering the angle (Fig 7-12).

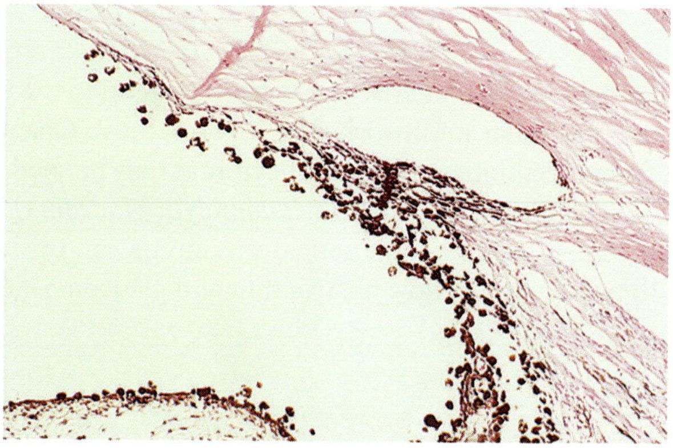

Figure 7-12 Melanomalytic glaucoma. The trabecular meshwork is obstructed by macrophages that have ingested pigment from a necrotic intraocular melanoma.

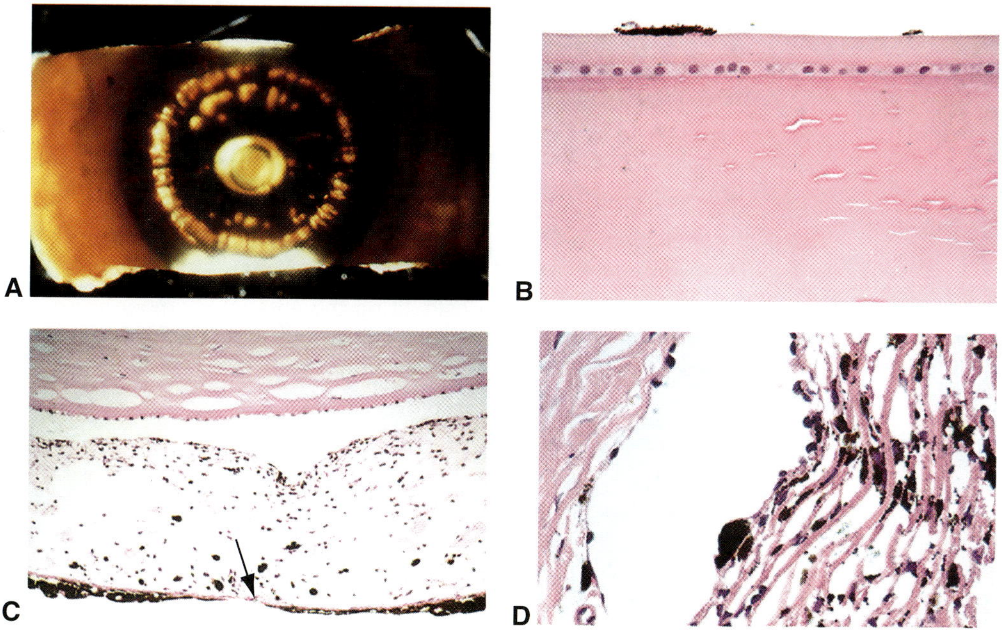

Figure 7-13 Pigment dispersion syndrome. **A,** Gross photograph demonstrating radially oriented transillumination defects in the iris. **B,** Melanin is present on the anterior surface of the lens. **C,** Note the focal loss of iris pigment epithelium *(arrow).* Chafing of the zonular fibers against the epithelium may release the pigment that is dispersed in this condition. **D,** Note the accumulation of pigment in the trabecular meshwork.

Pigment dispersion syndrome can lead to a secondary open-angle glaucoma (Fig 7-13) that is characterized by radially oriented defects in the midperipheral iris in addition to pigment in the trabecular meshwork, the corneal endothelium (*Krukenberg spindle*), and other anterior segment structures, such as the lens capsule. The dispersed pigment is presumed to be a result of iris pigment epithelium mechanically rubbing off via contact with lens zonular fibers. See also BCSC Section 10, *Glaucoma.*

Neoplasia

Melanocytic nevi and melanomas that arise in the iris or extend to the iris from the ciliary body may obstruct the trabecular meshwork (Fig 7-14). See also Chapter 17. In addition, pigment elaborated from melanomas and melanocytomas may be shed into the trabecular meshwork, producing secondary glaucoma *(melanomalytic glaucoma)* (see Fig 7-12). Occasionally, epibulbar tumors such as conjunctival carcinoma can invade the eye through the limbus, leading to trabecular outflow obstruction and glaucoma. See the section Neoplasia in Chapter 5.

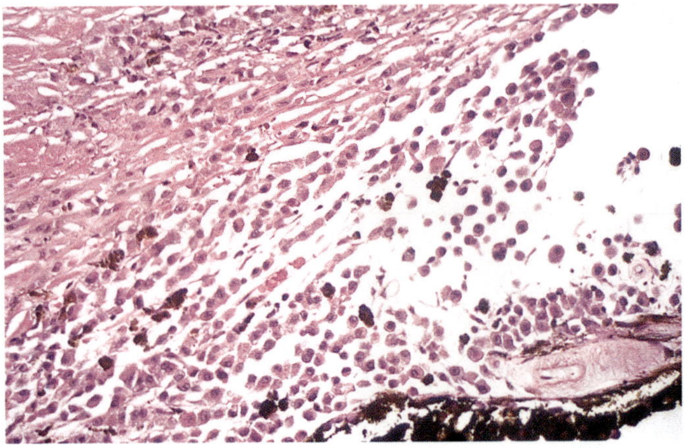

Figure 7-14 Photomicrograph shows melanoma cells filling the anterior chamber angle and obstructing the trabecular meshwork. Note the iris pigment epithelium in the lower right corner of the photomicrograph. *(Courtesy of Hans E. Grossniklaus, MD.)*

CHAPTER 8

Sclera

Topography

The sclera is the white, nearly opaque portion of the outer wall of the eye that covers from four-fifths to five-sixths of the eye's surface area. It is continuous anteriorly at the limbus with the corneal stroma. Posteriorly, the outer two-thirds of the sclera merge with the optic nerve dural sheath; the inner third continues as perforated sclera known as the lamina cribrosa, through which pass axonal fibers of the optic nerve (see Chapter 15, Fig 15-1). Histologically, the sclera is divided into 3 layers (from outermost inward): episclera, stroma, and lamina fusca (Fig 8-1). Embryologically, the sclera is derived predominantly from the neural crest. See BCSC Section 2, *Fundamentals and Principles of Ophthalmology,* for further discussion.

The episclera is a loose, thin fibrovascular tissue that covers the outer surface of the scleral stroma. The bulk of the sclera is made up of the stroma, a layer of sparsely vascularized, dense type I collagen fibers. In comparison to corneal stroma, scleral collagen fibers

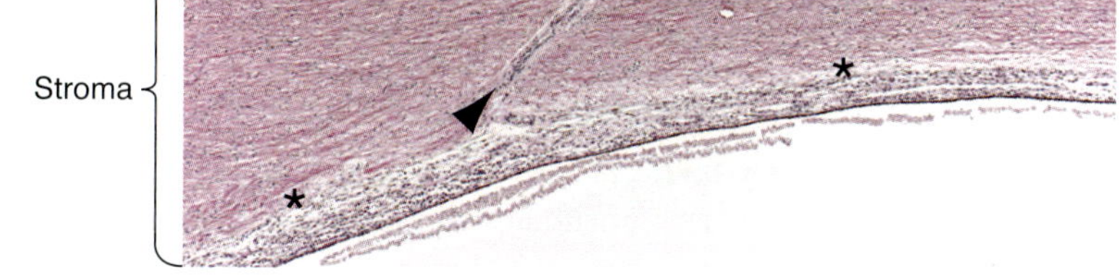

Figure 8-1 Normal sclera demonstrating the lamina fusca *(asterisks)* and emissary structures, including ciliary arteries *(black arrowheads)* and nerves *(red arrowheads)* entering and traversing the sclera (hematoxylin-eosin stain). *(Courtesy of Nasreen A. Syed, MD.)*

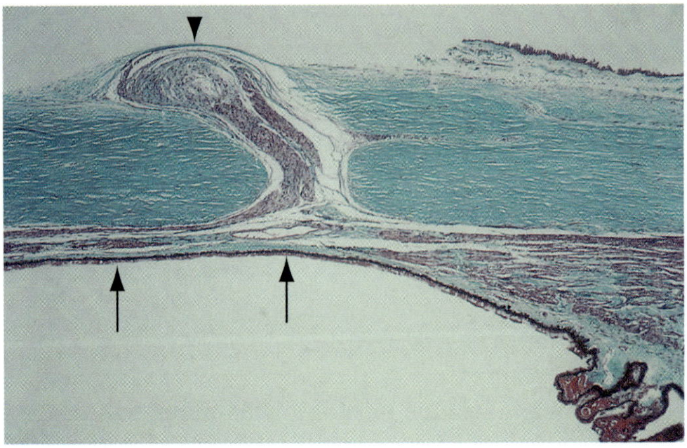

Figure 8-2 An emissary canal through the sclera with Axenfeld nerve loop *(arrowhead),* which is overlying the pars plana *(arrows)* (trichrome stain). *(Courtesy of Harry H. Brown, MD.)*

are thicker and more variable in thickness and orientation. Transmural emissary canals provide outlets within the stroma as follows (Fig 8-2; see also Fig 8-1):

- in the posterior region, for posterior ciliary arteries and nerves
- in the equatorial region, for vortex veins
- in the anterior regions, for anterior ciliary arteries and veins and long posterior ciliary nerves (Axenfeld nerve loops)

The lamina fusca is a delicate, pigmented fibrovascular tissue that loosely binds the uvea to the sclera. Sclerouveal attachments are strongest along the major emissary canals, the anterior base of the ciliary body, and the juxtapapillary region.

Congenital Anomalies

Choristoma

Epibulbar dermoids and episcleral osseous choristoma are discussed in Chapter 5.

Nanophthalmos

Nanophthalmos is a rare, usually bilateral, developmental disorder characterized by an eye with short axial length (<20 mm), a normal or slightly enlarged lens, thickened sclera, hyperopia, and a predisposition to uveal effusion and glaucoma. Most cases are sporadic, but both autosomal dominant and recessive inheritance patterns have been reported. Autosomal recessive cases have been linked to mutations in the MFRP gene that encodes a frizzle-related transmembrane protein, selectively expressed in retinal pigment epithelium and ciliary body.

In studies of patients with nanophthalmos, the collagen fibrils in the characteristic thick and nonelastic sclera demonstrated fraying and splitting, and abnormalities were found in the glycosaminoglycan matrix. These scleral changes may predispose the nanophthalmic eye to uveal effusion due to reduced protein permeability and impaired venous outflow through the vortex veins.

Nanophthalmic eyes are predisposed to angle-closure glaucoma due to a normal or enlarged lens in a small anterior segment.

See BCSC Section 10, *Glaucoma,* for additional discussion of nanophthalmos.

Stewart DH 3rd, Streeten BW, Brockhurst RJ, Anderson DR, Hirose T, Gass DM. Abnormal scleral collagen in nanophthalmos. An ultrastructural study. *Arch Ophthalmol.* 1991;109(7): 1017–1025.

Sundin OH, Dharmaraj S, Bhutto IA, et al. Developmental basis of nanophthalmos: MFRP is required for both prenatal ocular growth and postnatal emmetropization. *Ophthalmic Genet.* 2008; 29(1):1–9.

Microphthalmos

Microphthalmos refers to small eyes with associated developmental defects. Colobomas and cysts with associated scleral abnormalities are also common, due to failure of the fetal fissure to close properly.

See BCSC Section 6, *Pediatric Ophthalmology and Strabismus,* for additional discussion of microphthalmos.

Inflammations

See BCSC Section 8, *External Disease and Cornea,* for additional discussion of episcleritis and scleritis.

Episcleritis

Episcleritis is classified as simple or nodular. *Simple episcleritis* is a self-limited, often idiopathic condition. Histologic examination shows vascular congestion, stromal edema, and a chronic nongranulomatous perivascular inflammatory infiltrate that is composed primarily of lymphocytes.

Nodular episcleritis more often affects females and those with systemic illness, such as rheumatoid arthritis. It is characterized by tender, elevated, pink-red nodules on the anterior episclera. Histologically, the nodules are composed of a *necrobiotic granulomatous inflammatory infiltrate,* which is a palisading arrangement of epithelioid histiocytes around a central core of necrotic collagen. This light microscopic pattern is the same as that seen in rheumatoid nodules in subcutaneous tissue.

Scleritis

Scleritis can be infectious or noninfectious; infectious scleritis may be distinguished from noninfectious scleritis by appropriate laboratory testing. Special stains may aid in identifying causative organisms.

Noninfectious scleritis is often a painful, progressive ocular disease with potentially serious sequelae. Histologic examination of noninfectious scleritis reveals 2 main categories: necrotizing and nonnecrotizing inflammation. Either type may occur anteriorly or posteriorly, but anterior scleritis is more common (Fig 8-3). *Necrotizing scleritis* may be nodular or diffuse (also called brawny scleritis) (Fig 8-4). Both patterns demonstrate granulomas similar to those of episcleritis (Fig 8-5). A rim of lymphocytes and plasma cells is peripheral to the histiocytes. Multiple foci may show different stages of evolution. In the course of healing, the necrotic stroma is resorbed, leaving a thinned scleral remnant prone to staphyloma formation (Fig 8-6). Severe ectasia of the scleral shell predisposes the sclera to herniation of uveal tissue through the defect, a condition known as *scleromalacia perforans.*

Nonnecrotizing scleritis is characterized by a perivascular lymphocytic and plasmacytic infiltrate without a granulomatous inflammatory component. Vasculitis may be present in the form of fibrinoid necrosis of the vessel walls.

See BCSC Section 8, *External Disease and Cornea,* for additional discussion of episcleritis and scleritis.

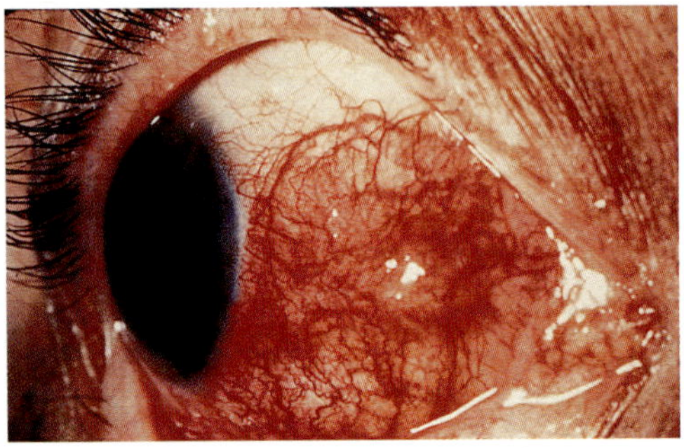

Figure 8-3 An eye with sectoral nodular anterior scleritis that causes severe ocular pain and photophobia. *(Courtesy of Harry H. Brown, MD.)*

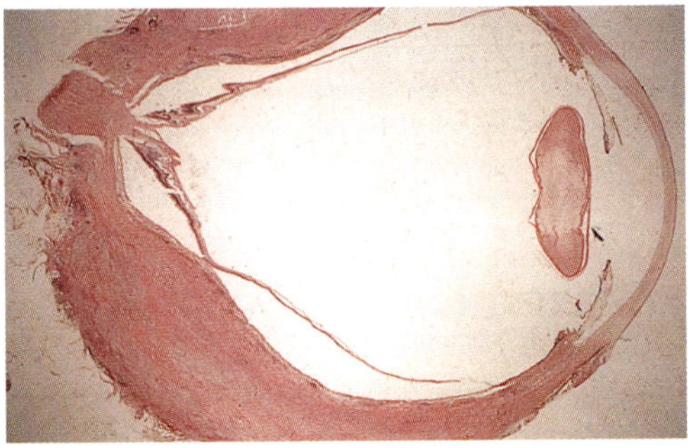

Figure 8-4 Diffuse posterior scleritis (brawny scleritis) that demonstrates marked thickening of the posterior sclera. *(Courtesy of Harry H. Brown, MD.)*

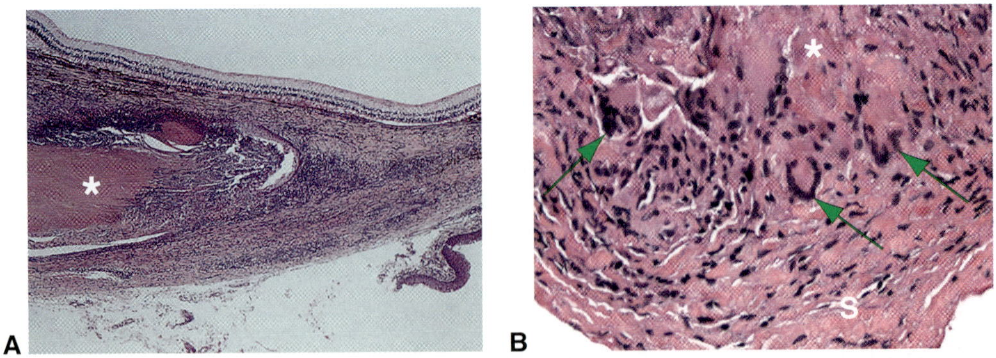

Figure 8-5 Necrotizing granulomatous scleritis. **A,** An area of necrobiotic sclera *(asterisk)* is sequestered by a zonal inflammatory reaction of histiocytes, lymphocytes, and plasma cells. **B,** High-magnification photomicrograph of scleral (S) biopsy illustrates palisading arrangement of histiocytes and multinucleated giant cells *(arrows)* around necrobiotic scleral collagen *(asterisk). (Part A courtesy of Harry H. Brown, MD; part B courtesy of Robert H. Rosa, Jr, MD.)*

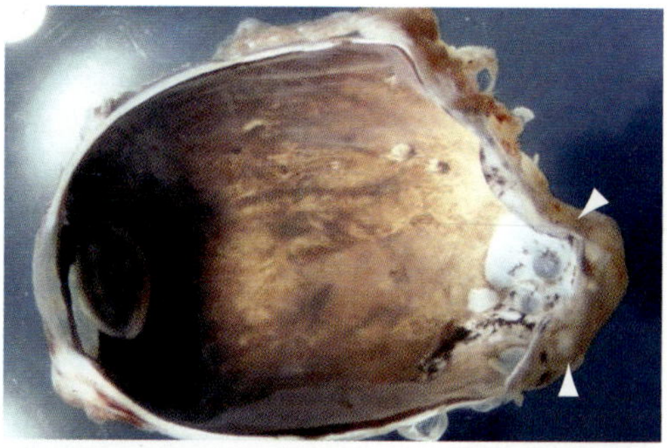

Figure 8-6 An eye with posterior staphyloma *(arrowheads)* as a sequela of scleritis. *(Courtesy of Hans E. Grossniklaus, MD.)*

Degenerations

Senile Calcific Plaque

Senile calcific plaques occur commonly in individuals over 70 years of age; they appear as flat, firm, sharply circumscribed, rectangular to ovoid gray scleral patches. The plaques, which appear bilaterally, are typically located anterior to the medial and lateral rectus muscle insertions (Fig 8-7A) in the interpalpebral fissure. The etiology is unknown; various causes, such as dehydration, actinic damage, and stress on scleral collagen exerted by rectus muscle insertions, have been proposed but not proven.

Histologic sections show that the calcium is present within the midportion of the scleral stroma. It begins as a finely granular deposition but may progress to a confluent plaque involving both superficial and deep sclera (see Fig 8-7B). Senile plaques may be highlighted by special stains for calcium, such as von Kossa and alizarin red.

Scleral Staphyloma

Scleral staphylomas are scleral ectasias that are lined internally by uveal tissue. Staphylomas may develop at points of weakness in the scleral shell, either in inherently thin areas

A
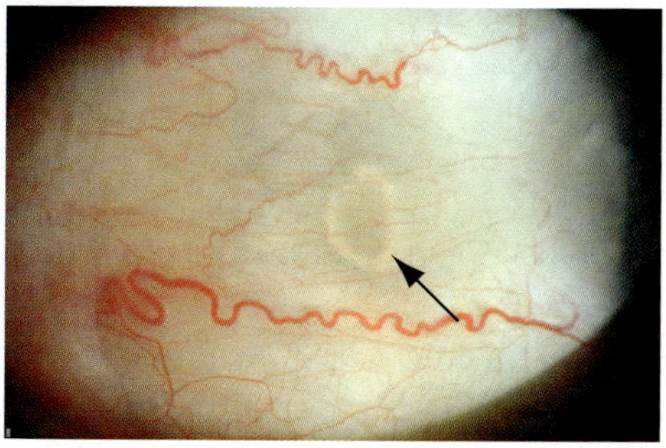

B
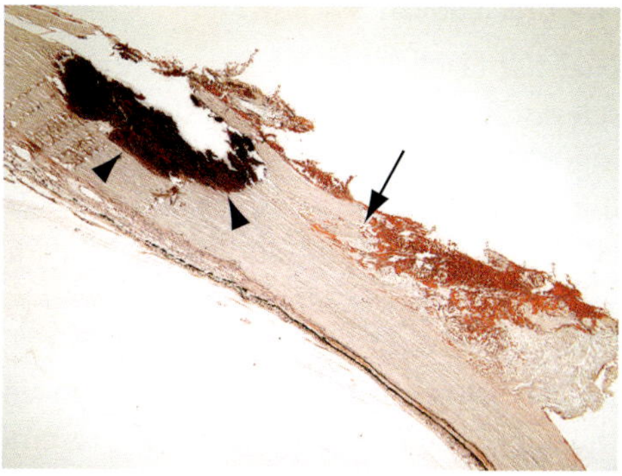

Figure 8-7 A calcific plaque of the sclera. **A,** Calcific plaques *(arrow)* are typically located just anterior to the insertion of the medial and lateral rectus muscles. **B,** Calcific deposits are noted in the sclera *(arrowheads)* anterior to the rectus muscle insertion *(arrow)* (von Kossa stain). *(Part A courtesy of Vinay A. Shah, MBBS; part B courtesy of Tatyana Milman, MD.)*

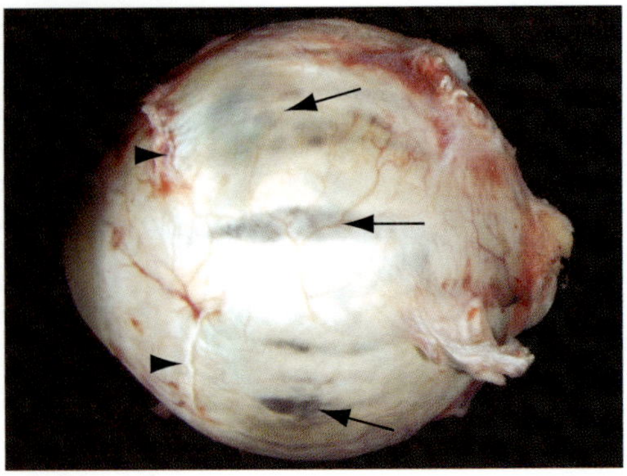

Figure 8-8 Scleral staphylomas. Several regions of scleral thinning *(arrows)*, which appear blue because of the underlying uveal tissue, are present posterior to the rectus muscle insertions *(arrowheads)* and in the equatorial sclera. *(Courtesy of Nasreen A. Syed, MD.)*

(such as posterior to the rectus muscle insertions; Fig 8-8) or in areas weakened by tissue destruction (as in scleritis; see Fig 8-6). In children, staphylomas may occur as a result of long-standing increased intraocular pressure or axial myopia, owing to the relative distensibility of the sclera in the young. Location and age at onset, therefore, vary according to the underlying etiology. Histologic examination invariably reveals thinned sclera, with or without fibrosis and scarring, depending on the cause.

Neoplasia

Neoplasms of the sclera are exceedingly rare. Tumors originate predominantly in the conjunctiva or uvea with secondary scleral involvement.

Fibrous Histiocytoma

Fibrous histiocytoma *(fibroxanthoma)* and its malignant variant *(pleomorphic undifferentiated sarcoma)* can occur in the sclera (Fig 8-9), although it is rare.

See Chapter 14 for further discussion of fibrous histiocytomas.

Nodular Fasciitis

Nodular fasciitis is a reactive process that may, in rare instances, cause a mass in the episclera. The disease usually affects young adults, 20 to 40 years of age, as a rapidly growing, round to oval, firm, white-gray nodule that measures 0.5–1.5 cm and appears at the limbus or anterior to a rectus muscle insertion. In other body sites, antecedent trauma has been implicated as an etiologic factor for the development of nodular fasciitis, but in the sclera such an association is infrequent. Though self-limited, nodular fasciitis is usually excised because of its rapid growth.

Histologic examination reveals a circumscribed spindle cell proliferation in which the appearance of individual cells resembles that of fibroblasts growing in tissue culture. These spindle cells aggregate in short fascicles (Fig 8-10). Older lesions may show foci of dense collagen deposition. Although mitotic figures may be present, atypical mitoses are absent. When diagnosing, the clinician should avoid the pitfall of misinterpreting nodular fasciitis histologically as sarcoma (soft-tissue malignancy); this can happen because of the cellular nature of the proliferations and the presence of mitotic figures.

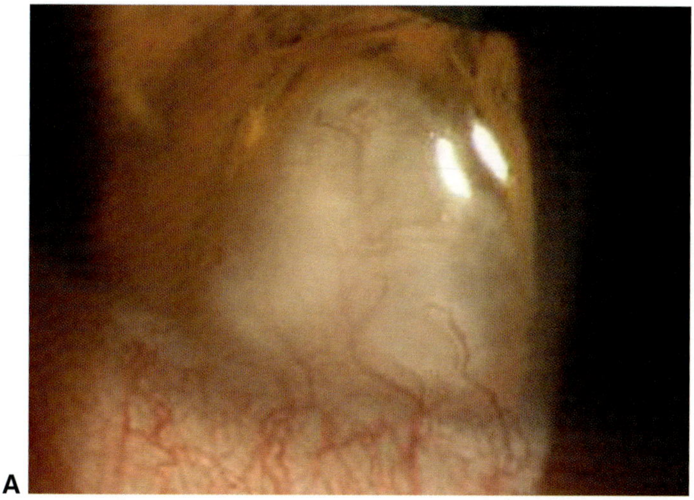

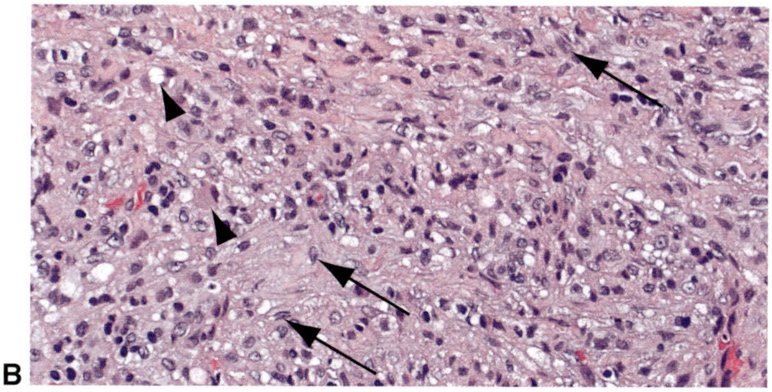

Figure 8-9 Fibrous histiocytoma of the corneoscleral limbus. **A,** A gelatinous, gray, vascularized, dome-shaped nodule that extends into the corneal stroma. **B,** Photomicrograph reveals spindle-shaped fibroblasts *(arrows)*, epithelioid and lipid-laden histiocytes *(arrowheads)*, and scattered lymphocytes. *(Part A courtesy of Ira J. Udell, MD; part B courtesy of Milton Boniuk, MD.)*

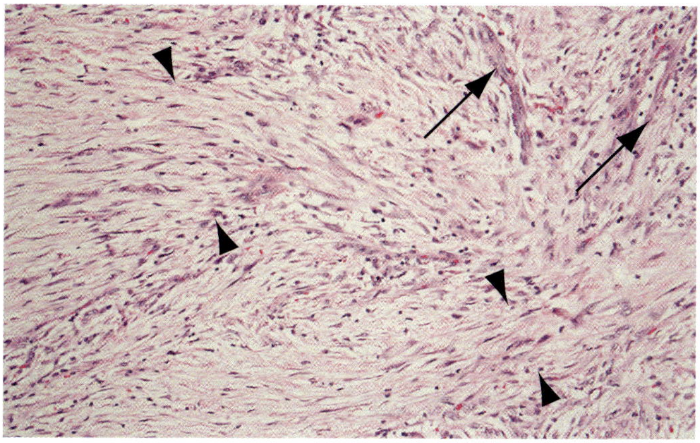

Figure 8-10 Nodular fasciitis. Activated spindled fibroblasts are loosely arranged in short fascicles *(between arrowheads)*. A prominent capillary network *(arrows)* and chronic inflammatory cell infiltrate are also observed. *(Courtesy of Tatyana Milman, MD.)*

CHAPTER 9

Lens

Topography

The crystalline lens is a soft, elastic, avascular, biconvex structure that measures approximately 9–10 mm in diameter and 5 mm anteroposteriorly in the adult eye (Fig 9-1). The lens is derived from surface ectoderm. See BCSC Section 11, *Lens and Cataract,* for discussion of the structure, embryology, and pathology of the lens.

Capsule

The capsule, which surrounds the entire lens, is a thick basement membrane elaborated by lens epithelial cells and is composed partly of type IV collagen fibers (Fig 9-2). The lens capsule is thickest anteriorly (12–21 µm) and peripherally near the equator and thinnest posteriorly (2–9 µm) (Fig 9-3). The zonular fibers insert into the capsule, which also has an important role in molding the lens shape for accommodation.

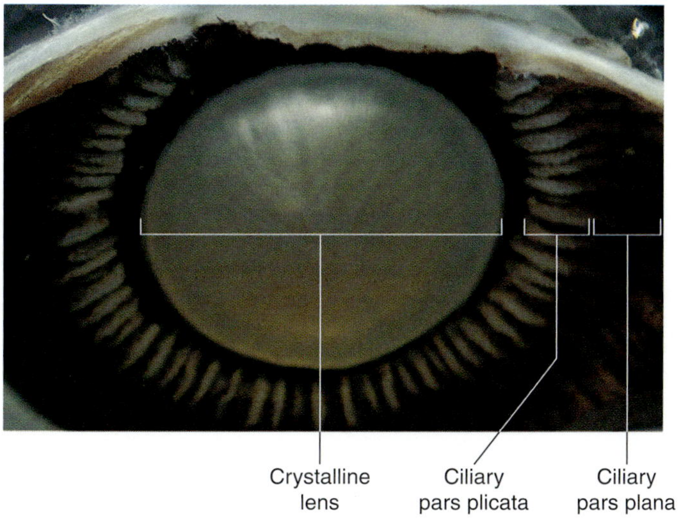

Figure 9-1 Posterior aspect of the crystalline lens, depicting its relationship to the peripheral iris and ciliary body. The zonular fibers are translucent and therefore not visible. *(Courtesy of Hans E. Grossniklaus, MD.)*

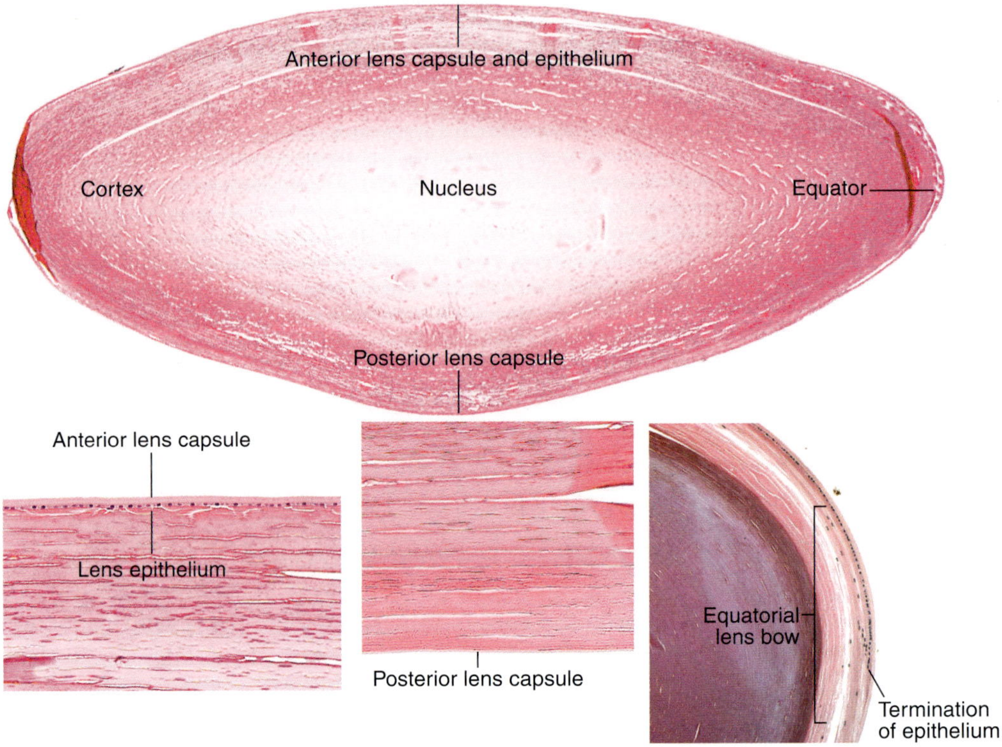

Figure 9-2 Microscopic appearance of the adult lens. *(Courtesy of Tatyana Milman, MD, except for lower right image, courtesy of Nasreen A. Syed, MD.)*

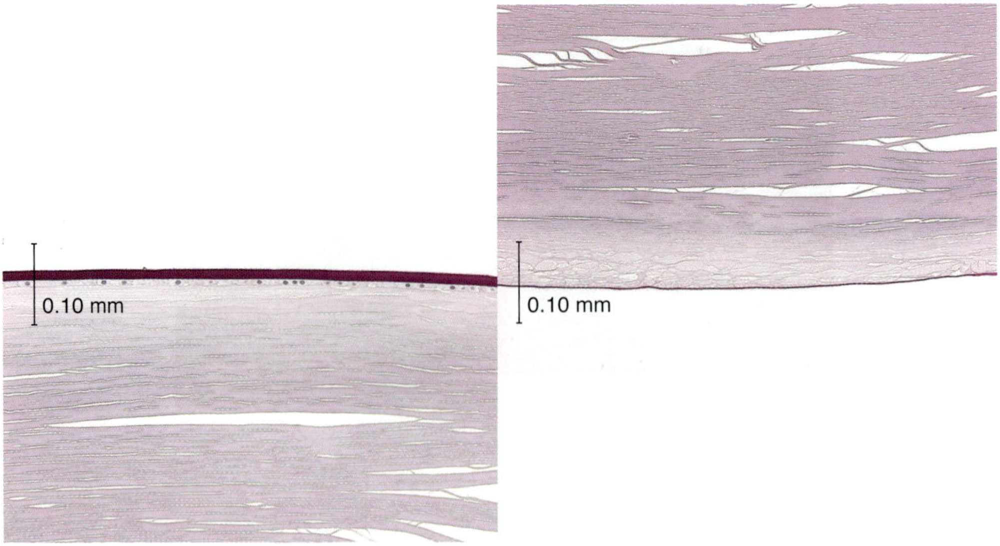

Figure 9-3 Lens capsule, periodic acid–Schiff (PAS) stain. Compare the thickness of the anterior capsule *(left)* with that of the posterior capsule *(right)*. Calibration bar = 0.01 mm. *(Courtesy of Nasreen A. Syed, MD.)*

Epithelium

The lens epithelium is derived from the cells of the original lens vesicle that did not differentiate into primary lens fibers. The anterior or axial lens epithelium forms a single layer of cuboidal cells; these cells' basilar surface is oriented toward the anterior lens capsule. In contrast, the equatorial, mitotically active cells appear more elongated as they differentiate into lens fibers. Epithelial cells are not typically observed posterior to the lens equator (see Fig 9-2).

Cortex and Nucleus

The center of the lens contains the oldest lens fibers, the *embryonic and fetal lens nucleus,* whereas the outer cortical fibers are derived from postnatally differentiated lens epithelial cells. As the lens epithelial cells differentiate, new lens fibers are continuously laid down from the outside. In the equatorial region, termed the *equatorial lens bow,* the lens epithelial cells move centrally, elongate, produce crystallins, lose organelles, and transform into cortical lens fibers. Clinically and histologically, the demarcation between the nucleus and cortex is not well defined (see Fig 9-2).

The overall shape of the lens changes over the first decade of life; with increasing age, the diameter of the lens nucleus and cortex increases from anterior to posterior.

Zonular Fibers

The lens is supported by zonular fibers that attach to the anterior and posterior lens capsule in the midperiphery (see Chapter 7, Fig 7-7). These fibers hold the lens in place through their attachments to the ciliary body processes. They are composed of an elastic type of glycoprotein known as fibrillin.

Congenital Anomalies

See BCSC Section 6, *Pediatric Ophthalmology and Strabismus,* and Section 11, *Lens and Cataract,* for discussion of lens coloboma, ectopia lentis, and congenital cataract, as well as additional discussion of the following topics.

Congenital Aphakia

Congenital aphakia is a rare anomaly that can be subdivided into 2 forms: primary and secondary. In primary congenital aphakia, the lens is absent histologically. Primary congenital aphakia results from failed induction of the surface ectoderm during embryogenesis and has been associated with homozygous mutations in the *FOXE3* gene and severe ocular and systemic developmental anomalies. The histologic findings of secondary congenital aphakia depend on the underlying etiology. In secondary congenital aphakia, the lens has developed but has been resorbed or extruded before or during birth. This form of aphakia is often associated with congenital infections such as rubella.

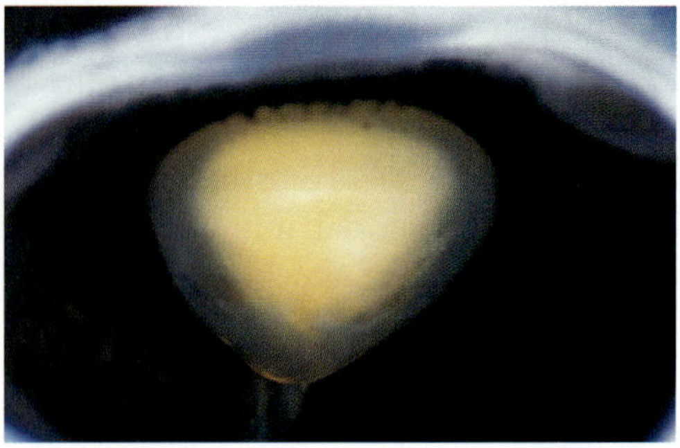

Figure 9-4 Posterior lenticonus. Macroscopic image. *(Courtesy of Hans E. Grossniklaus, MD.)*

Anterior Lenticonus and Lentiglobus

The anterior surface of the lens can assume an abnormal shape, either conical *(lenticonus)* or spherical *(lentiglobus).* Clinically, an "oil droplet" red reflex is present in both conditions. Anterior lenticonus may be unilateral or bilateral. Histologic examination reveals thinning of and dehiscences in the anterior lens capsule, a decrease in the number of anterior lens epithelial cells, and bulging of the anterior cortex. Ultrastructurally, alterations of lens capsule collagen and immunohistochemical abnormalities in type IV collagen have been observed.

Bilateral anterior lenticonus is usually associated with *Alport syndrome,* which is typically an autosomal dominant disease that is characterized by hemorrhagic nephritis, deafness, anterior polar cataract, retinal flecks, and retinal and iris neovascularization. Mutations in type IV collagen genes have been described in some forms of Alport syndrome.

Posterior Lenticonus (Lentiglobus)

Posterior lenticonus is characterized by a spherical deformity of the posterior surface of the lens (Fig 9-4). This condition usually occurs as a sporadic, unilateral anomaly and is associated with congenital cataract. Other, rare ocular associations include microphthalmos, microcornea, persistent anterior hyaloid vasculature, and uveal colobomas. Posterior lenticonus may also be a manifestation of Alport syndrome (due to mutations in the *COL4A3–5* genes) or *oculocerebrorenal syndrome (Lowe syndrome),* an X-linked condition characterized by systemic acidosis, renal rickets, hypotonia, and congenital cataracts, which histologically display focal, internally directed excrescences of the lens capsule. This syndrome may be due to mutations in the *OCRL1* gene.

Inflammations

Phacoantigenic Uveitis

Also known as *phacoanaphylactic endophthalmitis* or *lens-induced granulomatous endophthalmitis,* phacoantigenic uveitis is a type of lens-induced intraocular inflammation. It is thought to be precipitated by the deposition of antigen–antibody complexes (type III

Arthus-type reaction) that form following exposure of the immune system to lens antigens after violation of the lens capsule. The inflammation may follow accidental or surgical trauma to the lens.

Histologically, an eye with phacoantigenic uveitis shows a central nidus of degenerating lens material surrounded by concentric layers of inflammatory cells *(zonal granuloma)*. Multinucleated giant cells and neutrophils are present within the inner layer adjacent to the degenerating lens material. Lymphocytes and plasma cells make up the intermediate mantle of cells. These cells may be surrounded by fibrovascular connective tissue, depending on the duration of the inflammatory response (Fig 9-5). See also BCSC Section 9, *Intraocular Inflammation and Uveitis.*

Propionibacterium acnes Endophthalmitis

Chronic postoperative endophthalmitis caused by *P acnes* may have a delayed presentation following cataract surgery, usually 2 months to 2 years later. Histologic examination of the lens capsule reveals sequestration of the bacteria (Fig 9-6).

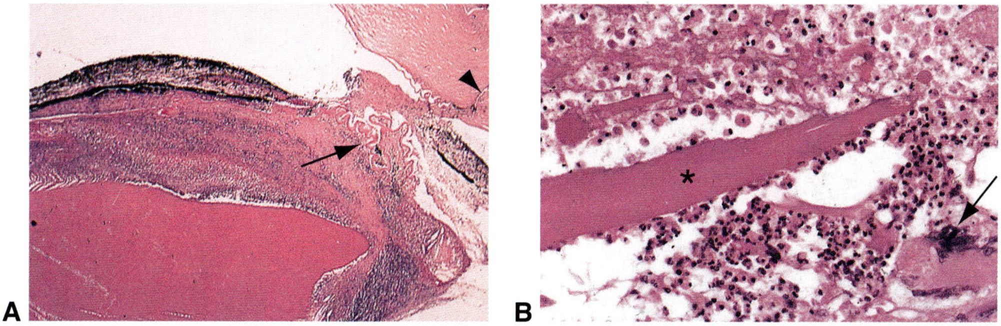

Figure 9-5 Phacoantigenic uveitis. **A,** Inflammatory reaction surrounds the lens *(lower left)*. The torn capsule is visible in the pupillary region *(arrow)*. Note the corneal scar *(arrowhead)*, representing the site of ocular penetration. **B,** Acute and granulomatous inflammation, including giant cells *(arrow)*, surrounds inciting lens fibers *(asterisk)*.

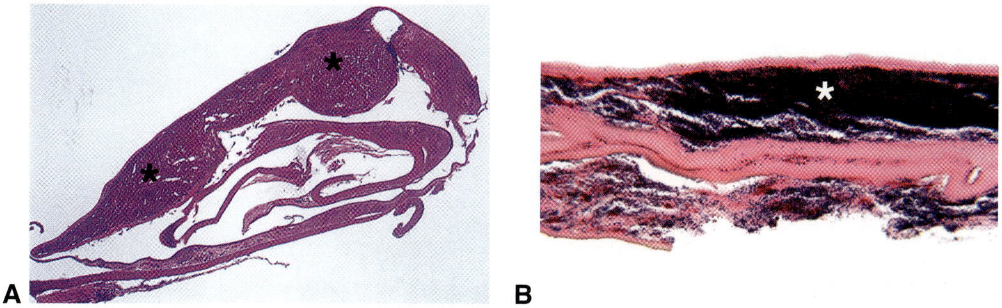

Figure 9-6 Lens capsule in a case of *Propionibacterium acnes* endophthalmitis. **A,** Colonies of bacteria are sequestered within the PAS-positive capsular bag *(asterisks)*. **B,** Gram-positive coccobacilli within the capsular bag *(asterisk)*. *(Part A courtesy of William C. Lloyd III, MD, and Ralph C. Eagle, Jr, MD; part B courtesy of Tatyana Milman, MD.)*

Degenerations

Cataract and Other Abnormalities

Capsule

Mild thickening of the lens capsule can be associated with pathologic proliferation of lens epithelium or with chronic inflammation of the anterior segment. Elements with an affinity for basement membranes, such as copper or silver, can form pigmented deposits in the anterior lens capsule, conditions known as chalcosis and argyrosis, respectively.

Epithelium

Severe elevation of intraocular pressure can injure the lens epithelial cells, leading to cell degeneration. Clinically, patches of white flecks *(glaukomflecken)* are observed beneath the lens capsule. Histologic examination shows focal areas of necrotic lens epithelial cells beneath the anterior lens capsule. Associated degenerated subepithelial cortical material is also present. See also BCSC Section 10, *Glaucoma.*

Inflammation, ischemia, or trauma can also cause injury to the lens epithelium, stimulating epithelial metaplasia and the formation of *anterior subcapsular fibrous plaques* (Fig 9-7A). In this situation, the epithelial cells have undergone a metaplastic transformation into fibroblast-like cells that are capable of producing collagen. Following resolution of the inciting stimulus, the lens epithelium may produce another capsule, thereby completely surrounding the fibrous plaque and creating a *duplication cataract* (Fig 9-7B).

Retention of iron-containing metallic foreign bodies in the eye may cause lens epithelial degeneration as a result of *siderosis.* The presence of iron within the epithelial cells can be demonstrated with Perls Prussian blue stain.

The most common abnormality involving the lens epithelium may be *posterior subcapsular cataract* (Fig 9-8A; see also Fig 9-7A). Histologically, development of this cataract begins with epithelial disarray at the equator, followed by posterior migration of the

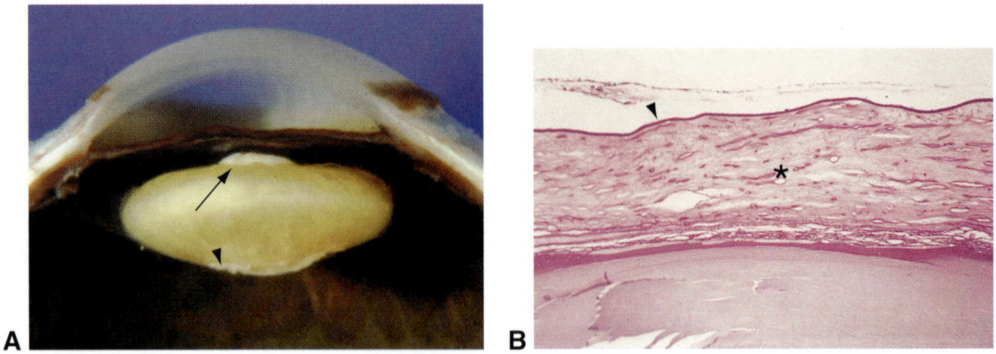

Figure 9-7 Anterior and posterior subcapsular cataracts. **A,** Gross photograph shows white anterior *(arrow)* and posterior *(arrowhead)* subcapsular plaques located centrally. **B,** Fibrous plaque *(asterisk)* is present posterior to the original lens capsule *(arrowhead)*. *(Part A courtesy of Tatyana Milman, MD; part B courtesy of Hans E. Grossniklaus, MD.)*

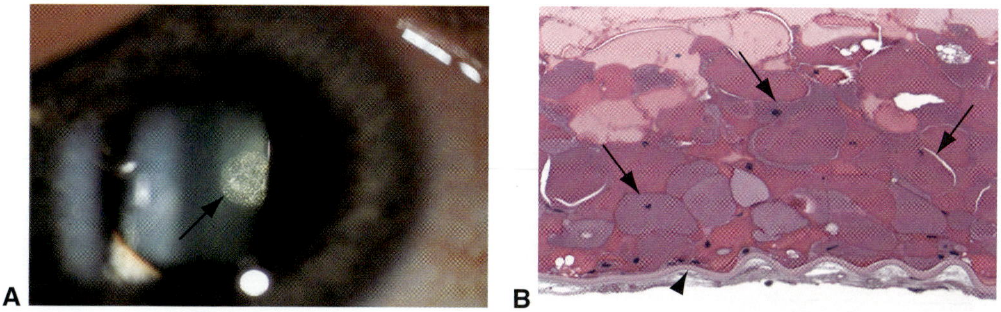

Figure 9-8 Posterior subcapsular cataract. **A,** Cataract *(arrow)* viewed at the slit lamp. **B,** Large, round, nucleated Wedl cells *(arrows)* and smaller lens epithelial cells line the posterior lens capsule *(arrowhead). (Part A courtesy of Alcon. Reproduced with permission from* Clinical Symposia. *Part B courtesy of Robert H. Rosa, Jr, MD.)*

lens epithelium along the capsule. As the cells migrate posteriorly, they may enlarge to 5–6 times their normal size. These swollen cells, referred to as *Wedl* or *bladder cells,* can cause significant visual impairment if they involve the axial portion of the lens (Fig 9-8B).

Disruption of the lens capsule often results in proliferation of lens epithelial cells. For example, following extracapsular cataract extraction, remaining epithelial cells can proliferate and cover the inner surface of the posterior lens capsule, resulting in clinically appreciable posterior capsule opacification. These accumulations of proliferating epithelial cells may form partially transparent globular masses, called *Elschnig pearls* (Fig 9-9), which are histologically identical to Wedl cells. Sequestration of proliferating lens fibers in the equatorial region may create a doughnut-shaped configuration that is referred to as a *Soemmering ring lens remnant* (Fig 9-10).

Cortex

Clinically, cortical degenerative changes fall into 2 broad categories: (1) generalized discolorations with loss of transparency and (2) focal opacifications. Generalized loss of transparency cannot reliably be diagnosed histologically; the histologic stains used to

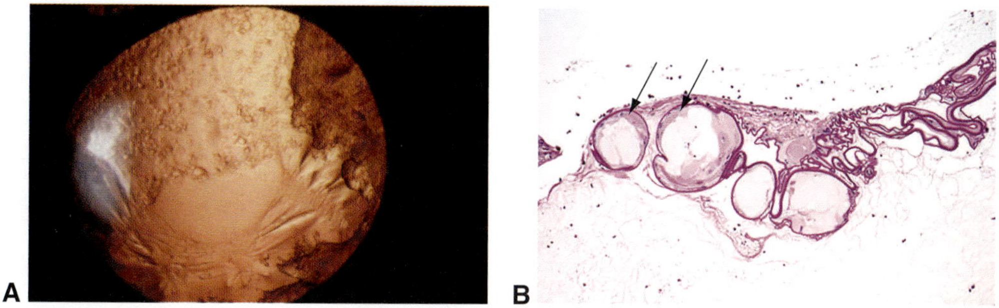

Figure 9-9 Elschnig pearls. **A,** Clinical appearance on retroillumination, demonstrating posterior capsule opacities. **B,** Photomicrograph depicts proliferating lens epithelium *(arrows)* on remnants of the posterior capsule (PAS stain). *(Part A courtesy of Sander Dubovy, MD; part B courtesy of Nasreen A. Syed, MD.)*

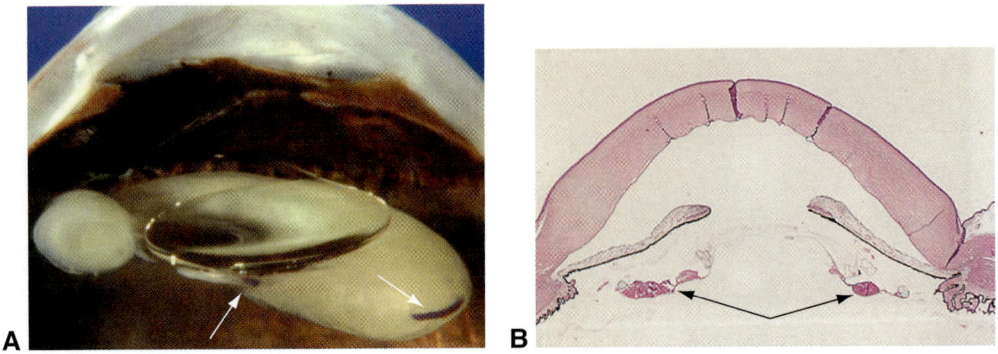

Figure 9-10 Soemmering ring cataract. **A,** Doughnut-shaped white cataractous material is present in the equatorial region of the lens capsule and surrounds a lens haptic *(arrows)*. The lens optic and a second haptic are positioned in front of the lens capsular bag, in the sulcus. **B,** Photomicrograph of a ring cataract *(arrows)*. *(Part A courtesy of Tatyana Milman, MD.)*

colorize the lens after it is processed prevent the assessment of lens clarity. The earliest sign of focal cortical degeneration is hydropic swelling of the lens fibers with decreased intensity of eosinophilic staining. Focal cortical opacities become more apparent when fiber degeneration is advanced enough to cause liquefactive change. Light microscopy shows the accumulation of eosinophilic globules *(morgagnian globules)* in slitlike spaces between the lens fibers (Fig 9-11; see Fig 9-12C). As focal cortical lesions progress, the slitlike spaces become confluent, forming globular collections of lens protein. Ultimately, the entire cortex can become liquefied, allowing the nucleus to sink downward and the capsule to wrinkle; this condition is referred to as *morgagnian cataract* (Fig 9-12).

Denatured lens protein can escape through an intact lens capsule and provoke an anterior chamber macrophagic inflammatory reaction, a condition known as *phacolytic glaucoma.* See Chapter 7 for a brief discussion of this topic, as well as BCSC Section 10, *Glaucoma.*

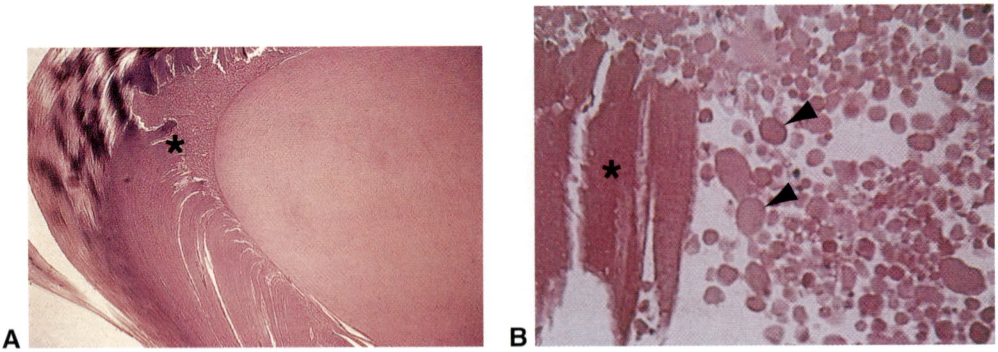

Figure 9-11 Cataract. **A,** Extensive cortical changes are present *(asterisk)*. **B,** Cortical degeneration. Lens cell fibers *(asterisk)* are swollen and fragmented. Note the morgagnian globules *(arrowheads)*. The lenticular fragments are opaque and increase osmotic pressure within the capsule. *(Courtesy of Hans E. Grossniklaus, MD.)*

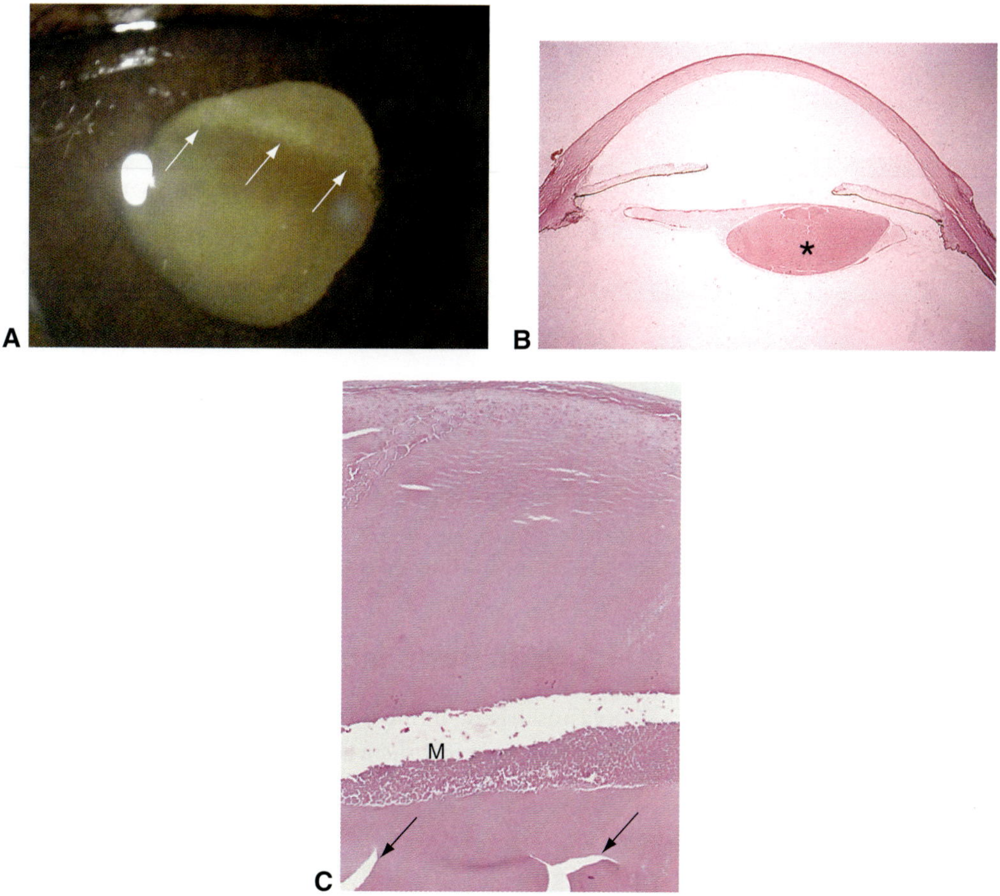

Figure 9-12 Morgagnian cataract. **A,** The brunescent nucleus has sunk inferiorly within the liquefied cortex. *Arrows* mark the superior edge of the nucleus. **B,** The lens cortex has liquefied, leaving the lens nucleus *(asterisk)* floating free within the capsular bag. **C,** Artifactitious, sharply angulated clefts *(arrows)* are present in this nuclear sclerotic cataract. A zone of morgagnian globules (M) is visible. *(Part A courtesy of Bradford Tannen, MD; part B courtesy of Debra J. Shetlar, MD.)*

Nucleus

In the adult lens, the continual production of lens fibers subjects the nucleus to the stress of mechanical compression, which causes hardening of the lens nucleus. Aging is also associated with alterations in the chemical composition of the nuclear fibers. The pathogenesis of nuclear discoloration is poorly understood and probably involves more than 1 mechanism, including accumulation of urochrome pigment. Clinically, the lens nucleus may appear yellow, brunescent, or deep brown.

Nuclear cataracts are difficult to assess histologically because they take on a subtle homogeneous eosinophilic appearance. Clinically, the loss of cellular laminations (artifactitious clefts) probably correlates better with nuclear firmness than it does with optical opacification (see Fig 9-12C). Occasionally, crystalline deposits, identified as calcium oxalate, may be observed within a nuclear cataract (Fig 9-13). These deposits are birefringent under polarized light.

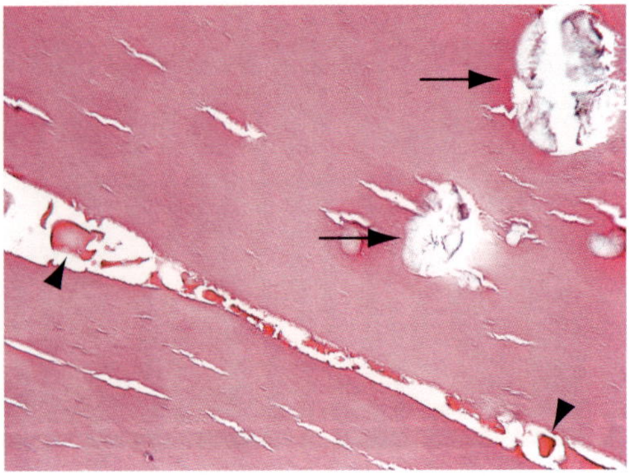

Figure 9-13 Crystalline deposits of calcium oxalate *(arrows)* are visible within the lens. Also apparent is a cortical cleft with morgagnian globules *(arrowheads). (Courtesy of Tatyana Milman, MD.)*

Zonular fibers

Deposition of protein on the lens zonular fibers in *pseudoexfoliation syndrome* (also called *exfoliation syndrome*) can lead to degeneration of the zonular fibers and their eventual dehiscence. See Chapter 7 in this volume for additional discussion.

Neoplasia and Associations With Systemic Disorders

There are no reported cases of neoplasms arising in the human lens. Premature opacification of the lens has been observed in many systemic disorders. See BCSC Section 11, *Lens and Cataract.*

Pathology in Intraocular Lenses

See BCSC Section 11, *Lens and Cataract,* for a discussion of this topic.

CHAPTER **10**

Vitreous

Topography

The vitreous humor makes up most of the volume of the globe and is important in many diseases that affect the eye. See BCSC Section 12, *Retina and Vitreous,* and Section 2, *Fundamentals and Principles of Ophthalmology,* for discussion of the anatomy of the vitreous. The strength of vitreoretinal adhesion or attachment is important in the pathogenesis of retinal tears and detachment, macular hole formation, and vitreous hemorrhage from neovascularization.

The embryologic development of the vitreous is generally divided into 3 stages: primary, secondary, and tertiary.

The *primary vitreous* consists of fibrillar material; mesenchymal cells; and vascular components: the hyaloid artery, vasa hyaloidea propria, and tunica vasculosa lentis (see Fig 4-3 in BCSC Section 11, *Lens and Cataract*). The *secondary vitreous* begins to form at approximately the ninth week of gestation and is destined to become the main portion of the vitreous in the postnatal and adult eye. The primary vitreous atrophies with formation of the secondary vitreous, leaving only a clear central zone through the vitreous (called the *hyaloid canal,* or the *Cloquet canal*) and, occasionally, the Bergmeister papilla and Mittendorf dot as vestigial remnants (discussed later). The secondary vitreous is relatively acellular and completely avascular. The cells present in the secondary vitreous are called *hyalocytes.* The lens zonular fibers (also referred to as the *zonules of Zinn*) represent the *tertiary vitreous.*

Congenital Anomalies

Persistent Fetal Vasculature

Persistent fetal vasculature (PFV; previously known as *persistent hyperplastic primary vitreous,* or *PHPV*) is characterized by the persistence of variable components of the primary vitreous and is most often unilateral. In most cases of clinically significant PFV, a fibrovascular plaque in the retrolental space extends laterally to involve the ciliary processes, which may be pulled centripetally by traction from the fibrovascular tissue. The clinical and gross appearance of elongated ciliary processes results. The anterior fibrovascular plaque is generally contiguous posteriorly with a remnant of the hyaloid artery that may attach to the optic nerve head (also called optic disc) (Fig 10-1). Involvement of the

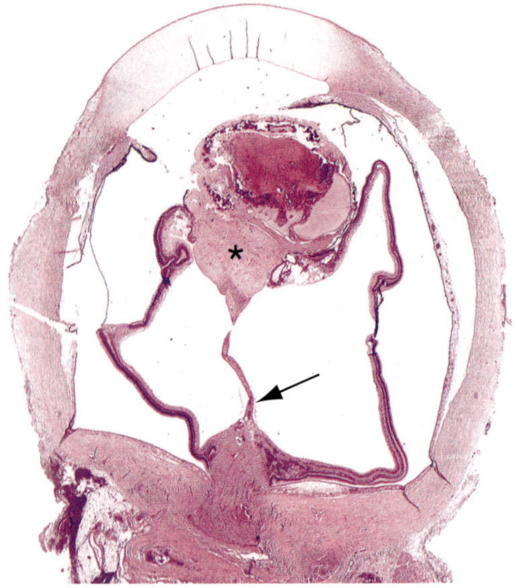

Figure 10-1 Photomicrograph of persistent fetal vasculature. Note the prominent anterior fibrovascular plaque *(asterisk)*. The posterior remnant of the persistent hyaloid artery is evident at the optic nerve head *(arrow)*. *(Courtesy of Nasreen Syed, MD.)*

posterior structures may be more extensive, with detachment of the peripapillary retina resulting from traction from preretinal membranes. The lens is often cataractous, and nonocular tissues such as adipose tissue and cartilage may be present in the retrolental mass. Eyes affected by PFV are often microphthalmic. See also Chapter 19 in this volume, BCSC Section 6, *Pediatric Ophthalmology and Strabismus,* and Section 12, *Retina and Vitreous.*

Bergmeister Papilla

As mentioned in the earlier Topography section, the persistence of a small part of the posterior portion of the hyaloid artery is referred to as a *Bergmeister papilla.* This anomaly generally takes the form of a veil-like structure or a fingerlike projection extending anteriorly from the surface of the optic nerve head (Fig 10-2). Retinal vessels may grow into a Bergmeister papilla and then return to the optic nerve head, creating prepapillary vascular loops. See Figure 16-6 in BCSC Section 12, *Retina and Vitreous.*

Mittendorf Dot

The hyaloid artery attaches to the tunica vasculosa lentis just inferior and nasal to the center of the lens. With regression of these vascular structures, development of a focal lens opacity at this site, referred to as a *Mittendorf dot,* is not uncommon (see Fig 2-41 in BCSC Section 2, *Fundamentals and Principles of Ophthalmology*).

Vitreous Cysts

Vitreous cysts generally occur in eyes with no other pathologic findings, but they have been seen in eyes with retinitis pigmentosa, those with uveitis, and eyes with remnants of

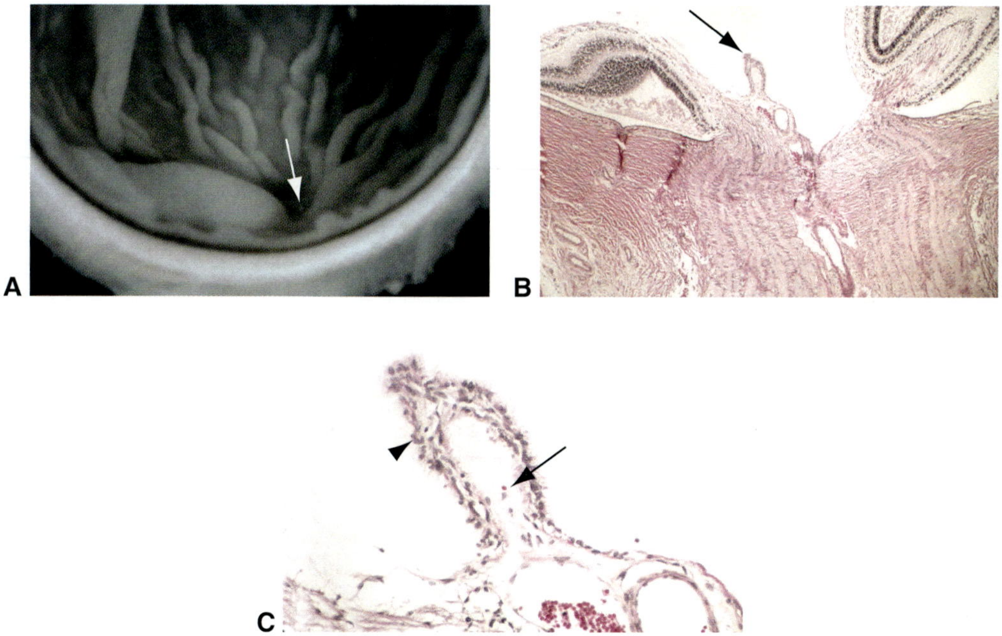

Figure 10-2 Bergmeister papilla. **A,** Gross photograph of infant eye showing fingerlike projection of whitish tissue *(arrow)* from the surface of the optic nerve head. **B,** Low-magnification photomicrograph of part **A** showing fibroglial tissue *(arrow)* projecting into the vitreous cavity from the optic nerve head. **C,** High-magnification photomicrograph of Bergmeister papilla demonstrating loose fibrous connective tissue with small capillary *(arrow),* surrounded by a thin layer of fibrous astrocyte-like cells *(arrowhead). (Courtesy of Robert H. Rosa, Jr, MD.)*

the hyaloid system. Histologic studies have suggested the presence of hyaloid remnants in the vitreous cysts. The exact origin of the cysts is not known.

Inflammations

As a relatively acellular and completely avascular structure, the vitreous is generally not a primary site for the initiation of inflammatory disorders. It does become involved secondarily in inflammatory conditions of adjacent tissues, however. The term *vitritis* is used to denote the presence of benign or malignant white blood cells in the vitreous. Vitreous inflammation associated with infectious agents, particularly bacteria and fungi, is clinically referred to as *infectious endophthalmitis.* Bacterial endophthalmitis is characterized by neutrophilic infiltration of the vitreous (Fig 10-3) that leads to liquefaction of the vitreous, with subsequent posterior vitreous detachment. Severe inflammation may be accompanied by formation of fibrocellular membranes, typically in the retrolental space; these may exert traction on the peripheral retina. The vitreous infiltrate in noninfectious uveitis is typically composed of chronic inflammatory cells, including T and B lymphocytes and histiocytes (Fig 10-4). See also BCSC Section 9, *Intraocular Inflammation and Uveitis.*

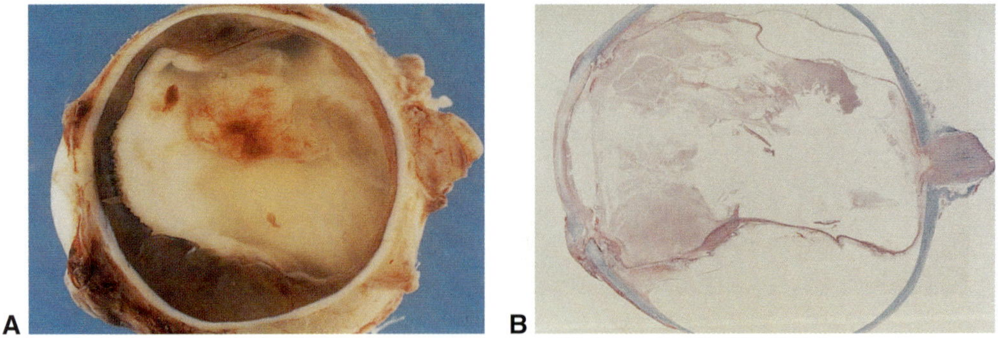

Figure 10-3 Endophthalmitis. **A,** Gross photograph of opacification and infiltration of the vitreous as a result of bacterial endophthalmitis. **B,** Photomicrograph of a section showing cellular infiltration of vitreous in endophthalmitis (retinal detachment is artifactitious). *(Courtesy of Hans E. Grossniklaus, MD.)*

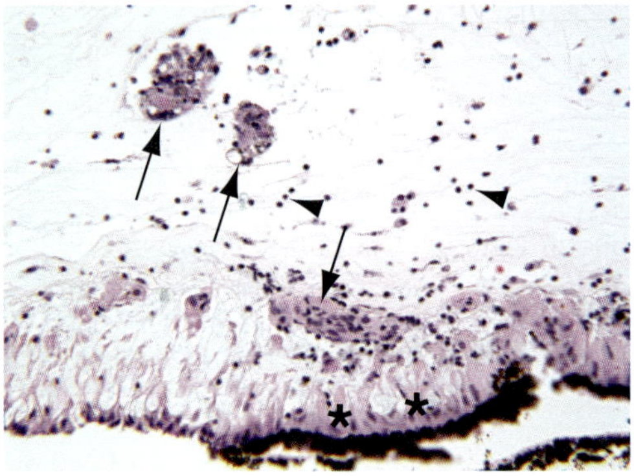

Figure 10-4 Noninfectious uveitis. Note the pigmented and nonpigmented ciliary epithelium *(asterisks)* and the aggregates of epithelioid histiocytes *(arrows)* and scattered lymphocytes *(arrowheads)* in the vitreous base in this evisceration specimen. *(Courtesy of Tatyana Milman, MD.)*

Degenerations

Syneresis and Aging

Syneresis of the vitreous is defined as liquefaction of the gel. Syneresis of the central vitreous is a nearly universal consequence of aging. It also occurs as a result of vitreous inflammation and hemorrhage and in the setting of pathologic myopia. The prominent lamellae and strands that develop in aging and following inflammation or hemorrhage are the result of abnormally aggregated collagenous vitreous fibers around syneretic areas (Fig 10-5). Syneresis is one of the contributing factors leading to vitreous detachment.

Posterior Vitreous Detachment

Posterior vitreous detachment (PVD) occurs when a dehiscence in the vitreous cortex allows fluid from a syneretic cavity to enter the potential subhyaloid space, causing the remaining cortex to be stripped from the internal limiting membrane (ILM) (Fig 10-6). As fluid drains out of the syneretic cavities under the newly formed posterior hyaloid, the

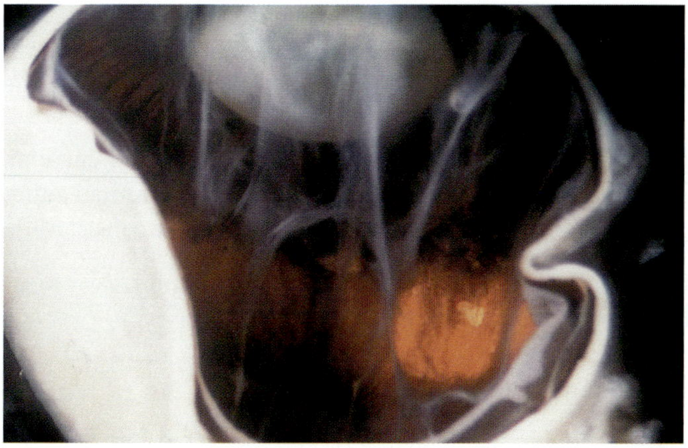

Figure 10-5 Gross photograph of vitreous condensations outlining syneretic cavities. *(Courtesy of Hans E. Grossniklaus, MD.)*

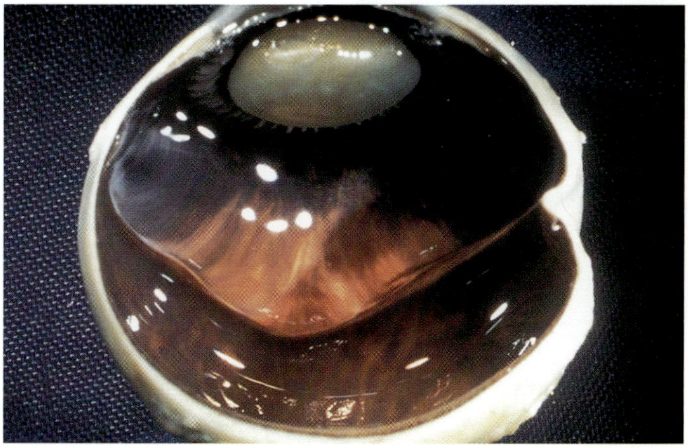

Figure 10-6 Gross photograph of posterior vitreous detachment. *(Courtesy of Hans E. Grossniklaus, MD.)*

vitreous body collapses anteriorly, remaining attached at its base. Vitreous detachment generally occurs rapidly over the course of a few hours to days.

An age-related weakening of the adherence of the cortical vitreous to the ILM also plays a role in PVDs. Clinical and pathologic studies have reported a prevalence of 50% or more of PVD in individuals aged 70 years and older. The incidence of PVD is increased in individuals with intraocular inflammation, aphakia or pseudophakia, trauma, myopia, and other vitreoretinal diseases. PVD is important in the pathogenesis of many conditions, including retinal tears and detachment, vitreous hemorrhage, and macular hole formation. See BCSC Section 12, *Retina and Vitreous,* for additional discussion.

Rhegmatogenous retinal detachment and proliferative vitreoretinopathy

Retinal tears form from vitreous traction on the retina during or after PVD or secondary to ocular trauma. Tears are most likely to occur at sites of greatest vitreoretinal adhesion, such as the vitreous base (Fig 10-7) or the margin of lattice degeneration. Histologic examination of retinal tears reveals that the vitreous adheres to the retina along the flap of the tear. In the area of retina separated from the underlying retinal pigment epithelium (RPE), there is loss of photoreceptors.

Retinal detachment occurs when vitreous traction and fluid currents resulting from eye movements combine to overcome the forces maintaining retinal adhesion to the RPE. The principal histopathologic findings in retinal detachment consist of the following:

- degeneration of the outer segments of the photoreceptors
- eventual loss of photoreceptor cells
- migration of Müller cells
- proliferation and migration of RPE cells

Small cystic spaces develop in the detached retina, and in chronic detachment, these cysts may coalesce into large macrocysts (Fig 10-8).

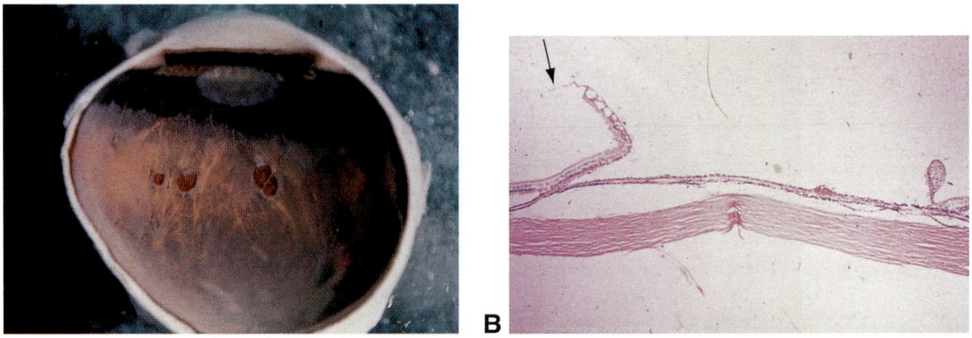

A B

Figure 10-7 Retinal tears. **A,** Gross photograph of retinal tears at vitreous base. **B,** Photomicrograph showing condensed vitreous *(arrow)* attached to the anterior flap of the retinal tear. *(Courtesy of W. Richard Green, MD.)*

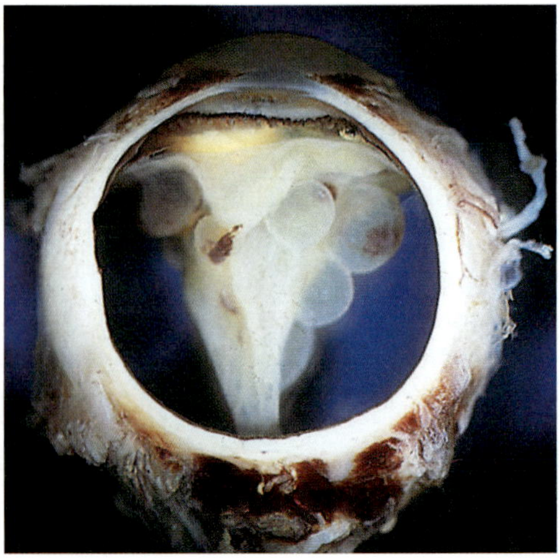

Figure 10-8 Long-standing total retinal detachment with macrocystic degeneration of the retina.

With rhegmatogenous retinal detachment, cellular membranes may form on either surface (anterior or posterior) of the retina (Fig 10-9). Clinically, this process is referred to as *proliferative vitreoretinopathy (PVR)*. These membranes form as a result of proliferation of RPE cells and other cellular elements, including glial cells (Müller cells, fibrous astrocytes), macrophages, fibroblasts, myofibroblasts, and possibly hyalocytes. The cell biology of PVR is complex and involves the interaction of various growth factors and integrins, as well as cellular proliferation. Studies have shown a significant association between clinical grades of PVR and the expression levels of specific cytokines and/or growth factors in the vitreous fluid.

Garweg JG, Tappeiner C, Halberstadt M. Pathophysiology of proliferative vitreoretinopathy in retinal detachment. *Surv Ophthalmol.* 2013;58(4):321–329.

Macular holes

Idiopathic macular holes most likely form as the result of degenerative changes in the vitreous. Optical coherence tomography (OCT) has greatly advanced our understanding of the anatomical features of full-thickness macular holes and early macular hole formation. These studies are most consistent with a focal vitreomacular traction mechanism. Localized perifoveal vitreous detachment (an early stage of age-related PVD) appears to be the primary pathogenetic event in idiopathic macular hole formation (Fig 10-10). Detachment of the posterior hyaloid from the pericentral retina exerts anterior traction on the foveola and localizes the dynamic vitreous traction associated with ocular rotations into the perifoveolar region.

OCT has clarified the pathoanatomy of early macular hole stages, beginning with a foveal pseudocyst (stage 1a), typically followed by disruption of the outer retina (stage 1b), before progressing to a full-thickness dehiscence (stage 2). Histologically, full-thickness macular holes are similar to holes in other locations. A full-thickness retinal defect with rounded tissue margins (stage 3) is accompanied by loss of the photoreceptor outer segments in adjacent retina that is separated from the RPE by subretinal fluid (see Fig 10-10C).

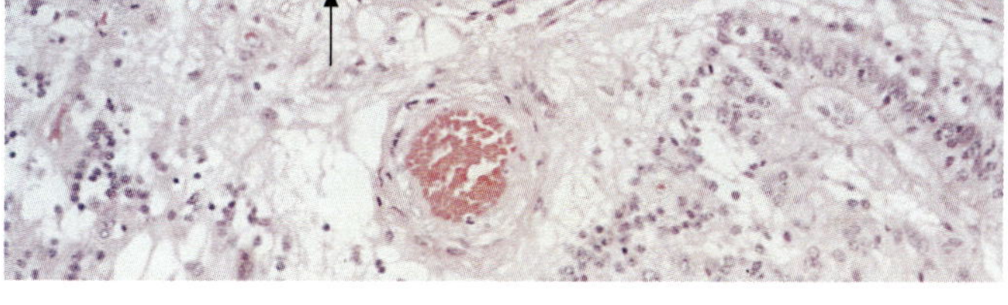

Figure 10-9 Preretinal membrane *(between arrows)* on the surface of the retina, secondary to proliferative vitreoretinopathy. *(Courtesy of David J. Wilson, MD.)*

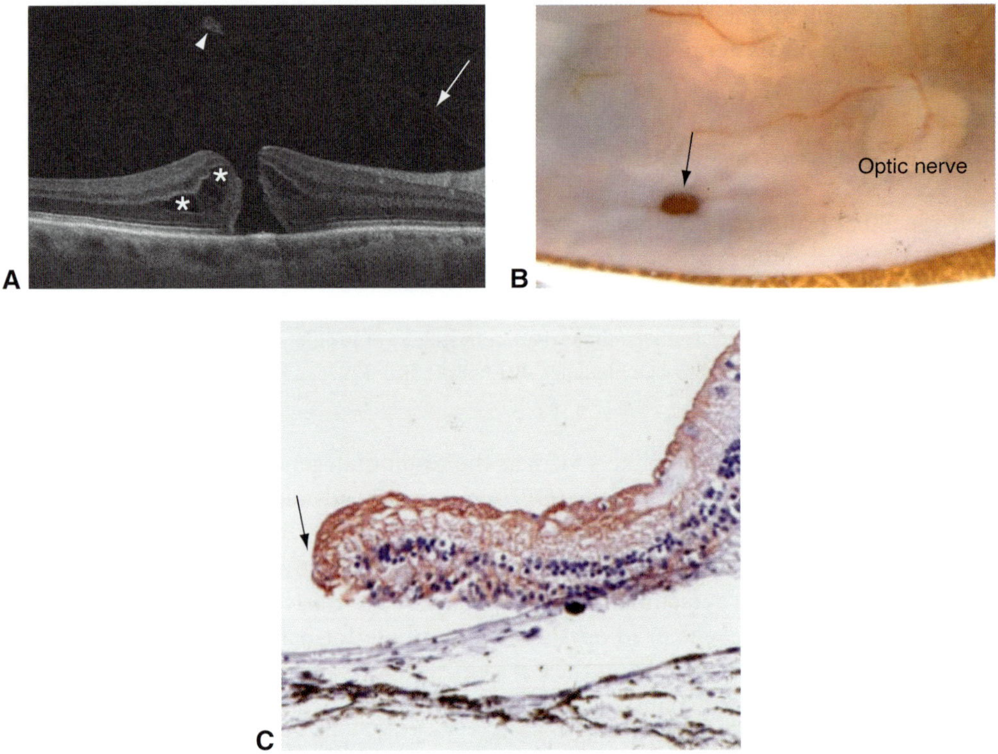

Figure 10-10 Macular holes. **A,** Spectral domain optical coherence tomography (OCT) showing stage 3 macular hole with full-thickness retinal defect, rounded margins, cystoid macular edema *(asterisks),* and operculum *(arrowhead).* Note the posterior hyaloid face *(arrow)* tethered to the peripapillary retina near the optic nerve head. **B,** Gross photograph of full-thickness macular hole *(arrow).* **C,** Photomicrograph of full-thickness macular hole showing rounded gliotic margin *(arrow)* with positive staining for glial fibrillary acidic protein (GFAP), highlighting the Müller cells and fibrous astrocytes. *(Part A courtesy of Robert H. Rosa, Jr, MD; parts B and C courtesy of Patricia Chévez-Barrios, MD.)*

An epiretinal membrane composed of Müller cells, fibrous astrocytes, and fibroblasts with myoblastic differentiation is often present on the surface of the retina adjacent to the macular hole. Cystoid macular edema in the parafoveal retina adjacent to the full-thickness macular hole is relatively common. Following surgical repair of macular holes, closer apposition of the remaining photoreceptors and variable glial scarring close the macular defect. See BCSC Section 12, *Retina and Vitreous,* for further discussion.

Smiddy WE, Flynn HW Jr. Pathogenesis of macular holes and therapeutic implications. *Am J Ophthalmol.* 2004;137(3):525–537.

Steel DHW, Lotery AJ. Idiopathic vitreomacular traction and macular hole: a comprehensive review of pathophysiology, diagnosis, and treatment. *Eye.* 2013;27(Suppl 1):S1–S21.

Hemorrhage

A constellation of pathologic features may develop in the vitreous following vitreous hemorrhage. After 3–10 days, red blood cell clots undergo fibrinolysis, and red blood cells may diffuse throughout the vitreous cavity. At this time, breakdown of the red blood cells also occurs. Loss of hemoglobin from the red blood cells produces ghost cells (see Chapter 7, Fig 7-10) and hemoglobin spherules. Obstruction of the trabecular meshwork by these cells may lead to *ghost cell glaucoma.* See also BCSC Section 10, *Glaucoma.*

The process of red blood cell dissolution attracts macrophages, which phagocytose the effete red blood cells. Iron (Fe^{3+}) is released during hemoglobin breakdown. This can occur intracellularly in macrophages with iron storage as ferritin or hemosiderin, or extracellularly with iron binding to vitreous proteins such as lactoferrin and transferrin. In massive hemorrhages, cholesterol crystals caused by the breakdown of red blood cell membranes may be present, often surrounded by a foreign body giant cell reaction. Cholesterol appears clinically as refractile crystals in the vitreous cavity; the crystals are typically not attached to vitreous fibrils (synchysis scintillans). Syneresis of the vitreous and PVD are common after vitreous hemorrhage.

Asteroid Hyalosis

Asteroid hyalosis is a condition with a spectacular clinical appearance (see Fig 16-9 in BCSC Section 12, *Retina and Vitreous*) but little clinical significance. Histologically, asteroid bodies are rounded structures measuring 10–100 nm, typically attached to vitreous fibrils, that stain positively with alcian blue and with stains for neutral fats, phospholipids, and calcium (Fig 10-11). The bodies stain metachromatically and exhibit birefringence. Occasionally, asteroid bodies will be surrounded by a foreign body giant cell reaction, but the condition is not generally associated with vitreous inflammation.

The exact mechanism of formation of asteroid bodies is not known; however, element mapping by electron spectroscopic imaging has revealed a homogeneous distribution of calcium, phosphorus, and oxygen. Thus, asteroid bodies exhibit structural and elemental similarity to hydroxyapatite, and proteoglycans and their glycosaminoglycan side chains appear to play a role in regulating the biomineralization process.

Fawzi AA, Vo B, Kriwanek Ret al. Asteroid hyalosis in an autopsy population: The University of California at Los Angeles (UCLA) experience. *Arch Ophthalmol.* 2005;123(4):486–490.

Winkler J, Lünsdorf H. Ultrastructure and composition of asteroid bodies. *Invest Ophthalmol Vis Sci.* 2001;42(5):902–907.

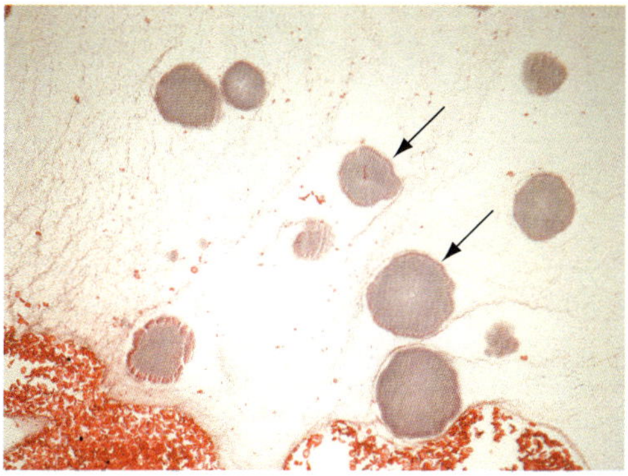

Figure 10-11 Asteroid bodies *(arrows)* and erythrocytic debris within the vitreous. *(Courtesy of Tatyana Milman, MD.)*

Vitreous Amyloidosis

The term *amyloidosis* refers to a group of diseases that lead to extracellular deposition of amyloid. Amyloid is composed of various types of proteins that have a characteristic ultrastructural appearance of nonbranching fibrils with variable length and a diameter of 75–100 Å. The proteins forming amyloid are able to form a tertiary structure characterized as a β-pleated sheet, which enables the proteins to bind Congo red stain and show birefringence in polarized light (Fig 10-12).

Amyloid's protein of origin is characteristic for different forms of amyloidosis. Amyloid deposits occur in the vitreous when the protein forming the amyloid is *transthyretin.* There are multiple genetic mutations that can result in various amino acid substitutions in the transthyretin protein. The most common mutations were originally described in *familial amyloid polyneuropathy (FAP).* Systemic manifestations in patients with FAP include vitreous opacities and perivascular infiltrates (Fig 10-13), peripheral neuropathy, cardiomyopathy, and carpal tunnel syndrome.

The mechanism by which the vitreous becomes involved is not known with certainty. Because amyloid deposits are found within the walls of retinal vessels and in the RPE and ciliary body, amyloid may gain access to the vitreous through these tissues. In addition,

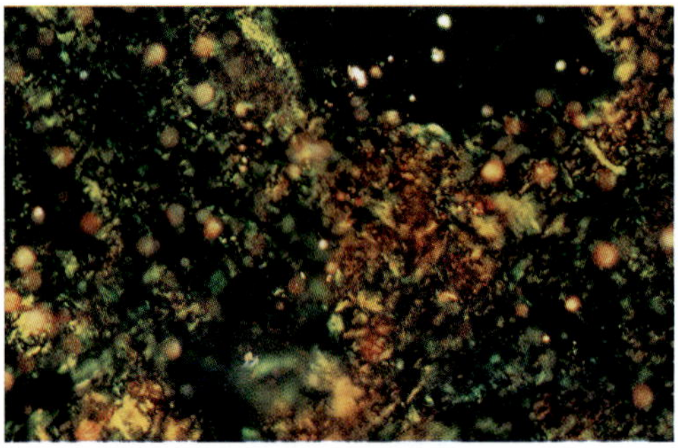

Figure 10-12 Polarized light photomicrograph of the Congo red–stained vitreous from a patient with familial amyloid polyneuropathy. *(Courtesy of David J. Wilson, MD.)*

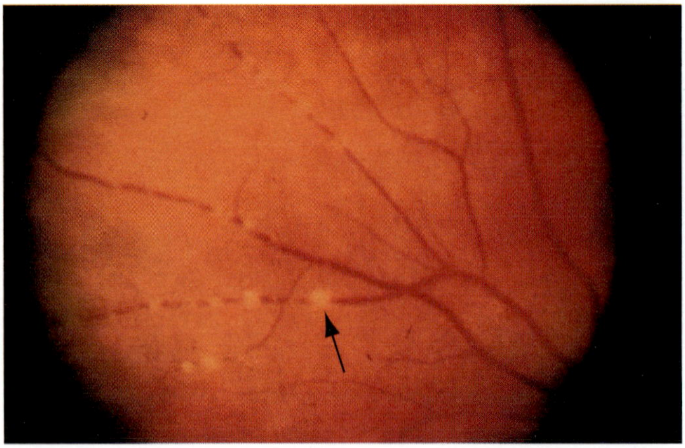

Figure 10-13 Perivascular sheathing *(arrow)* associated with vitreous amyloidosis. *(Courtesy of Hans E. Grossniklaus, MD.)*

because transthyretin is a blood protein, it may gain access to the vitreous by crossing the blood–aqueous or blood–retina barrier.

Neoplasia

Intraocular Lymphoma

Primary neoplastic involvement of the vitreous is uncommon because of the relatively acellular nature of the vitreous. However, the vitreous can be the site of primary involvement in cases of B-cell lymphoma. This type of lymphoma has been referred to as *primary intraocular/central nervous system lymphoma, large cell lymphoma,* and *vitreoretinal/retinal lymphoma.* Immunohistochemical and molecular genetic studies have confirmed that this entity is typically a B-cell lymphoma; however, T-cell lymphomas may occur in rare instances.

Clinically, *primary intraocular lymphoma (PIOL)* presents most commonly as a vitritis. Some patients have sub-RPE infiltrates (Fig 10-14) with a very characteristic speckled pigmentation overlying tumor detachments of the RPE. The sub-RPE infiltrates are present in a minority of patients with intraocular lymphoma. Recent evidence suggests that the lymphoma cells may be attracted to the RPE by B-cell chemokines and subsequently migrate from the sub-RPE space into the vitreous. More than half of patients presenting with ocular findings have or will develop involvement of the central nervous system.

The diagnosis of intraocular lymphoma can be challenging and relies primarily on cytologic analysis of vitreous and/or subretinal specimens. Cytologically, the vitreous infiltrate in intraocular lymphoma is heterogeneous. The atypical cells are large lymphoid cells, frequently with a convoluted nuclear membrane and multiple, conspicuous nucleoli. An accompanying infiltrate of small lymphocytes almost always appears, and the normal cells may obscure the neoplastic cell population. These small round lymphocytes are

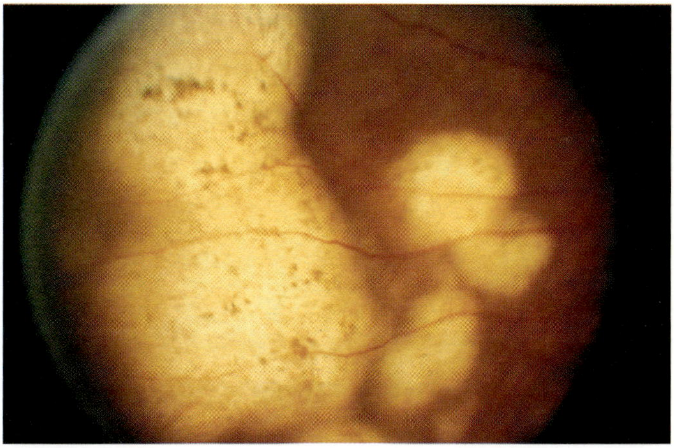

Figure 10-14 Sub-RPE infiltrates in a patient with primary intraocular lymphoma. Note the characteristic speckled pigmentation over the tumor detachments of the RPE. *(Courtesy of Robert H. Rosa, Jr, MD.)*

mostly reactive T cells. Numerous necrotic cells are usually present, and this feature is very suggestive of a diagnosis of intraocular lymphoma (Fig 10-15). Immunohistochemically, the viable tumor cells can be labeled as a monoclonal population of B cells. Flow cytometry is helpful in demonstrating a monoclonal population. Other laboratory tests that may be useful in the diagnosis and follow-up of patients with intraocular lymphoma are determination of the interleukin-10 to interleukin-6 ratio and the use of microdissection and polymerase chain reaction (PCR) for the detection of immunoglobulin gene rearrangement and translocation.

The subretinal/sub-RPE infiltrates are composed of neoplastic lymphoid cells (Fig 10-16). With or without treatment, the subretinal infiltrates may resolve, leaving a

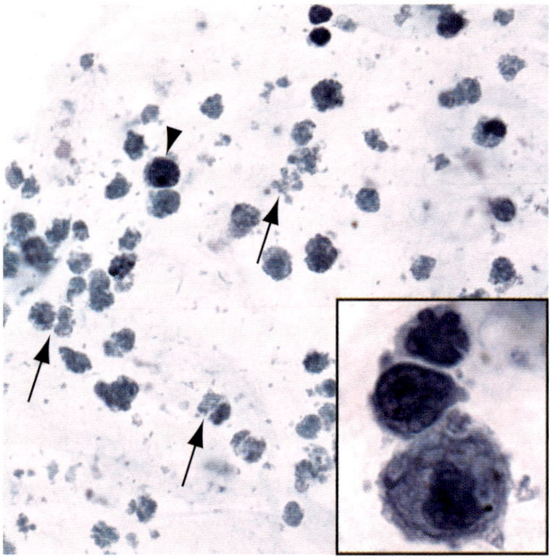

Figure 10-15 Cytologic preparation of vitreoretinal lymphoma. Note the atypical cells with hyperchromatic nuclei, prominent nucleoli, and scant cytoplasm *(arrowhead).* Numerous necrotic, smudgy cells *(arrows)* are present. Inset shows atypical lymphoid cells with nuclear membrane abnormalities. *(Courtesy of Robert H. Rosa, Jr., MD.)*

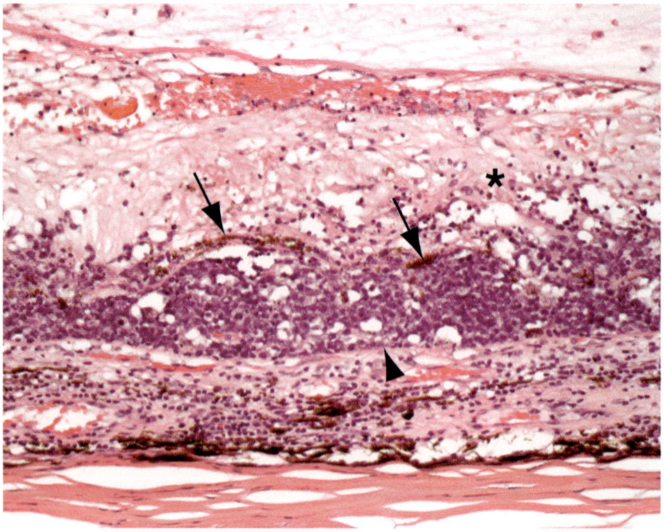

Figure 10-16 Primary intraocular lymphoma. Note the detachment of the RPE by tumor *(arrows)* overlying retinal gliosis *(asterisk),* and intact Bruch membrane *(arrowhead).* Secondary chronic inflammation is present in the choroid. *(Courtesy of Robert H. Rosa, Jr, MD.)*

focal area of RPE atrophy. Optic nerve and retinal infiltration may also be present. Infiltrates in these locations tend to be perivascular and may lead to ischemic retinal or optic nerve damage. The choroid is typically free of lymphoma cells; however, secondary chronic inflammation may be present in the choroid. In the setting of systemic lymphoma with ocular involvement, the choroid (rather than the vitreous, retina, or subretinal space) is the primary site of involvement (see Chapter 12 for more on choroidal lymphoma).

Chan CC, Rubenstein JL, Coupland SE, et al. Primary vitreoretinal lymphoma: a report from an International Primary Central Nervous System Lymphoma Collaborative Group symposium. *Oncologist.* 2011;16(11):1589–1599.

Coupland SE. Molecular pathology of lymphoma. *Eye.* 2013;27:180–189.

CHAPTER **11**

Retina and Retinal Pigment Epithelium

Topography

Two distinct layers form the inner lining of the posterior two-thirds of the globe:

1. The neurosensory retina, which is a delicate, transparent layer derived from the inner layer of the optic cup.
2. The retinal pigment epithelium (RPE), which is a pigmented layer derived from the outer layer of the optic cup.

Anteriorly, the RPE is continuous with the pigmented ciliary body epithelium, and the neurosensory retina is continuous with the nonpigmented ciliary body epithelium. Posteriorly, the RPE terminates at the optic nerve, just prior to the termination of Bruch membrane. The nuclear, photoreceptor, and synaptic layers of the retina gradually taper at the optic nerve head, and only the nerve fiber layer (NFL) continues on to form the optic nerve. See BCSC Section 2, *Fundamentals and Principles of Ophthalmology,* and Section 12, *Retina and Vitreous,* for additional discussion.

Neurosensory Retina

The topographic variation in the structures of the retina is striking, with regional variation in the neural structures as well as the retinal vasculature. The neurosensory retina has 10 layers (Fig 11-1).

The arrangement of the retina (in tissue sections that are perpendicular to the retinal surface) is vertical from outer to inner layers, except for the NFL, where the axons run horizontally toward the optic nerve head. Consequently, deposits and hemorrhages in the deep retinal layers have a round appearance clinically, whereas those in the NFL have a feathery or splinter-shaped appearance.

Two sources supply the retina with blood, with a watershed zone inside the inner nuclear layer of the retina. The *retinal blood vessels* supply the NFL, ganglion cell layer, inner plexiform layer, and inner two-thirds of the inner nuclear layer. The *choroidal vasculature* supplies the outer one-third of the inner nuclear layer, outer plexiform layer, outer nuclear layer, photoreceptors, and RPE. Because of this division of the blood

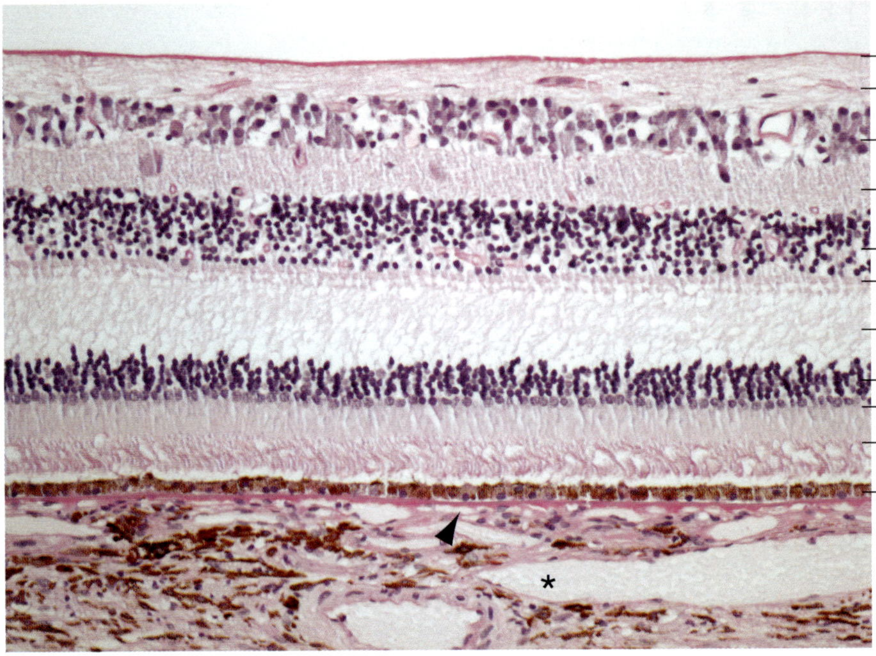

Figure 11-1 Normal retinal layers (periodic acid–Schiff [PAS] stain). From vitreous to choroid: ILM = internal limiting membrane, NFL = nerve fiber layer, GCL = ganglion cell layer, IPL = inner plexiform layer, INL = inner nuclear layer, MLM = middle limiting membrane, OPL = outer plexiform layer, ONL = outer nuclear layer, ELM = external limiting membrane, P = photoreceptors (inner/outer segments) of rods and cones, RPE = retinal pigment epithelium. Bruch membrane, *arrowhead;* choroid, *asterisk.* *(Courtesy of Robert H. Rosa, Jr, MD.)*

supply, ischemic choroidal vascular lesions and ischemic lesions attributed to the retinal vasculature produce different histologic pictures. Ischemic retinal injury produces inner retinal atrophy (see Fig 11-14), and choroidal ischemia produces outer retinal atrophy (see Fig 11-15).

Histologically, the term *macula* refers to the area of the retina where the ganglion cell layer is thicker than a single cell (Fig 11-2). Clinically, this area corresponds approximately with the area of the retina bound by the inferior and superior vascular arcades. The macula is subdivided into the *foveola,* the *fovea,* the *parafovea,* and the *perifovea.* The central foveola contains only cone photoreceptor cells; ganglion cells, other nucleated cells (including Müller cells), and blood vessels are not present. The concentration of cones is greater in the macula than in the peripheral retina, and only cones are present in the fovea.

Nerve fibers in the outer plexiform layer of the macula (nerve fiber layer of Henle) run obliquely (see Fig 11-2A). This morphologic feature results in the "flower petal" appearance of cystoid macular edema (CME) observed on fluorescein angiography, as well as the star-shaped configuration of hard exudates observed ophthalmoscopically in conditions that cause macular edema. Xanthophyll pigment gives the macula its yellow appearance clinically and grossly (macula lutea), but the xanthophyll dissolves during tissue processing and is not present in histologic sections.

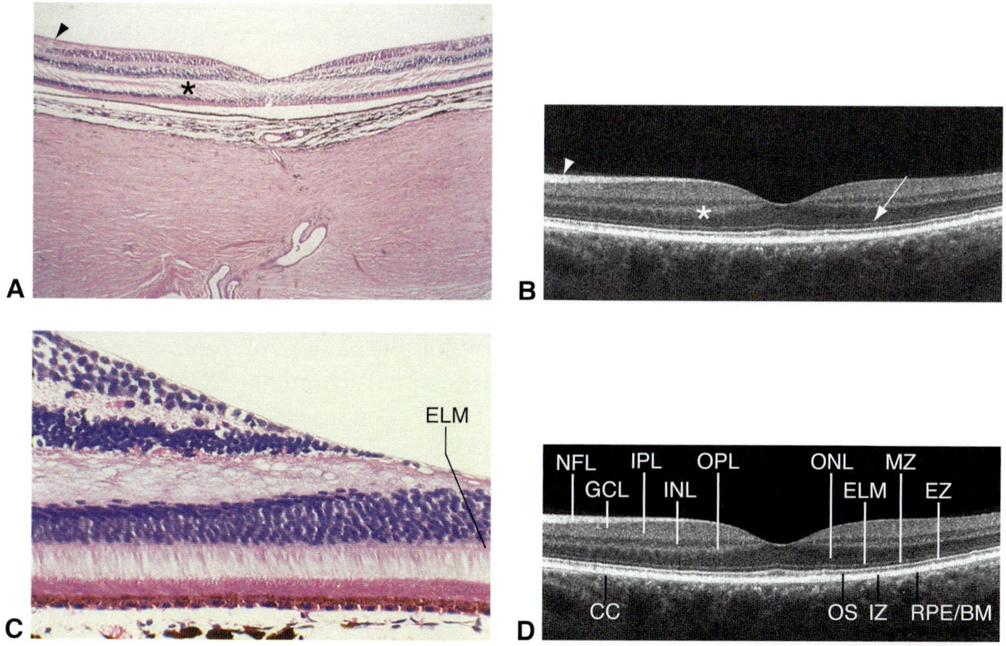

Figure 11-2 Macula. **A,** The normal macula is identified histologically by a multicellular, thick ganglion cell layer and an area of focal thinning, the foveola. Note the nerve fiber layer (NFL, *arrowhead*) in the nasal macular region and the oblique orientation of the nerve fiber layer of Henle (outer plexiform layer, *asterisk*) (hematoxylin-eosin [H&E] stain). Clinically, the macula lies between the inferior and superior vascular arcades. **B,** Spectral domain optical coherence tomography (SD-OCT) of the macula showing in vivo histologic assessment with tremendous details of the lamellar architecture of the retina. Note the NFL *(arrowhead)* in the nasal macular region, the nerve fiber layer of Henle (outer plexiform layer, *asterisk*), and the external limiting membrane *(arrow)*. **C,** In the region of the foveola, the inner cellular layers are absent, with an increased density of pigment in the retinal pigment epithelium (RPE). Note the external limiting membrane (ELM) (PAS stain). The incident light falls directly on the photoreceptor outer segments, reducing the potential for distortion of light by overlying tissue elements. **D,** SD-OCT of the macula. NFL = nerve fiber layer, GCL = ganglion cell layer, IPL = inner plexiform layer, INL = inner nuclear layer, OPL = outer plexiform layer, ONL = outer nuclear layer, ELM = external limiting membrane, MZ = myoid zone, EZ = ellipsoid zone, OS = outer segments, IZ = interdigitation zone between outer segments and RPE, RPE/BM = retinal pigment epithelium/Bruch membrane, CC = choriocapillaris. *(Parts B and D courtesy of Robert H. Rosa, Jr, MD; part D adapted from Staurenghi G, Sadda S, Chakravarthy U, Spaide RF; International Nomenclature for Optical Coherence Tomography (IN-OCT) Panel. Proposed lexicon for anatomic landmarks in normal posterior segment spectral-domain optical coherence tomography: the IN-OCT consensus.* Ophthalmology. *2014;121(8):1572–1578.)*

Retinal Pigment Epithelium

The RPE consists of a monolayer of hexagonal cells with apical microvilli and a basement membrane at the base of the cells. In contrast to the retina, the topographic variation of the RPE is subtle. In the macula, the RPE is taller, narrower, and more heavily pigmented, and it forms a regular hexagonal array. In the equatorial and midperipheral areas, RPE cells are larger in diameter and thinner. Variability in the diameter of RPE cells increases in the peripheral retina. The amount of cytoplasmic pigment, primarily lipofuscin, increases with age, particularly in the macular region.

Congenital Anomalies

Albinism

The term *albinism* refers to a congenital dilution of the pigment of the skin, the eyes, or both. This condition results from genetic mutations that cause abnormalities in the biosynthesis of melanin pigment. True albinism has been subdivided into *oculocutaneous albinism* and *ocular albinism.* Clinically, this distinction is somewhat helpful, but in reality all cases of ocular albinism have some degree of mild cutaneous involvement. The 2 types of albinism do have a pathophysiologic difference: in oculocutaneous albinism, transmission is commonly autosomal recessive, and the amount of melanin in each melanosome is reduced; in ocular albinism, transmission is commonly X-linked recessive, and the number of melanosomes is reduced (Fig 11-3). See BCSC Section 6, *Pediatric Ophthalmology and Strabismus,* and Section 12, *Retina and Vitreous,* for further discussion of albinism.

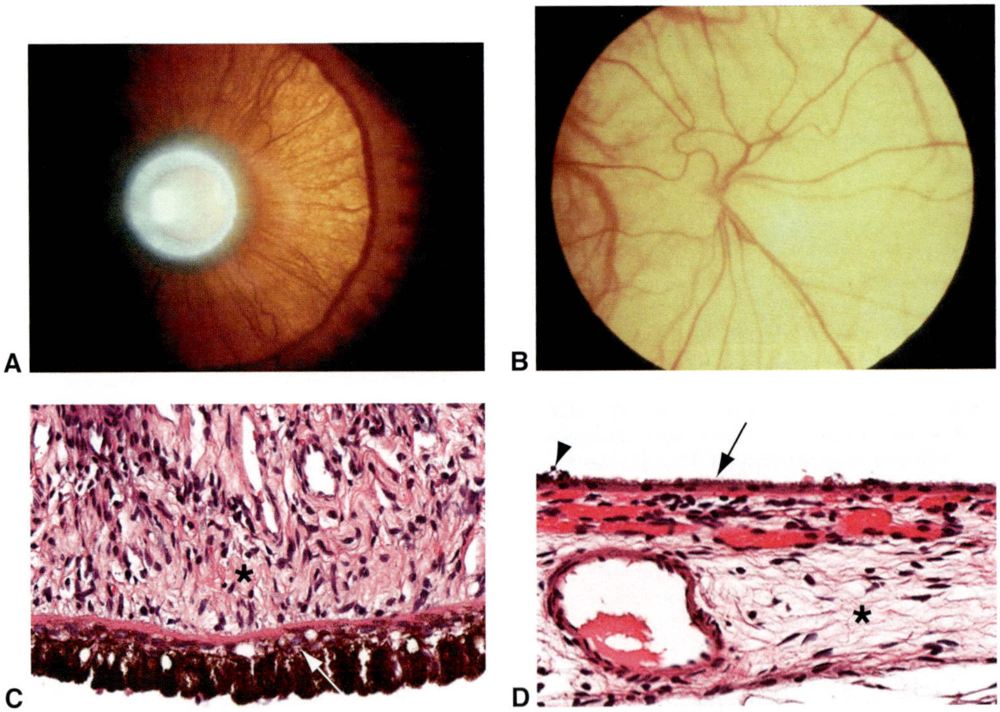

Figure 11-3 Albinism. **A,** Iris transillumination. **B,** Fundus hypopigmentation. **C,** Photomicrograph illustrates decreased pigmentation in the iris pigment epithelium (smaller melanosomes) allowing visualization of the nuclei *(white arrow).* No appreciable pigmentation is present in the iris stroma *(asterisk)* (H&E stain). **D,** Photomicrograph shows RPE and choroid in an albino eye. Note the apical distribution of melanin granules and overall decreased pigmentation in the RPE *(arrow),* rare giant melanosomes *(arrowhead)* in the RPE, and lack of appreciable pigmentation in the choroidal stroma *(asterisk)* (H&E stain). *(Parts A and B courtesy of Robert H. Rosa, Jr, MD; parts C and D courtesy of Tatyana Milman, MD, and Ralph C. Eagle, Jr, MD.)*

Myelinated Nerve Fibers

Generally, myelination of the nerve fibers in the optic pathways terminates at the lamina cribrosa. However, oligodendroglial cells in the NFL can produce a myelin sheath around nerve fibers in the retina (see Fig 26-7 in BCSC Section 6, *Pediatric Ophthalmology and Strabismus*). Though it is usually contiguous with the optic nerve head, myelination may also occur in isolation away from the optic nerve head and, if large, can produce a clinically significant scotoma. Myelinated nerve fibers have been associated with myopia, amblyopia, strabismus, and nystagmus.

Vascular Anomalies

There are numerous congenital anomalies of the retinal vasculature, including cavernous hemangioma, parafoveal telangiectasia, and Coats disease. In Coats disease, exudative retinal detachment occurs as a result of leakage from abnormalities in the peripheral retina, including telangiectatic vessels, microaneurysms, and saccular dilations of retinal vessels (Fig 11-4). Histologically, retinal detachments secondary to Coats disease are characterized by the presence of "foamy" macrophages and cholesterol crystals in the subretinal space.

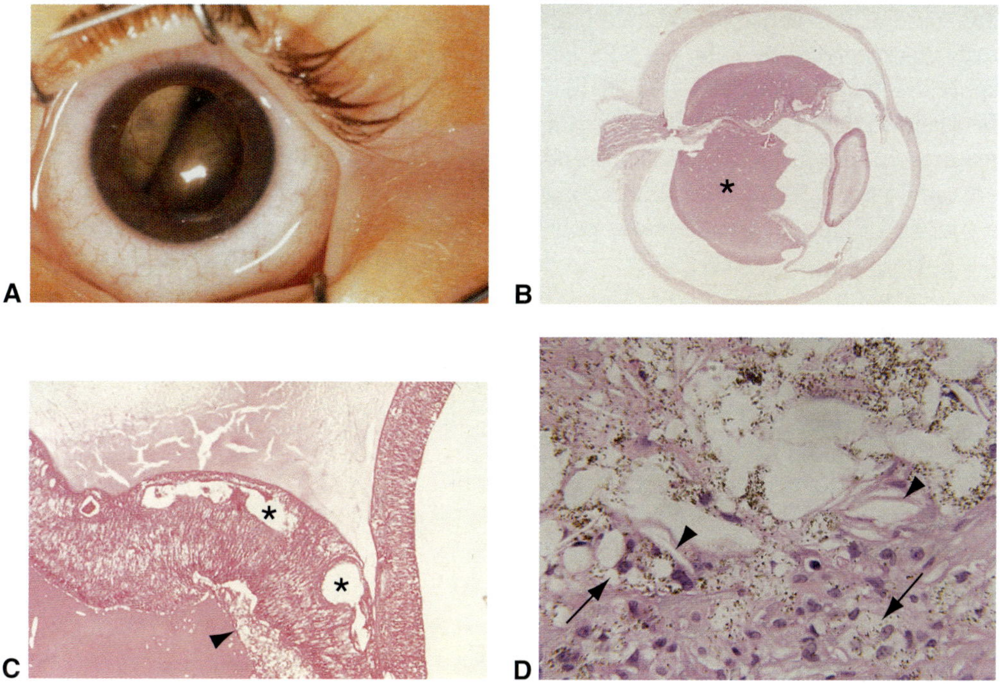

Figure 11-4 Coats disease. **A,** Leukocoria as a result of Coats disease. **B,** Total exudative retinal detachment in Coats disease. Note the dense subretinal proteinaceous fluid *(asterisk)* (H&E stain). **C,** Telangiectatic vessels *(asterisks)* and "foamy" macrophages *(arrowhead)* typical of Coats disease (H&E stain). **D,** High magnification of subretinal exudate showing lipid-laden and pigment-laden macrophages *(arrows)* and cholesterol clefts *(arrowheads)* (H&E stain). *(Parts A–C courtesy of Hans E. Grossniklaus, MD; part D courtesy of George J. Harocopos, MD.)*

Retinal hemangioblastoma is a "vascular" tumor that may be observed in patients with von Hippel–Lindau (VHL) syndrome (see Chapter 18 and BCSC Section 12, *Retina and Vitreous*). Histologically, retinal and optic nerve hemangioblastomas are similar to hemangioblastomas of the central nervous system. These tumors are composed of many abnormal, capillary-like, fenestrated channels surrounded by vacuolated, foamy stromal cells and reactive glial cells (Fig 11-5). Loss of heterozygosity of the *VHL* gene has been clearly identified in the vacuolated stromal cells but not in the vascular endothelial or reactive glial cells of retinal and optic nerve hemangioblastomas. Thus, the vacuolated, foamy stromal cells are the actual tumor cells of retinal hemangioblastomas.

See BCSC Section 12, *Retina and Vitreous,* for further discussion of these vascular anomalies and their clinical features.

Chan CC, Collins AB, Chew EY. Molecular pathology of eyes with von Hippel–Lindau (VHL) disease: a review. *Retina.* 2007;27(1):1–7.

Congenital Hypertrophy of the RPE

Congenital hypertrophy of the RPE (CHRPE), a relatively common congenital lesion, is characterized clinically by a flat, black lesion that can vary in size from a few mm to 10 mm in diameter (see Chapter 17, Fig 17-10). Frequently, central lacunae and a peripheral zone of less dense pigmentation appear within the lesion. This lesion is histologically characterized by enlarged RPE cells with densely packed and larger-than-normal, spherical melanin granules (Fig 11-6). This benign congenital condition can generally be distinguished from choroidal nevi and melanoma on the basis of ophthalmoscopic features. In rare instances, adenoma and adenocarcinoma of the RPE may develop in an area of CHRPE. RPE lesions mimicking CHRPE may be present in Gardner syndrome, a subtype of familial adenomatous polyposis (FAP). Histologic study of RPE changes in Gardner syndrome reveals that they are more consistent with hyperplasia of the RPE than

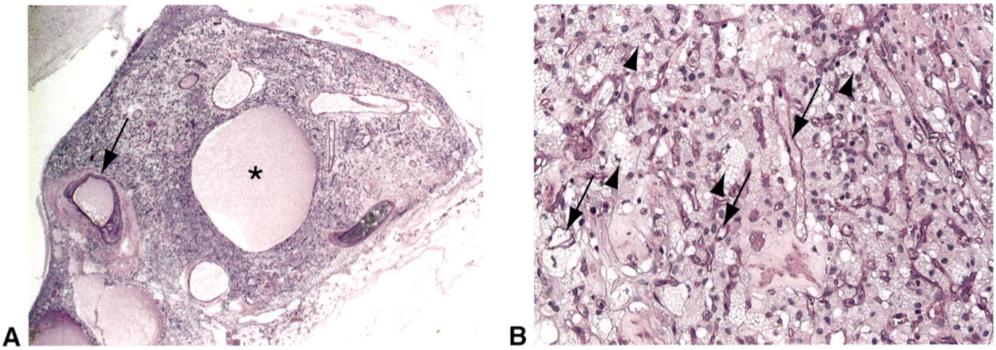

Figure 11-5 Retinal hemangioblastoma in von Hippel–Lindau syndrome. **A,** Low-magnification photomicrograph (PAS stain) showing a retinal tumor with a thick-walled feeder vessel *(arrow)* and a cystic area filled with proteinaceous material *(asterisk).* Note the prominent vascularity and areas of denser cellularity. **B,** Higher magnification (PAS stain) shows the numerous small, capillary-like vascular channels *(arrows).* The vacuolated, foamy stromal cells *(arrowheads)* are tumor cells that express the *VHL* gene mutation. *(Courtesy of Robert H. Rosa, Jr, MD.)*

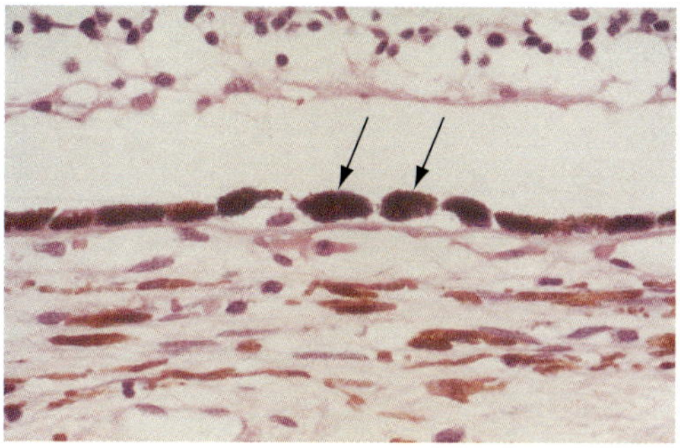

Figure 11-6 In congenital hypertrophy of the RPE (CHRPE), the RPE cells are larger than normal and contain more densely packed melanin granules *(arrows)* (H&E stain). For clinical images of CHRPE, see Chapter 17, Figure 17-10. *(Courtesy of Hans E. Grossniklaus, MD.)*

with hypertrophy. The RPE changes in Gardner syndrome are probably more appropriately termed *hamartomas,* consistent with the loss of regulatory control of cell growth that results in other soft-tissue lesions in this syndrome. A mutation in the *APC* gene, which is linked to Gardner syndrome, gives a person an increased lifetime risk of developing colon polyps, benign tumors, and cancer.

Traboulsi EI. Ocular manifestations of familial adenomatous polyposis (Gardner syndrome). *Ophthalmol Clin North Am.* 2005;18(1):163–166.

Inflammations

Infectious

Viral

Multiple viruses may cause retinal infections, including rubella, measles, human immunodeficiency virus (HIV), herpes simplex virus (HSV), varicella-zoster virus (VZV, or herpes zoster), and cytomegalovirus (CMV). Two of the most frequent clinical presentations of retinal viral infection, acute retinal necrosis (ARN) and CMV retinitis, are discussed here.

Acute retinal necrosis is a rapidly progressive, necrotizing retinitis caused by infection with HSV types 1 and 2, VZV, and, in rare instances, CMV. ARN can occur in healthy or immunocompromised individuals. The histologic findings include inflammation in the vitreous and anterior chamber, with a prominent obliterative retinal vasculitis and retinal necrosis (Fig 11-7). Electron microscopy has demonstrated viral inclusions in retinal cells. Polymerase chain reaction (PCR) analysis of aqueous or vitreous biopsy specimens can be used to rapidly demonstrate the viral cause of ARN, reducing the need for other diagnostic techniques such as viral culture, intraocular antibody analysis, or immunohistochemistry.

CMV retinitis is an opportunistic infection that occurs in immunosuppressed patients (Fig 11-8). This infection is histologically characterized by retinal necrosis, which leads to a thin fibroglial scar with healing. Acute lesions show large neurons (20–30 μm) that contain large eosinophilic intranuclear or intracytoplasmic inclusion bodies. At the cellular level, CMV may infect vascular endothelial cells, retinal neurons, RPE, and macrophages.

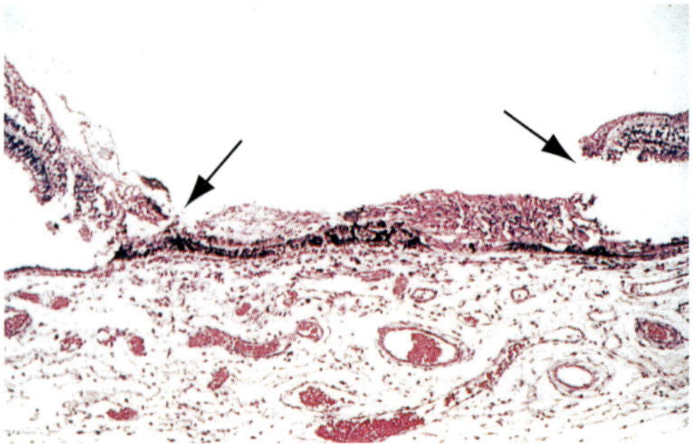

Figure 11-7 Acute retinal necrosis (ARN) is characterized by full-thickness necrosis of the retina *(between arrows)* (H&E stain). *(Courtesy of Hans E. Grossniklaus, MD.)*

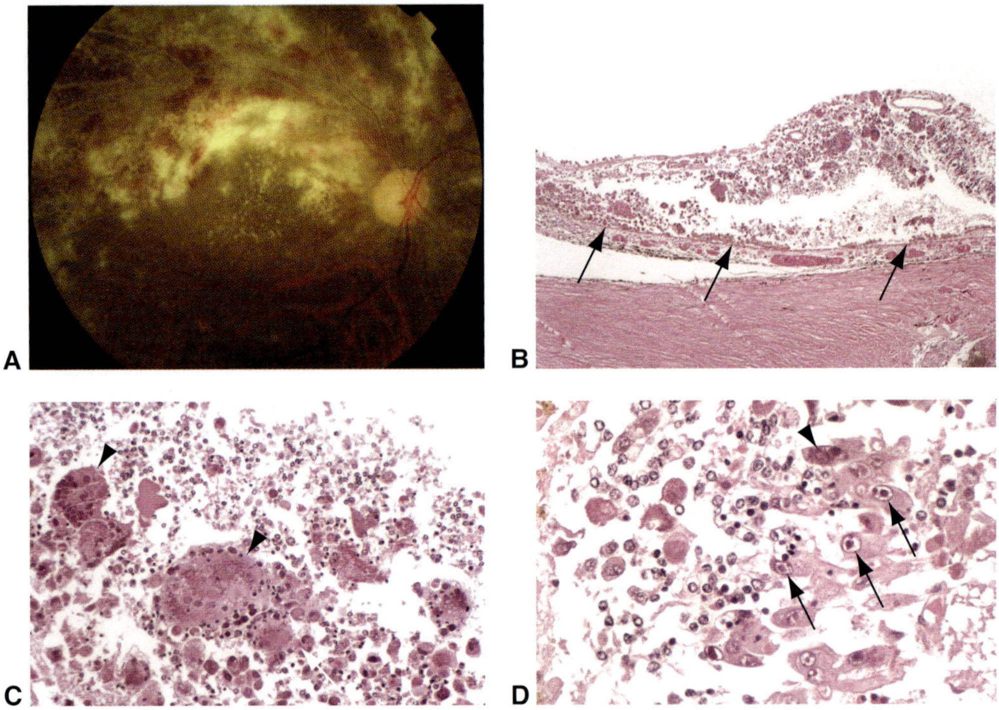

Figure 11-8 Cytomegalovirus (CMV) retinitis. **A,** Retinal hemorrhages and areas of opaque retina are present. Note the vascular sheathing in the superotemporal arcade and hard exudates in the macular region. **B,** Histologically, full-thickness retinal necrosis is present. Note loss of the normal lamellar architecture of the retina, including disruption of the RPE *(arrows)* (H&E stain). **C,** Large syncytial cells *(arrowheads)* are present in areas of necrosis, characteristic of CMV retinitis (H&E stain). **D,** Intranuclear "owl's eye" inclusions *(arrows)* and intracytoplasmic inclusions *(arrowhead)* are present in CMV-infected cells (H&E stain). *(Courtesy of Robert H. Rosa, Jr, MD.)*

Bacterial

See the discussion of endophthalmitis in Chapter 10 and in BCSC Section 9, *Intraocular Inflammation and Uveitis.*

Fungal

Fungal infections of the retina are uncommon, occurring most often in immunosuppressed patients and in patients with fungemia (eg, from parenteral nutrition or intravenous drug use). These infections usually begin as single or multiple foci of choroidal and retinal infection (Fig 11-9). The most common causative fungi are *Candida* species, particularly *C. albicans*. Less common agents include *Aspergillus* species and *Cryptococcus neoformans*.

Histologically, fungal infections are characterized by necrotizing granulomatous inflammation. A central zone of necrosis is typically surrounded by granulomatous inflammation, and an outer layer of lymphocytes is common. With treatment, the lesions heal with a fibrous scar. Evaluation of histologic material may demonstrate a causative agent; however, culture and/or molecular studies are required for definitive identification of the organism.

Protozoal

Toxoplasmosis Ocular toxoplasmosis, which is the most common infectious retinitis, may occur because of reactivation of congenitally acquired disease or as the result of an acquired *Toxoplasma* infection in healthy or immunocompromised individuals. In patients with reactivated disease, ocular toxoplasmosis typically presents as a posterior uveitis or panuveitis with marked vitritis and focal retinochoroiditis adjacent to a pigmented chorioretinal scar. The absence of prior chorioretinal scarring suggests newly acquired disease. Microscopic examination of active toxoplasmic retinitis reveals necrosis of the retina, a prominent infiltrate of neutrophils and lymphocytes, and *Toxoplasma* organisms in the form of tissue cysts and tachyzoites (Fig 11-10). There is generally a prominent lymphocytic infiltrate of the vitreous and the anterior segment and, not uncommonly,

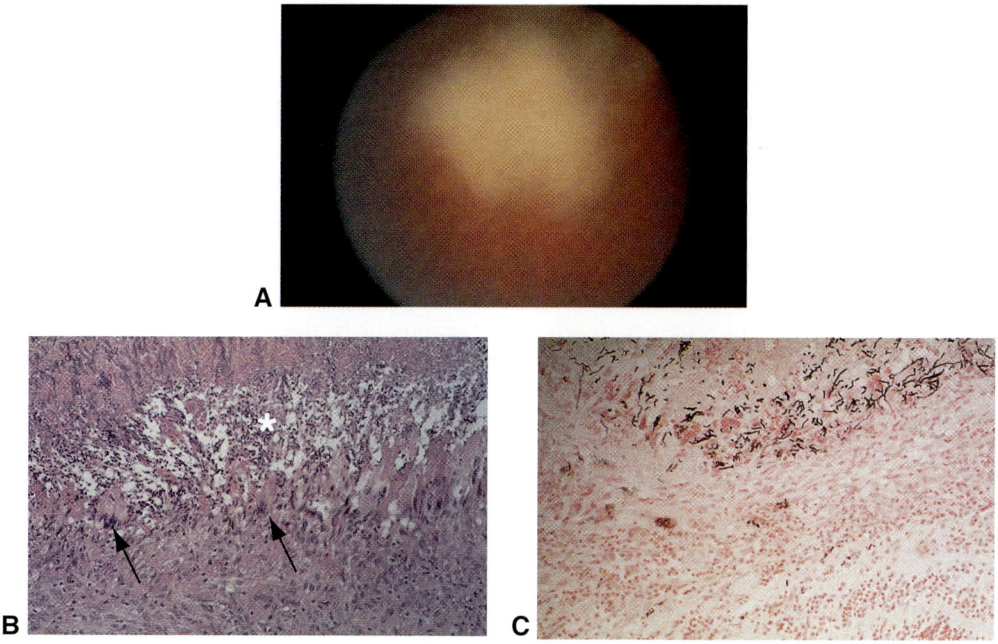

Figure 11-9 Fungal chorioretinitis. **A,** Vitreous, retinal, and choroidal infiltrate in a patient with fungal chorioretinitis. **B,** Granulomatous infiltration surrounding central area of necrosis *(asterisk)*. Note multinucleated giant cells *(arrows)* (H&E stain). **C,** Grocott-Gomori methenamine–silver nitrate stain of section parallel to that shown in part **B** demonstrates numerous fungal hyphae (black staining). *(Courtesy of David J. Wilson, MD.)*

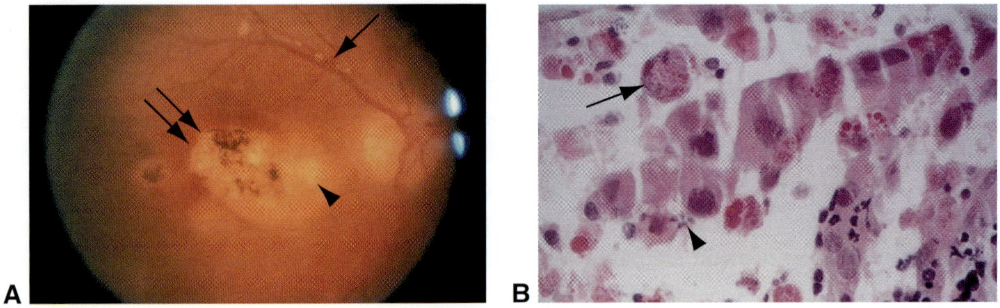

Figure 11-10 Toxoplasmic chorioretinitis. **A,** Chorioretinal scars with pigmentation *(double arrow)* typical of prior infection with toxoplasmosis. Active retinitis *(arrowhead)* and perivascular sheathing *(arrow)* are present. **B,** Cysts *(arrow)* and released organisms (tachyzoites, *arrowhead*) in active toxoplasmosis (H&E stain). *(Courtesy of Hans E. Grossniklaus, MD.)*

granulomatous inflammation in the inner choroid. Healing brings resolution of the inflammatory cell infiltrate with encystment of the organisms in the retina adjacent to the chorioretinal scar.

Noninfectious

Noninfectious (autoimmune) inflammatory conditions involving the retina are discussed in BCSC Section 9, *Intraocular Inflammation and Uveitis,* and Section 12, *Retina and Vitreous.*

Degenerations

Typical and Reticular Peripheral Cystoid Degeneration and Retinoschisis

In *typical peripheral cystoid degeneration (TPCD),* which is a universal finding in the eyes of individuals older than 20 years, cystic spaces develop in the outer plexiform layer of the retina. In *reticular peripheral cystoid degeneration (RPCD),* which is less common, the cystic spaces develop in the NFL, posterior to areas of TPCD (Fig 11-11). Coalescence of the cystic spaces of TPCD forms *typical degenerative retinoschisis,* which is usually inferotemporal in location. In *reticular degenerative retinoschisis,* the splitting of retinal layers occurs in the NFL.

Lattice Degeneration

Lattice degeneration (Fig 11-12), which may be a familial condition, is found in up to 10% of the general population, but retinal detachment develops in only a small number of affected individuals. In contrast, lattice degeneration is seen in up to 40% of all rhegmatogenous detachments. The most important histologic features of lattice degeneration include

- discontinuity of the internal limiting membrane (ILM) of the retina
- an overlying pocket of liquefied vitreous
- focal sclerosis of retinal vessels, which remain physiologically patent
- condensation and adherence of vitreous at the margins of the lesion
- variable degrees of atrophy of the inner layers of the retina

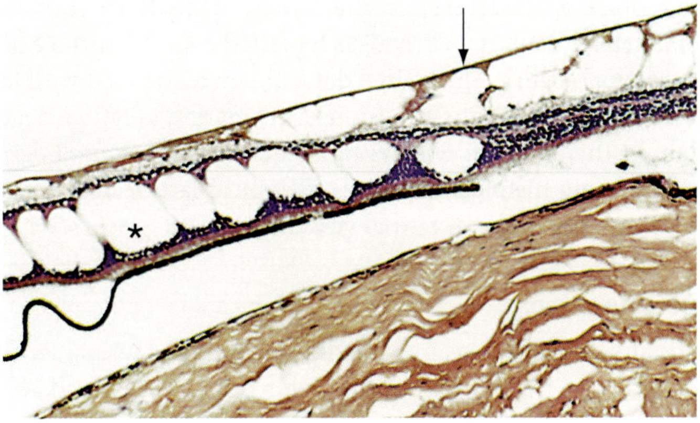

Figure 11-11 Typical peripheral cystoid degeneration consists of cystoid spaces in the outer plexiform layer *(asterisk)* on the lower left (anterior retina). In the upper right (posterior retina), reticular peripheral cystoid degeneration *(arrow)* is present (H&E stain).

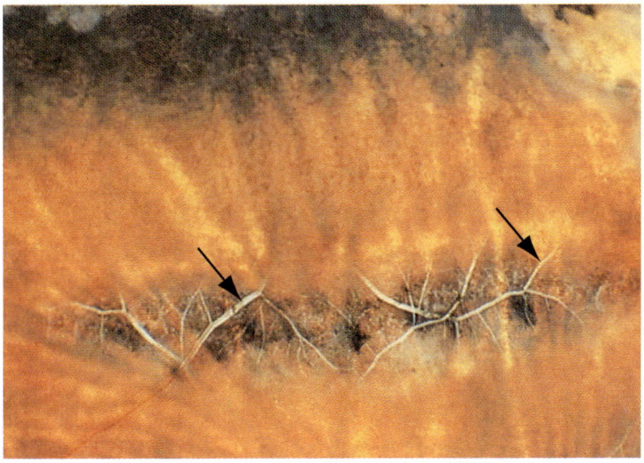

A

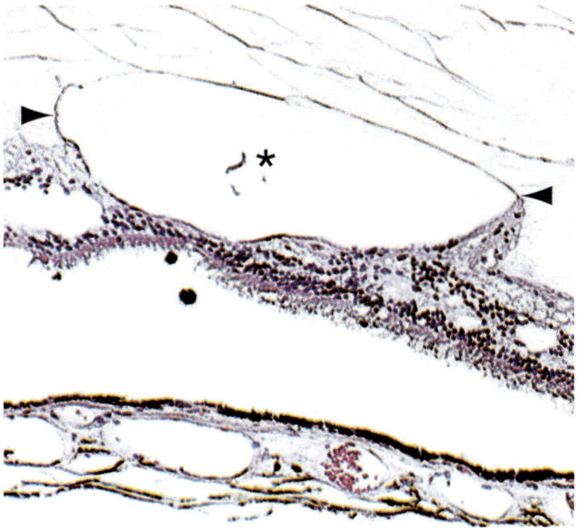

B

Figure 11-12 Retinal lattice degeneration. **A,** Lattice degeneration may present as prominent sclerotic vessels *(arrows)* in a wicker or lattice pattern. **B,** The vitreous directly over lattice degeneration is liquefied *(asterisk),* but formed vitreous remains adherent at the margins *(arrowheads)* of the degenerated area. The internal limiting membrane is discontinuous, and the inner retinal layers are atrophic (H&E stain).

Although atrophic holes often develop in the center of the lattice lesion, they are rarely the cause of retinal detachment; the vitreous is liquefied over the surface of the lattice, and thus no vitreous traction occurs. The retinal detachment associated with lattice degeneration is generally the result of vitreous adhesion at the margin of lattice degeneration, leading to retinal tears in this location with vitreous detachment. *Radial perivascular lattice degeneration* has the same histologic features as typical lattice degeneration but occurs more posteriorly along the course of retinal vessels.

Paving-Stone Degeneration

In contrast to retinal vascular occlusion, which leads to inner retinal ischemia, occlusion of the choriocapillaris can lead to loss of the outer retinal layers and RPE. This type of atrophy, called *paving-stone* or *cobblestone degeneration,* is very common in the retinal periphery. The well-demarcated, flat, pale lesions seen clinically correspond to circumscribed areas of outer retinal and RPE atrophy and loss of the choriocapillaris, with adherence of the inner nuclear layer to Bruch membrane (Fig 11-13). These histologic findings are similar to those found in geographic atrophy in age-related macular degeneration.

Ischemia

Retinal ischemia can be caused by many conditions, including diabetes mellitus, retinal artery and vein occlusions, radiation retinopathy, retinopathy of prematurity, sickle cell retinopathy, vasculitis, and carotid occlusive disease. The specific aspects of some of these diseases are discussed later in this chapter. However, certain histologic findings are common to all the disorders that result in retinal ischemia. The retinal changes that result from ischemia can be divided into cellular responses and vascular responses.

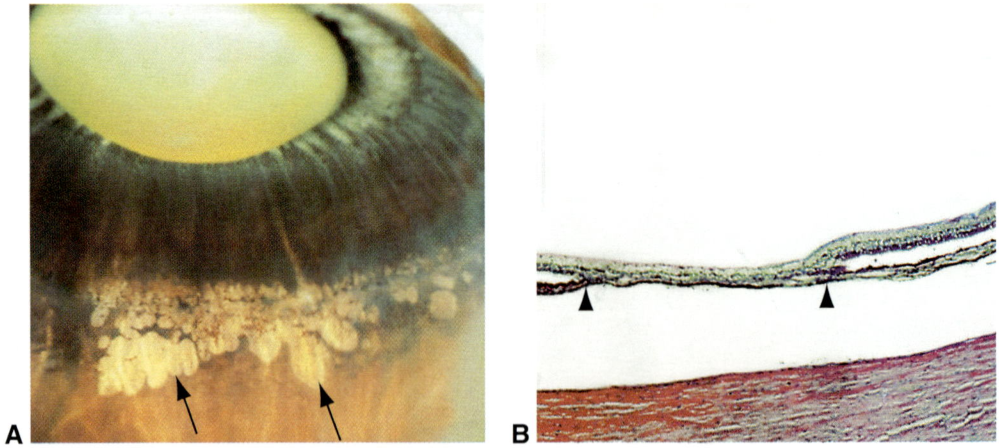

Figure 11-13 Paving-stone degeneration. **A,** Paving-stone degeneration appears as areas of depigmentation *(arrows)* in the periphery of the retina near the ora serrata. **B,** Histologically, paving-stone degeneration consists of atrophy of the outer retinal layers and adhesion of the remaining inner retinal elements to Bruch membrane. A sharp boundary *(arrowheads)* exists between normal and atrophic retina, corresponding to the clinical appearance of paving-stone degeneration.

Retinal changes

Cellular responses The neurons in the retina are highly active metabolically, requiring large amounts of oxygen for production of adenosine triphosphate (ATP) (see also BCSC Section 2, *Fundamentals and Principles of Ophthalmology,* Part IV, Biochemistry and Metabolism). This makes them highly sensitive to interruption of their blood supply. With prolonged oxygen deprivation (>90 minutes in experimental studies), the neuronal cell nuclei become pyknotic (ie, hyperchromatic and shrunken); they are subsequently phagocytosed, and they disappear. The extent and the location of atrophic retina resulting from ischemia depend on the size of the occluded vessel and on whether it is a retinal or a choroidal blood vessel. As described earlier, the retinal circulation supplies the inner retina, and the choroidal circulation supplies the outer retina and RPE. Infarctions of the retinal circulation lead to *inner ischemic retinal atrophy* (Fig 11-14), and infarctions of the choroidal circulation lead to *outer ischemic retinal atrophy* (Fig 11-15).

The neuronal cells of the retina have no capacity for regeneration after ischemic damage. Following ischemic damage to the nerve fibers of the ganglion cells, *cytoid bodies*

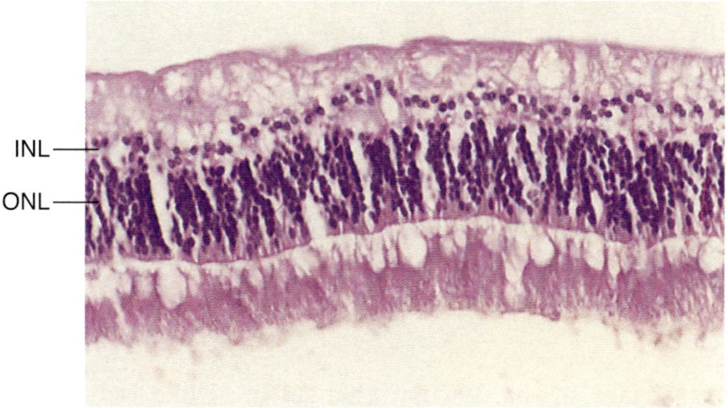

Figure 11-14 Inner ischemic retinal atrophy. The photoreceptor nuclei (outer nuclear layer, ONL) and the outer portion of the inner nuclear layer (INL) are identifiable. The inner portion of the inner nuclear layer is absent. There are no ganglion cells, and the NFL is absent (H&E stain). This pattern of ischemia corresponds to the supply of the retinal arteriolar circulation and may be observed after healing from arterial and venular occlusions.

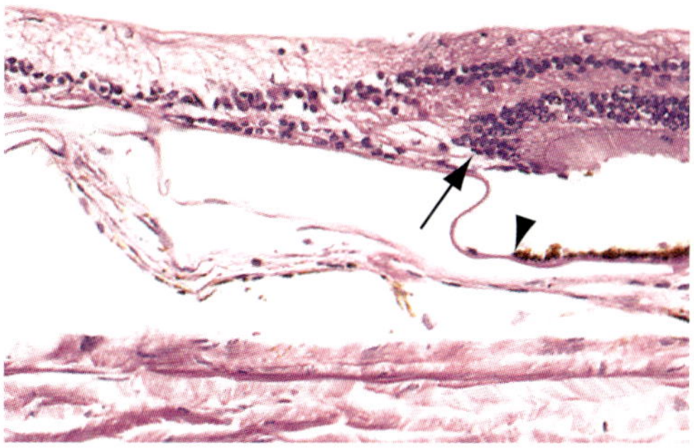

Figure 11-15 Outer ischemic retinal atrophy. Begin at the right edge of the photograph and trace the ganglion cell and the inner nuclear layer toward the left. In this case, there is loss of the nuclei of the photoreceptor layer (outer nuclear layer, *arrow*), the photoreceptor inner and outer segments, and the RPE *(arrowhead)* (H&E stain). This is the pattern of outer retinal atrophy, secondary to interruption in the choroidal vascular blood supply. Compare with Figure 11-14.

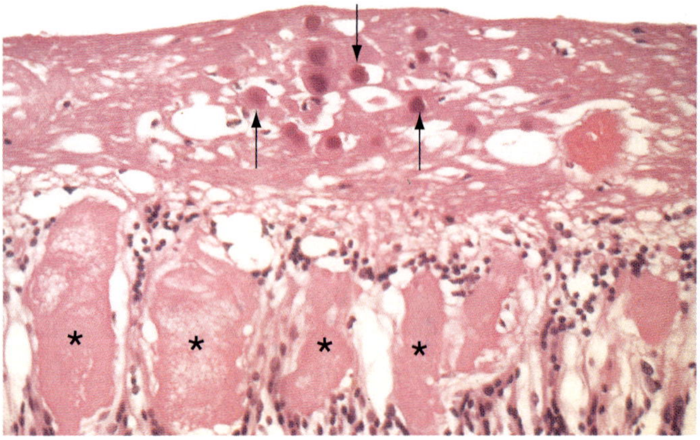

Figure 11-16 Cytoid bodies *(arrows)* within the NFL. Cystoid spaces *(asterisks)* are filled with proteinaceous fluid (H&E stain). *(Courtesy of W. Richard Green, MD.)*

(swollen axons) become apparent histologically (Fig 11-16). These are localized accumulations of axoplasmic material that are present in ischemic infarcts of the NFL. *Cotton-wool spots* are the clinical correlate of ischemic infarcts of the NFL; they resolve over 4–12 weeks, leaving an area of inner ischemic retinal atrophy.

Glial cells, like neurons, degenerate in areas of infarction. Glial cells may proliferate adjacent to local areas of infarction or in areas of ischemia without infarction, resulting in a glial scar.

Microglial cells are actually tissue macrophages rather than true glial cells. These cells are involved in the phagocytosis of necrotic cells, as well as of extracellular material, such as lipid or blood, that accumulates in areas of ischemia. Microglial cells are fairly resistant to ischemia.

Vascular responses Many of the vascular changes in retinal ischemia are mediated by vascular endothelial growth factor (VEGF), which is a potent stimulus of vascular permeability and angiogenesis.

Edema, one of the earliest manifestations of retinal ischemia, is a result of transudation across the inner blood–retina barrier. Fluid and serum components accumulate in the extracellular space, and the fluid pockets are delimited by the surrounding neurons and glial cells, resulting in CME (Fig 11-17; see also Fig 5-3, Fig 6-5C, and Fig 6-12A in BCSC Section 12, *Retina and Vitreous*). As previously mentioned, exudate accumulation in the outer plexiform layer of the macula (Henle layer) produces a star figure because of the orientation of the nerve fibers in this layer (Fig 11-18). Histologically, retinal exudates appear as eosinophilic, sharply circumscribed spaces within the retina (Fig 11-19).

Intravitreally administered triamcinolone acetonide and biologic agents that inhibit VEGF (eg, bevacizumab, ranibizumab, and aflibercept) are employed in the treatment of various retinal diseases associated with macular edema and choroidal neovascularization. Improvement in vision, which is mostly secondary to a decrease in macular edema and subretinal fluid, has been demonstrated in studies in which these treatments were

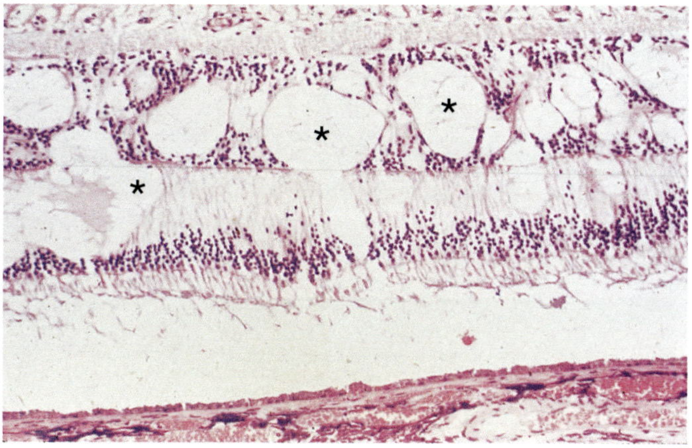

Figure 11-17 Cystoid macular edema. Cystoid spaces in inner nuclear and outer plexiform layers *(asterisks)* (H&E stain). *(Courtesy of W. Richard Green, MD.)*

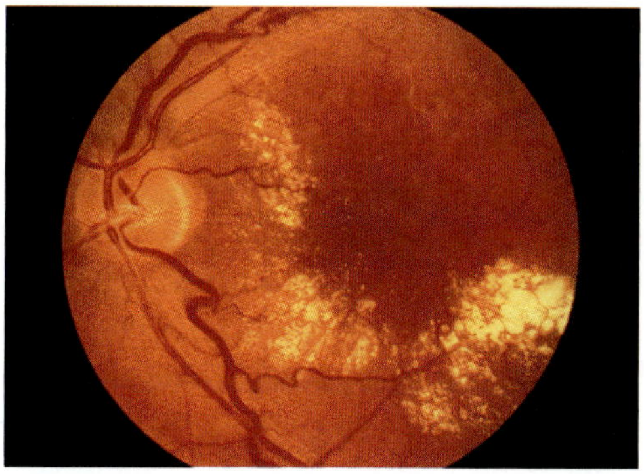

Figure 11-18 Intraretinal lipid deposits, or hard exudates. *(Courtesy of David J. Wilson, MD.)*

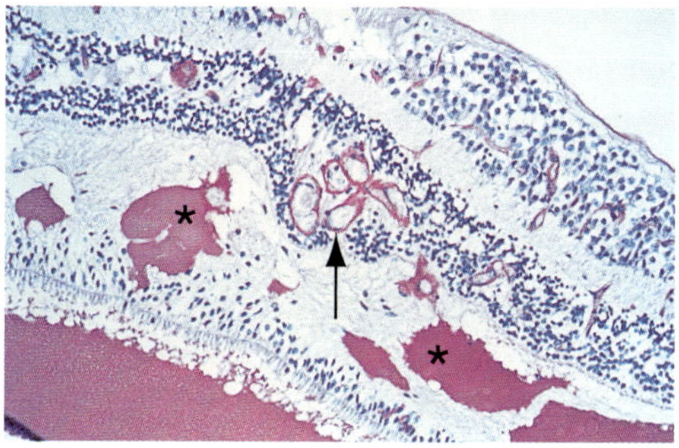

Figure 11-19 PAS stain showing intraretinal exudates *(asterisks)* surrounding intraretinal microvascular abnormalities *(arrow)*. *(Courtesy of W. Richard Green, MD.)*

used for diabetic macular edema, retinal vein occlusion, and choroidal neovascularization (Fig 11-20).

Retinal hemorrhages may also develop as a result of ischemic damage to the inner blood–retina barrier. As with edema and exudates, the shape of the hemorrhage conforms to the surrounding retinal tissue. Consequently, hemorrhages in the NFL are flame-shaped, whereas those in the nuclear or inner plexiform layers are circular, or "dot and blot"

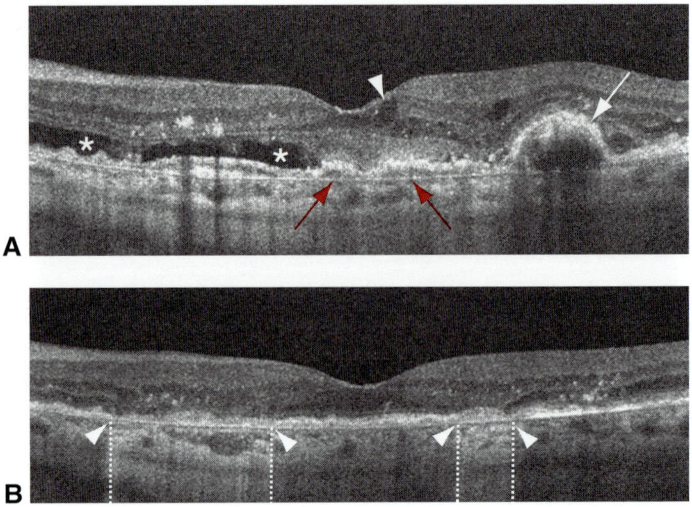

Figure 11-20 Cystoid macular edema and anti-VEGF therapy. **A,** SD-OCT shows mild cystoid macular edema *(arrowhead),* subretinal fluid *(asterisks),* and irregular elevation and detachment of the RPE *(white arrow)* secondary to exudative age-related macular degeneration. Note the outer aspect of Bruch membrane *(red arrows).* **B,** SD-OCT after anti–vascular endothelial growth factor therapy shows resolution of the cystoid macular edema and detachment of the RPE. Focal areas of geographic atrophy of the RPE with attenuation of the photoreceptor cell layer are more apparent *(between arrowheads).* Note the hyperreflectivity *(between dashed lines)* in the choroid corresponding to the areas of geographic atrophy. *(Courtesy of Robert H. Rosa, Jr, MD.)*

(Fig 11-21). Subhyaloid hemorrhages have a boat-shaped configuration. White-centered hemorrhages *(Roth spots)* may be present in a number of conditions. The white centers of these hemorrhages can have a number of causes, including aggregates of white blood cells, platelets and fibrin, microorganisms, or neoplastic cells, or they may be due to retinal light reflexes.

Chronic retinal ischemia leads to architectural changes in the retinal vessels. The capillary bed becomes acellular in an area of vascular occlusion. Adjacent to acellular areas, dilated irregular vascular channels known as *intraretinal microvascular abnormalities (IRMA)* (Fig 11-22; see also Fig 11-19) and microaneurysms often appear (Fig 11-23). *Microaneurysms* are fusiform or saccular outpouchings of the retinal capillaries best seen clinically with fluorescein angiography and histologically with trypsin digest preparations stained with periodic acid–Schiff (PAS) reagent (see Fig 11-23). The density of the endothelial cells that line the microaneurysms and IRMA is frequently variable. Microaneurysms evolve from being thin-walled and hypercellular to hyalinized and hypocellular.

In some retinal ischemia cases, neovascularization of the retina and the vitreous may occur, most commonly in diabetes mellitus and central retinal vein occlusion. Retinal neovascularization arises from existing retinal blood vessels and penetrates the ILM, extending into the vitreous (Fig 11-24). Hemorrhage may develop from retinal neovascularization as the vitreous exerts traction on the fragile new vessels.

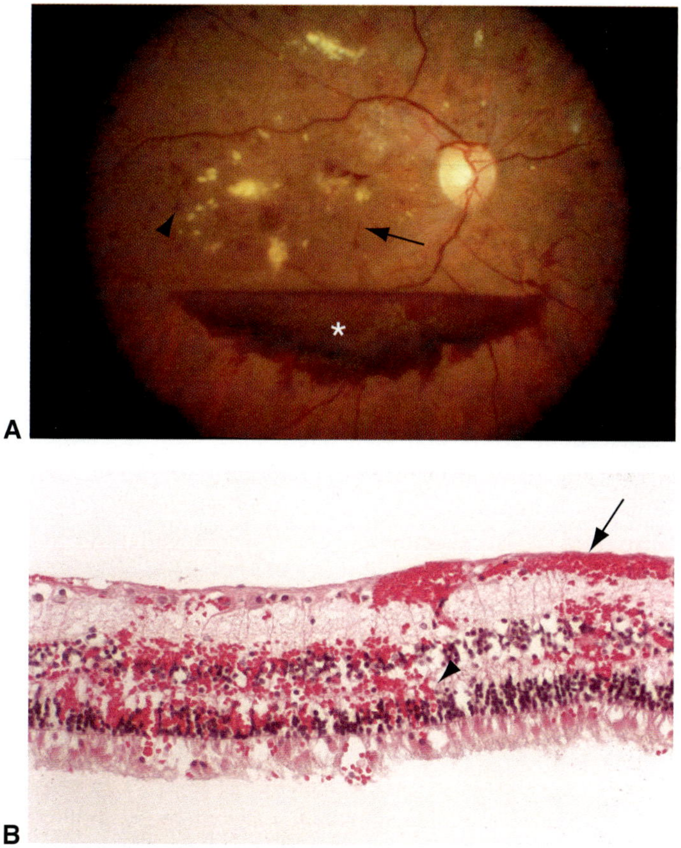

Figure 11-21 Intraretinal hemorrhage. **A,** Fundus photograph showing dot-blot *(arrowhead),* flame-shaped *(arrow),* and boat-shaped *(asterisk)* hemorrhages in diabetic retinopathy. **B,** Histologically, the dot-blot hemorrhage corresponds to blood in the middle layers (inner nuclear and outer plexiform layers) of the retina *(arrowhead).* The flame-shaped hemorrhage corresponds to blood in the NFL *(arrow),* and the boat-shaped hemorrhage corresponds to subhyaloid blood (H&E stain). *(Courtesy of Robert H. Rosa, Jr, MD.)*

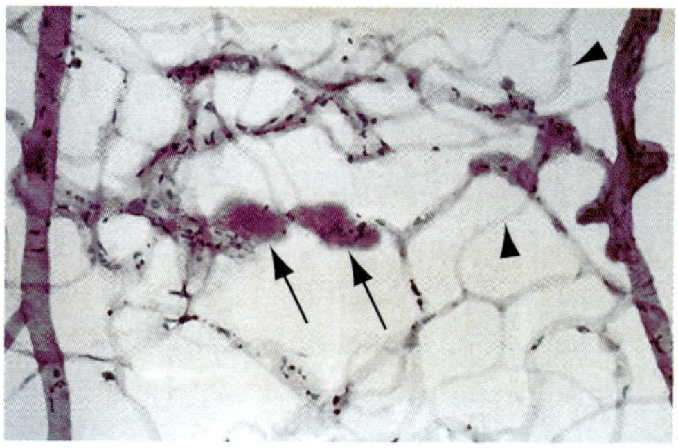

Figure 11-22 Trypsin digest preparation shows acellular capillaries *(arrowheads)* adjacent to intraretinal microvascular abnormalities (IRMA, *arrows*) (PAS stain). *(Courtesy of W. Richard Green, MD.)*

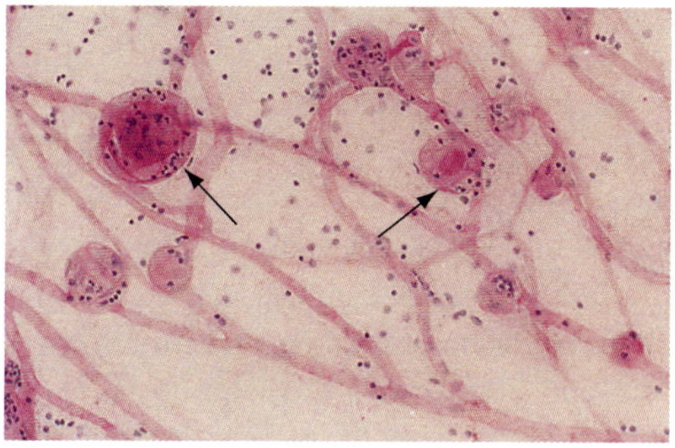

Figure 11-23 Retinal trypsin digest preparation (PAS stain) showing diabetic microaneurysms *(arrows).*

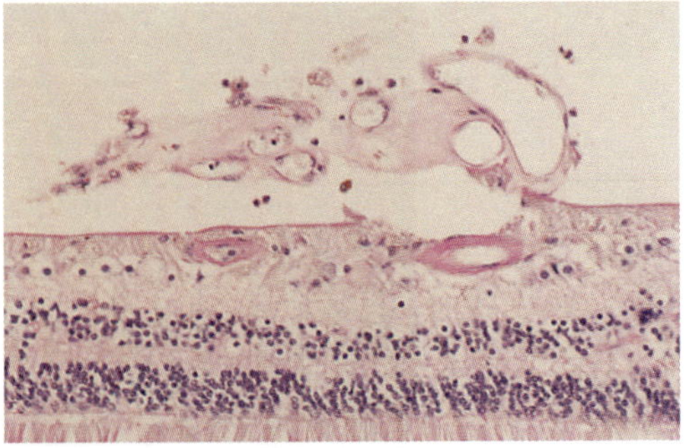

Figure 11-24 Retinal neovascularization. New blood vessels have broken through the ILM (PAS stain).

Specific ischemic retinal disorders

Central and branch retinal artery and vein occlusions *Central retinal artery occlusion (CRAO)* results from localized arteriosclerotic changes, an embolic event, and, in rare instances, vasculitis (as in temporal arteritis). As the retina becomes ischemic, it swells and loses its transparency. This swelling is best seen clinically and histologically in the posterior pole, where the NFL and the ganglion cell layer are thickest (Fig 11-25). Because the ganglion cell layer and the NFL are thickest in the macula and absent in the fovea, the normal color of the choroid shows through in the fovea and produces a cherry-red spot, ophthalmoscopically suggesting CRAO. The retinal swelling eventually clears, leaving the classic histologic picture of inner ischemic retinal atrophy (see Fig 11-14). Scarring and neovascularization following CRAO are rare.

Branch retinal artery occlusion (BRAO) is usually the result of an embolus that lodges at the bifurcation of a retinal arteriole. *Hollenhorst plaques,* which are cholesterol emboli within retinal arterioles, seldom occlude the vessel. Emboli may be the first or most important clue to a significant systemic disorder such as carotid vascular disease (Hollenhorst plaques), cardiac valvular disease (calcific emboli), or thromboembolism (platelet-fibrin emboli).

The histology of the acute phase of BRAO is characterized by swelling of the inner retinal layers with early cell death. As the edema resolves, a classic picture emerges of inner ischemic atrophy in the distribution of the retina supplied by the occluded arteriole, with loss of cells in the NFL, ganglion cell layer, inner plexiform layer, and inner nuclear layer (see Fig 11-14). Arteriolar occlusions result in infarcts with complete postnecrotic atrophy of the affected layers.

Central retinal vein occlusion (CRVO) occurs at the lamina cribrosa level. The pathophysiology of CRVO is the same as that of hemiretinal vein occlusion, but different from that of branch retinal vein occlusion (see the following discussion). CRVOs develop as a result of structural changes in the central retinal artery and the lamina cribrosa that lead to compression of the central retinal vein. This compression creates turbulent flow in the vein and predisposes to thrombosis. These structural changes occur in arteriosclerosis, hypertension, diabetes mellitus, and glaucoma.

CRVO is recognized clinically by the presence of retinal hemorrhages in all 4 quadrants. Usually, prominent edema of the optic nerve head is observed, along with dilation and tortuosity of the retinal veins, variable numbers of cotton-wool spots, and macular edema. CRVO occurs in 2 forms: a milder, perfused type and a more severe, nonperfused (ischemic) type.

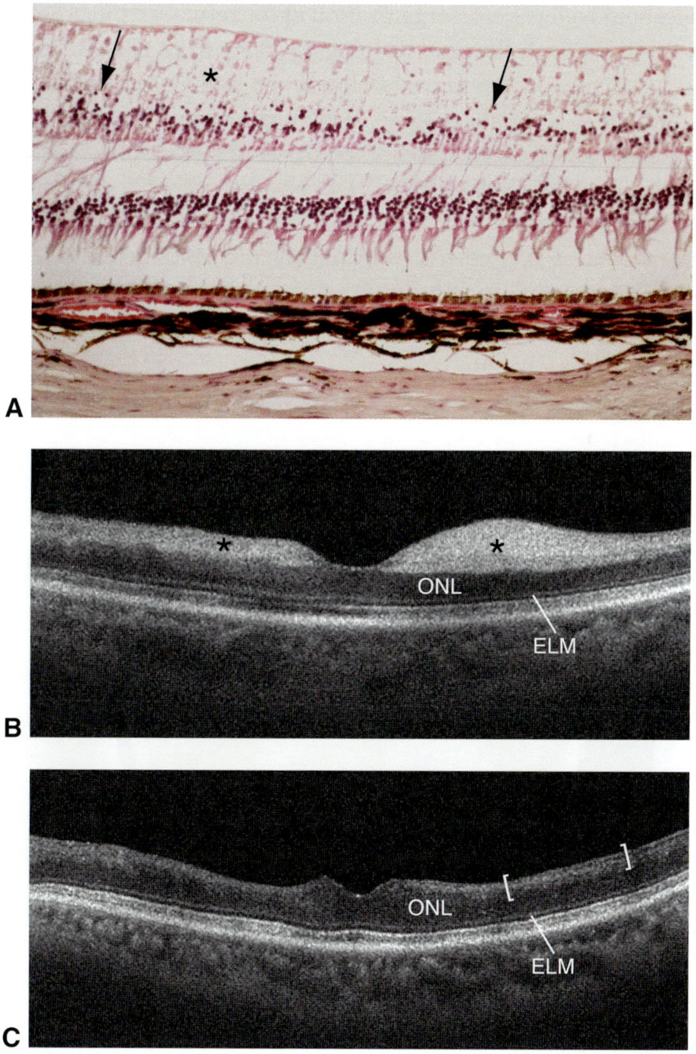

Figure 11-25 Central retinal artery occlusion (CRAO). **A,** Histologically, necrosis occurs in the inner retina *(asterisk)* corresponding to the retinal whitening observed on ophthalmoscopic examination. Note the pyknotic nuclei *(arrows)* in the inner aspect of the inner nuclear layer (H&E stain). **B,** SD-OCT reveals increased reflectivity in the area of retinal necrosis *(asterisks).* **C,** SD-OCT in remote CRAO in the same patient shown in **B** reveals attenuation of the inner retina *(in brackets)* with loss of the normal lamellar architecture up to the outer plexiform layer–outer nuclear layer junction. ELM = external limiting membrane, ONL = outer nuclear layer. *(Courtesy of Robert H. Rosa, Jr, MD.)*

The Central Vein Occlusion Study (CVOS) defined *nonperfused CRVO* as a CRVO in which more than 10 disc areas showed nonperfusion on fluorescein angiography. Nonperfused CRVOs typically have extensive retinal edema and hemorrhage, marked venular dilation, and numerous cotton-wool spots on ophthalmoscopic examination.

Acute ischemic CRVO is characterized histologically by marked retinal edema, focal retinal necrosis, and extensive intraretinal hemorrhage. With long-standing CRVO, glial cells respond to the insult by replication and intracellular deposition of filaments *(gliosis).*

The hemorrhage, hemosiderosis, disorganization of the retinal architecture, and gliosis seen in vein occlusions distinguish the final histologic picture from CRAO (Fig 11-26). Following CRVO, numerous microaneurysms develop in the retinal capillaries, and acellular capillary beds are present to a variable degree. With time, dilated collateral vessels develop at the optic nerve head. Neovascularization of the iris is common following ischemic CRVO.

In *branch retinal vein occlusion (BRVO),* occlusion of a tributary retinal vein occurs at the site of an arteriovenous crossing. At the crossing of a branch retinal artery and vein, the 2 vessels share a common adventitial sheath. With arteriosclerotic changes in the arteriole, the retinal venule may become compressed, leading to turbulent flow, which predisposes the vessel to thrombosis. This condition is more common in patients with arteriosclerosis and hypertension.

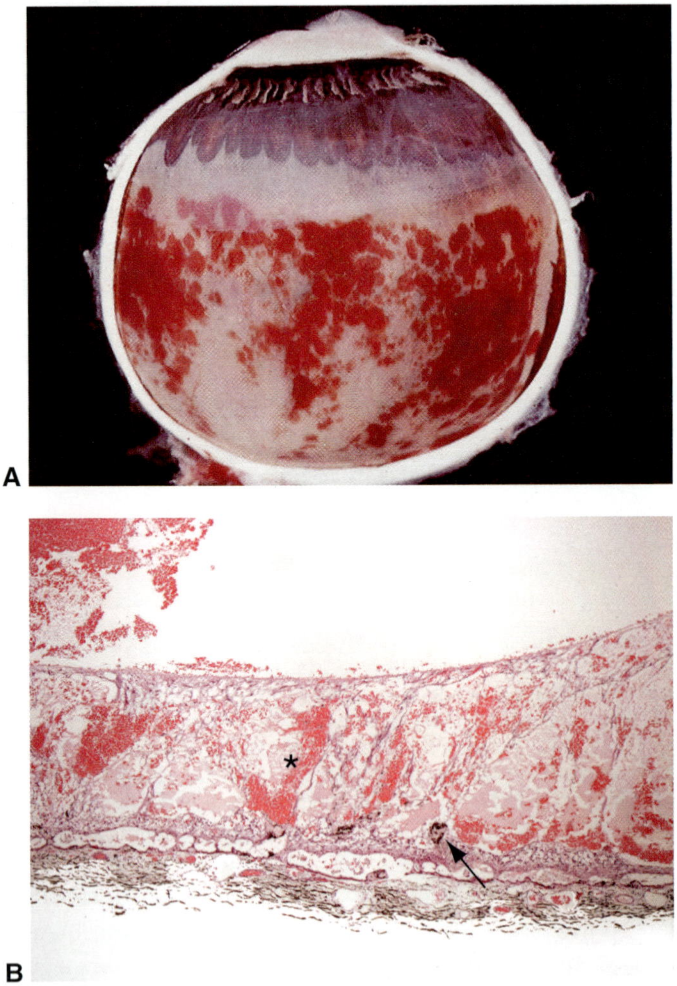

Figure 11-26 Central retinal vein occlusion (CRVO). **A,** Diffuse retinal hemorrhage following CRVO. The damaged retina will be replaced by gliosis. **B,** Histology of long-standing CRVO shows loss of the normal lamellar architecture of the retina, marked edema with cystic spaces *(asterisk)* containing blood and proteinaceous exudate, vitreous hemorrhage, and nodular hyperplasia of the RPE *(arrow)* (H&E stain). *(Part B courtesy of Robert H. Rosa, Jr, MD.)*

BRVO leads to retinal hemorrhages and cotton-wool spots. Because BRVO does not always result in total inner retinal ischemia and death of all tissue, neovascularization is unlikely unless the ischemia is extensive (>5 disc diameters). Findings in eyes with permanent vision loss from BRVO include CME, retinal nonperfusion, macular edema with hard lipid exudates, late pigmentary changes in the macula, subretinal fibrosis, and epiretinal membrane formation.

The histologic picture of BRVO resembles that of CRVO but is localized to the area of the retina in the distribution of the occluded vein. Inner ischemic retinal atrophy is a characteristic late histologic finding in both retinal arterial and venous occlusions (see Fig 11-14). Numerous microaneurysms and dilated collateral vessels may be present. Acellular retinal capillaries are present to a variable degree, correlating with retinal capillary nonperfusion on fluorescein angiography.

Baseline and early natural history report. The Central Vein Occlusion Study. *Arch Ophthalmol.* 1993;111(8):1087–1095.

Natural history and clinical management of central retinal vein occlusion. The Central Vein Occlusion Study Group. *Arch Ophthalmol.* 1997;115(4):486–491.

Diabetic retinopathy

Diabetic retinopathy is 1 of the 4 most frequent causes of new blindness in the United States and is the leading cause among 20- to 60-year-olds. Early in the course of diabetic retinopathy, certain physiologic abnormalities occur:

- impaired autoregulation of the retinal vasculature
- alterations in retinal blood flow
- breakdown of the blood–retina barrier

Histologically, the primary changes occur in the retinal microcirculation. These changes include

- thickening of the retinal capillary basement membrane
- selective loss of pericytes compared with retinal capillary endothelial cells
- microaneurysm formation (see Fig 11-23)
- retinal capillary closure (see Fig 11-22) (histologically recognized as acellular capillary beds)

Dilated intraretinal telangiectatic vessels, or IRMA, may develop, as shown in Figures 11-19 and 11-22, and neovascularization may follow (see Fig 11-24). Intraretinal edema, hemorrhages, exudates, and microinfarcts of the NFL may develop secondary to the primary retinal vascular changes. Acutely, microinfarcts of the NFL (see Fig 11-16) manifest as cotton-wool spots. Subsequently, focal inner ischemic atrophy appears (see Fig 11-14).

Other histologic changes in diabetes mellitus In diabetes mellitus, the corneal epithelial basement membrane thickens. This change is associated with inadequate adherence of the epithelium to the underlying Bowman layer, predisposing diabetic patients to corneal abrasions and poor corneal epithelial healing. Lacy vacuolation of the iris pigment epithelium (Fig 11-27) occurs in association with hyperglycemia; histologically, the intraepithelial vacuoles contain glycogen, which is PAS-positive and diastase-sensitive. Thickening of the pigmented ciliary epithelial basement membrane (see Fig 11-27) is almost universally present in diabetic eyes. The incidence of cataract formation is increased.

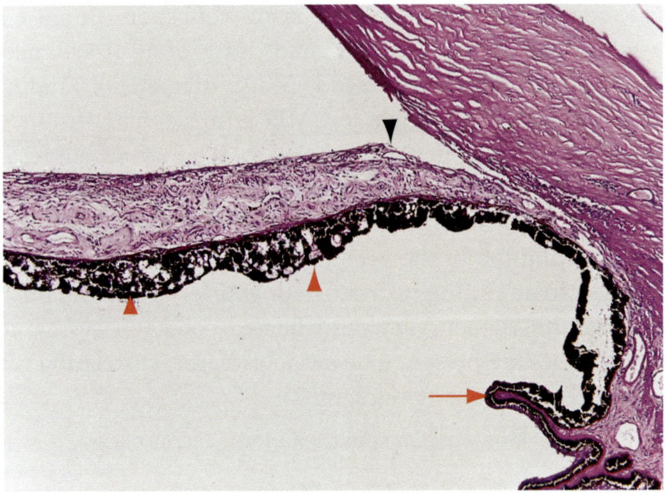

Figure 11-27 Histologic changes in diabetes mellitus. Photomicrograph (PAS stain) showing iris neovascularization *(black arrowhead),* lacy vacuolation of the iris pigment epithelium *(red arrowheads),* and thickening of the basement membrane of the pigmented ciliary epithelium *(red arrow).* These histologic findings are typically found in the eyes of patients with diabetes mellitus. *(Courtesy of Tatyana Milman, MD.)*

Argon laser photocoagulation, used in diabetic retinopathy, results in variable destruction of the retina and RPE and occlusion of the choriocapillaris (Fig 11-28). These lesions heal by proliferation of the adjacent RPE and glial scarring.

Age-Related Macular Degeneration

Age-related macular degeneration (AMD) is the leading cause of new blindness in the United States. Although the etiology of AMD remains unknown, evidence suggests that both genes and environmental factors play a role in its pathogenesis. Genome-wide and candidate association studies have identified risk loci for AMD and implicated certain genes, particularly *CFH* and *HTRA1/LOC387715/ARMS2.* Older age, tobacco use, positive family history, and cardiovascular disease increase the risk of AMD development. In addition, randomized clinical trials showing the benefit of antioxidant supplementation in AMD provide support for the role of oxidative stress in progression of the disease. See BCSC Section 12, *Retina and Vitreous,* for additional discussion.

Several characteristic changes in the retina, RPE, Bruch membrane, and choroid occur in AMD. The first detectable pathologic change is the appearance of deposits between the basement membrane of the RPE and the elastic portion of Bruch membrane (basal linear deposits) and similar deposits between the plasma membrane of the RPE and the basement membrane of the RPE (basal laminar deposits). Electron microscopy may be required to distinguish between these types of deposits; in advanced cases, the deposits may become confluent and visible with light microscopy without being clinically apparent (Fig 11-29). This histologic appearance has been described as *diffuse drusen.*

The first clinically detectable feature of AMD is the appearance of drusen. The clinical term *drusen* has been correlated pathologically to large, extracellular PAS-positive deposits between the RPE and Bruch membrane. Histochemical and molecular/biologic

A B

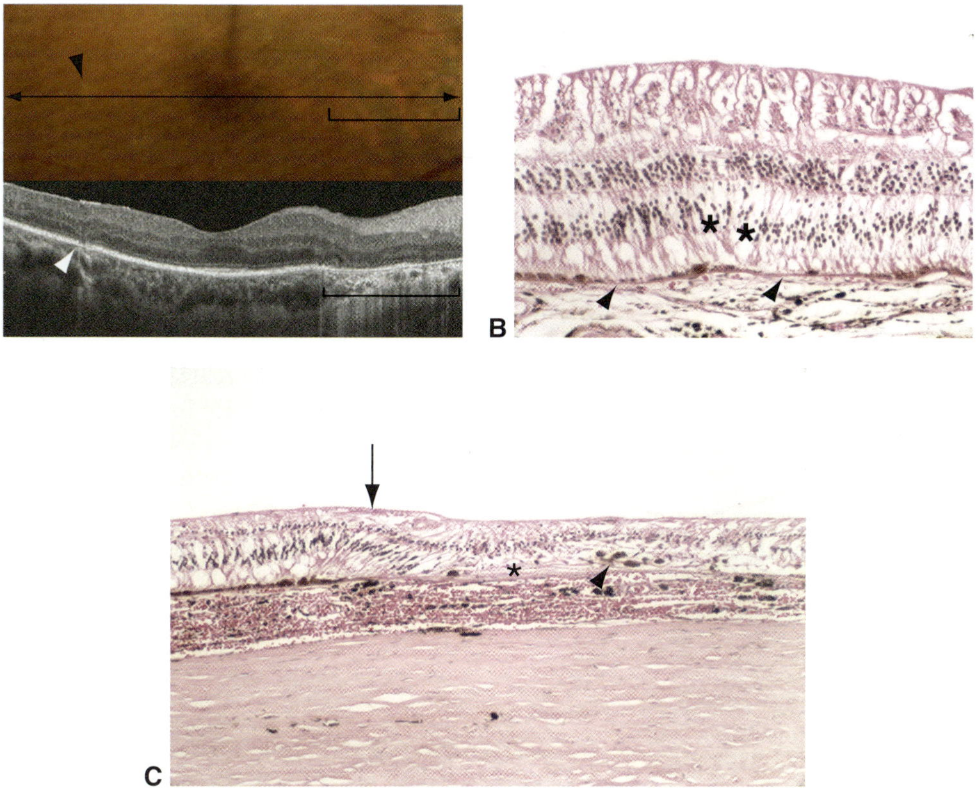

C

Figure 11-28 Laser photocoagulation scars. **A,** Clinical photograph (upper panel) and SD-OCT (lower panel) showing focal laser scar *(arrowheads)* and area of peripapillary atrophy *(brackets)*. The double-headed arrow in upper panel indicates macular region scanned with SD-OCT. In lower panel, note the disruption of the outer plexiform layer, outer nuclear layer, ellipsoid zone, and RPE in the region of the focal laser scar. **B,** In light applications of laser photocoagulation, focal disruption and attenuation of the outer nuclear layer *(asterisks)*, inner/outer segments, and RPE *(arrowheads)* may occur (H&E stain). **C,** In more intense laser applications, loss of the photoreceptor cell layer and RPE and closure of the choriocapillaris *(right of arrow)* may occur (H&E stain). Note the thin subretinal fibrosis *(asterisk)* in the laser scar. Variable RPE hypertrophy, hyperplasia, and migration into the retina *(arrowhead)*, as well as breaks in Bruch membrane, can occur. *(Courtesy of Robert H. Rosa, Jr, MD.)*

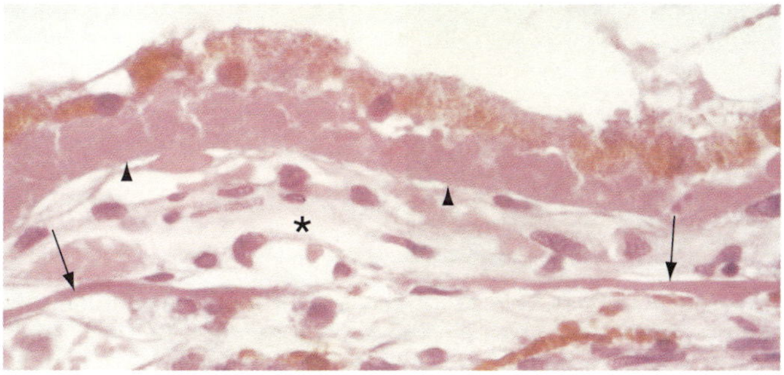

Figure 11-29 Diffuse drusen. Note the diffuse deposition of eosinophilic material *(arrowheads)* beneath the RPE. Choroidal neovascularization *(asterisk)* is present between the diffuse drusen and the elastic portion of Bruch membrane *(arrows)* (PAS stain). *(Courtesy of Hans E. Grossniklaus, MD.)*

analyses have demonstrated that the major constituents of human drusen include albumin, apolipoproteins, complement factors and related proteins, immunoglobulins, lipids, and amyloid-β. *Reticular pseudodrusen (RPD),* also known as *subretinal drusenoid deposits,* are extracellular material interposed between the photoreceptor inner/outer segments and the RPE; they may be associated with progression to advanced AMD (geographic atrophy and choroidal neovascularization). RPD contain membranous debris, unesterified cholesterol, complement factors and related proteins, and apolipoproteins but lack opsins. Many eyes with clinically apparent drusen (especially soft drusen) are found to have basal laminar and/or basal linear deposits and diffuse drusen on histologic analysis. Drusen, which may be transient, have been classified clinically as follows:

- *hard (hyaline) drusen:* typical discrete, yellowish lesions that are PAS-positive nodules composed of hyaline material between the RPE and Bruch membrane (Fig 11-30)
- *soft drusen:* drusen with amorphous, poorly demarcated boundaries, usually >63 μm in size; histologically, they represent cleavage of the RPE and basal laminar or linear deposits from Bruch membrane (Fig 11-31)
- *basal laminar,* or *cuticular, drusen:* diffuse, small, regular, and nodular deposits of drusenlike material in the macula

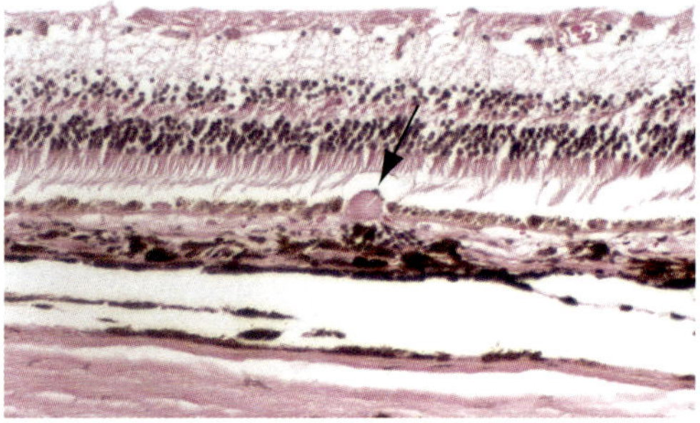

Figure 11-30 Hard drusen *(arrow).* Note the dome-shaped, nodular, hard druse and attenuation of the overlying RPE (H&E stain). *(Courtesy of Robert H. Rosa, Jr, MD.)*

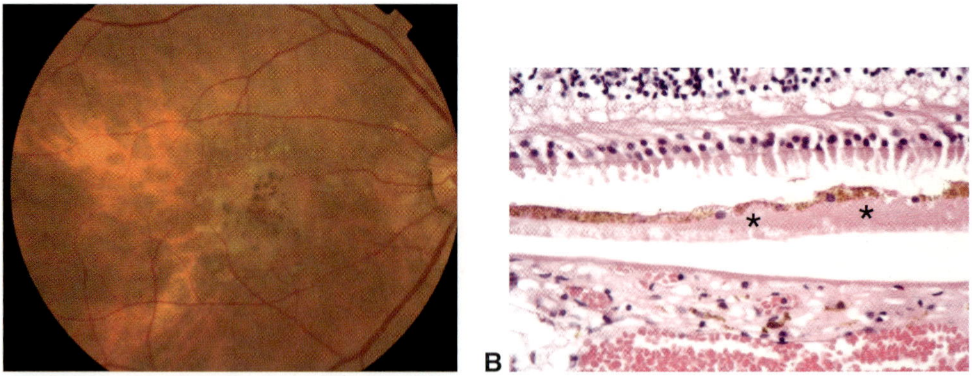

Figure 11-31 Confluent drusen. **A,** Clinical photograph of confluent drusen. Note the pigment clumping overlying the confluent drusen in the central macula. **B,** Thick eosinophilic deposits *(asterisks)* between the RPE and Bruch membrane (H&E stain). The separation between the retina and RPE and the RPE and Bruch membrane is artifact. Note the marked attenuation of the photoreceptor cell nuclei in the outer nuclear layer and loss of the outer segments over the confluent drusen. *(Part A courtesy of Robert H. Rosa, Jr, MD; part B courtesy of Nasreen A. Syed, MD.)*

- *calcific drusen:* sharply demarcated, glistening, refractile lesions usually associated with RPE atrophy
- *reticular pseudodrusen:* ill-defined, yellowish, reticular pattern in the superior and temporal macula with enhanced visibility when viewed with blue light, near-infrared imaging, or fundus autofluorescence; histologically, RPD are located between the photoreceptor inner/outer segments and the RPE (Fig 11-32)

Photoreceptor atrophy occurs to a variable degree in macular degeneration. This atrophy may be a primary abnormality of the photoreceptors or may be secondary to the

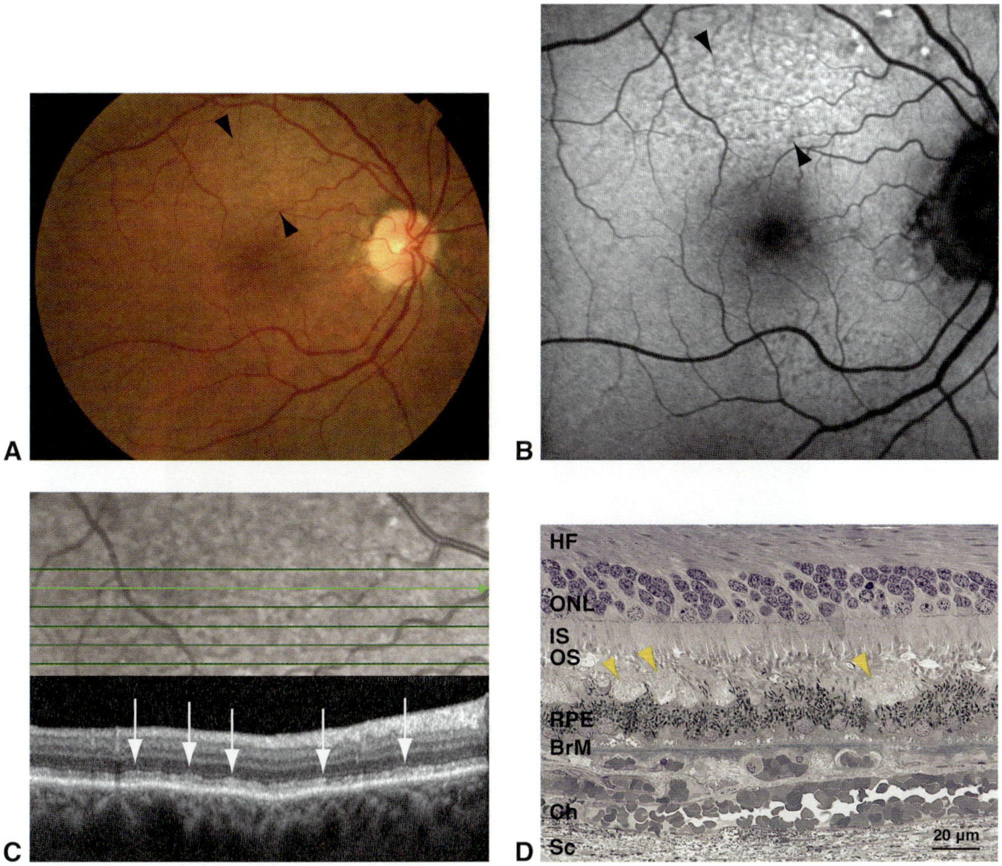

Figure 11-32 Reticular pseudodrusen. **A,** Color photograph shows ill-defined, yellowish, reticular pattern *(between arrowheads)* in the superior macula. **B,** Fundus autofluorescence (FAF) image shows corresponding region *(between arrowheads)* with dotlike areas of decreased and increased FAF. **C,** Near-infrared image (upper panel) shows similar dotlike areas of decreased reflectance, which, on SD-OCT (lower panel), correspond to deposits *(arrows)* interposed between the photoreceptor outer segments and RPE with focal disruption of the ellipsoid zone. **D,** Subretinal drusenoid deposits *(yellow arrowheads)* are the histologic correlate of reticular pseudodrusen. Note their location in the region of the outer segments. HF = Henle fiber layer; ONL = outer nuclear layer; IS = inner segments; OS = outer segments; RPE = retinal pigment epithelium; BrM = Bruch membrane; Ch = choroid; Sc = sclera. Submicrometer epoxy section, toluidine blue stain, osmium paraphenylenediamine post-fixation. *(Parts A–C courtesy of Robert H. Rosa, Jr, MD; Part D courtesy of Christine A. Curcio, PhD.)*

underlying changes in the RPE, Bruch membrane, and choriocapillaris. In addition to photoreceptor atrophy, large zones of RPE atrophy may appear. When RPE atrophy occurs in the macular region, it is termed *geographic atrophy* (Fig 11-33). Drusen, photoreceptor atrophy, and RPE atrophy may all be present to varying degrees in *dry,* or *nonexudative, AMD.*

In eyes with choroidal neovascularization *(neovascular, wet,* or *exudative AMD),* fibrovascular tissue is present between the inner and outer layers of Bruch membrane, beneath the RPE, and/or in the subretinal space (Fig 11-34). The new blood vessels leak fluid and may rupture easily, producing the exudative consequences of neovascular AMD, including macular edema, serous retinal detachment, and subretinal and intraretinal hemorrhages. VEGF inhibition achieved with intravitreally administered anti-VEGF agents has been shown to reduce the macular edema, slow the progression of the choroidal neovascularization, and improve the visual outcomes of patients with neovascular AMD (also see the previous section Vascular responses).

A

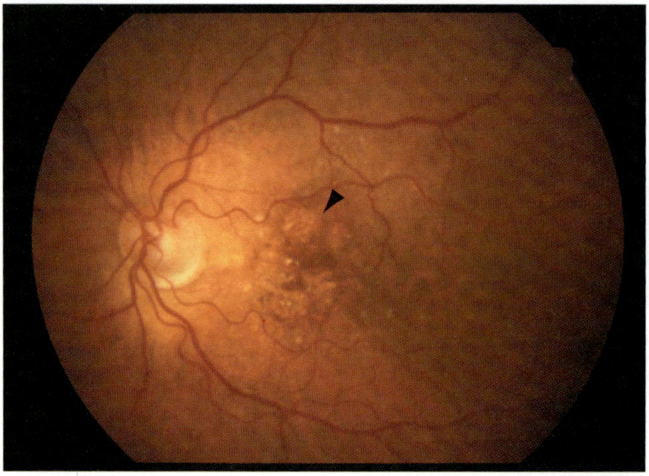

B

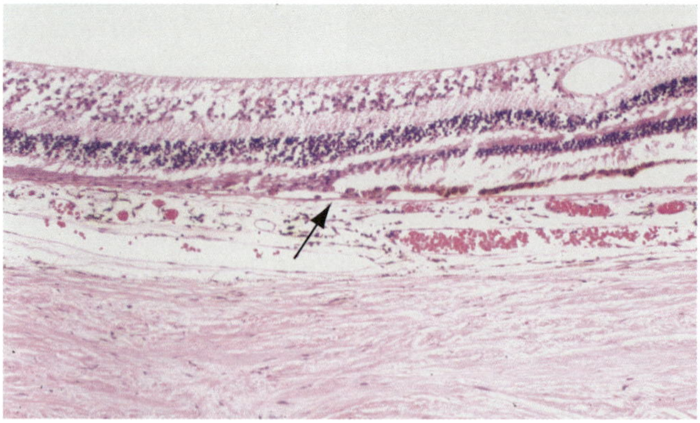

Figure 11-33 Geographic atrophy of the RPE. **A,** Fundus photograph shows focal geographic atrophy of the RPE *(arrowhead)* and drusen in nonexudative age-related macular degeneration. **B,** Histologically, there is loss of the photoreceptor cell layer, RPE, and choriocapillaris *(left of arrow)* with an abrupt transition zone *(arrow)* to a more normal-appearing retina and RPE *(right of arrow).* Note the multicellular, thick ganglion cell layer identifying the macular region (H&E stain). *(Courtesy of Robert H. Rosa, Jr, MD.)*

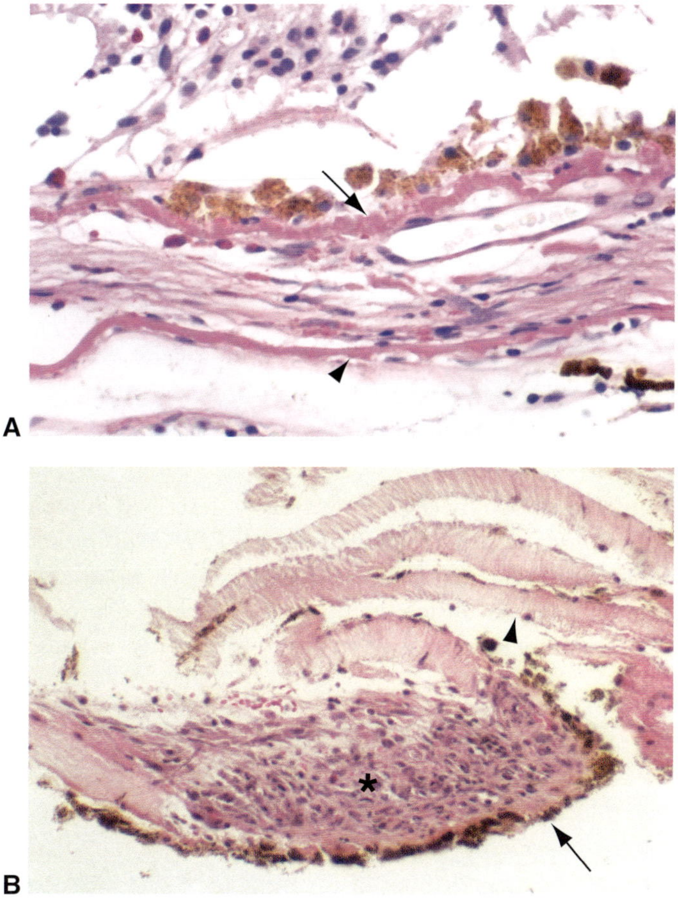

Figure 11-34 Choroidal neovascularization (CNV). **A,** CNV located between the inner *(arrow)* and outer *(arrowhead)* layers of Bruch membrane (sub-RPE, type 1 CNV). Note loss of the overlying photoreceptor inner and outer segments, RPE hyperplasia, and the PAS-positive basal laminar deposit *(arrow)*. **B,** Surgically excised CNV (subretinal, type 2 CNV) composed of fibrovascular tissue *(asterisk)* lined externally by RPE *(arrow)* with adherent photoreceptor outer segments *(arrowhead)* (H&E stain). *(Courtesy of Robert H. Rosa, Jr, MD.)*

Choroidal neovascular membranes are classified as type 1 or type 2, based on their pathologic and clinical features. *Type 1 neovascularization* (see Fig 11-34A) is typically associated with the presence of basal laminar deposits and diffuse drusen and is characterized by neovascularization within Bruch membrane in the sub-RPE space. RPE atrophy and/or hyperplasia may be present overlying type 1 neovascularization. *Type 2 neovascularization* (see Fig 11-34B) occurs in the subretinal space and generally features only a small defect in the RPE. Type 1 neovascularization is more characteristic of AMD, whereas type 2 is more characteristic of ocular histoplasmosis. Type 2 membranes are more amenable to surgical removal than type 1 membranes, because native RPE would be excised with a type 1 membrane, leaving an atrophic lesion (without RPE) in the area of membrane excision.

Though surgical excision is not routinely performed, surgically excised choroidal neovascular membranes (see Fig 11-34B) are composed of vascular channels, RPE, and various other components of the RPE–Bruch membrane complex, including photoreceptor outer segments, basal laminar and linear deposits, and inflammatory cells.

Curcio CA, Messinger JD, Sloan KR, McGwin G, Medeiros NE, Spaide RF. Subretinal drusenoid deposits in non-neovascular age-related macular degeneration: morphology, prevalence, topography, and biogenesis model. *Retina.* 2013;33(2):265–276.

Grossniklaus HE, Gass JD. Clinicopathologic correlations of surgically excised type 1 and type 2 submacular choroidal neovascular membranes. *Am J Ophthalmol.* 1998;126(1):59–69.

Grossniklaus HE, Miskala PH, Green WR, et al. Histopathologic and ultrastructural features of surgically excised subfoveal choroidal neovascular lesions: submacular surgery trials report no. 7. *Arch Ophthalmol.* 2005;123(7):914–921.

Ratnapriya R, Chew EY. Age-related macular degeneration—clinical review and genetics update. *Clin Genet.* 2013;84(2):160–166.

Polypoidal Choroidal Vasculopathy

Polypoidal choroidal vasculopathy (PCV), previously described as *posterior uveal bleeding syndrome* and *multiple recurrent serosanguineous RPE detachments,* is a disorder in which dilated, thin-walled vascular channels (Figs 11-35, 11-36) are interposed between the RPE and the outer aspect of Bruch membrane. Associated choroidal neovascularization is often present in these lesions, as observed in several histologic specimens. PCV is

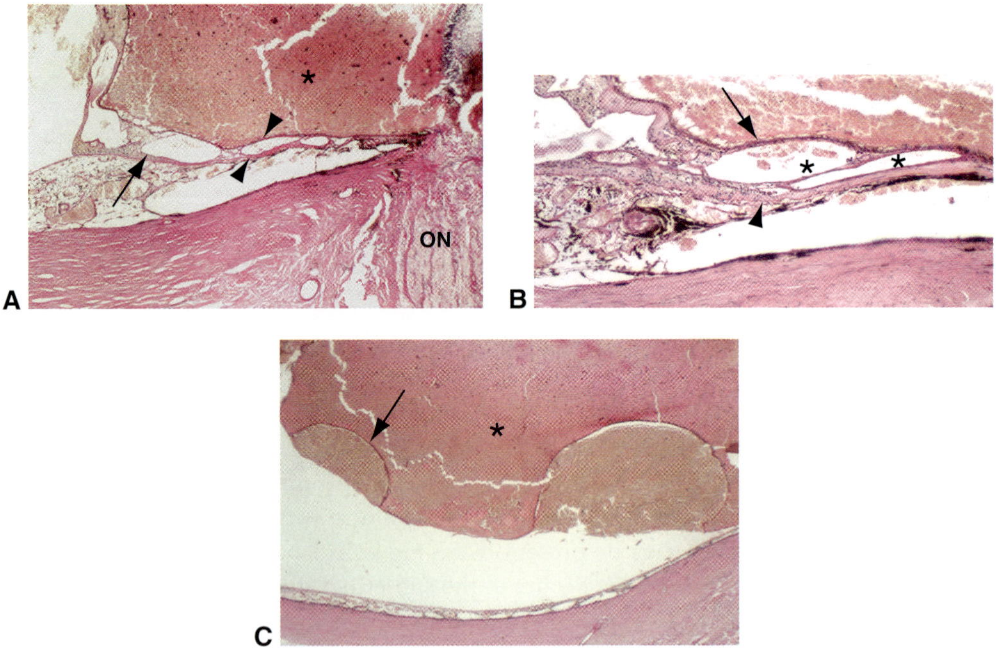

Figure 11-35 Polypoidal choroidal vasculopathy (PCV). **A,** Peripapillary dilated vascular channels *(arrow)* between the RPE and outer aspect of Bruch membrane *(arrowheads).* Note the dense subretinal hemorrhage *(asterisk)* (PAS stain). ON = optic nerve. **B,** Higher-magnification view of thin-walled vascular channels *(asterisks)* interposed between the RPE *(arrow)* and Bruch membrane *(arrowhead)* (PAS stain). **C,** Hemorrhagic RPE detachments *(arrows)* and serosanguineous subretinal fluid *(asterisk)* (PAS stain). *(Courtesy of Robert H. Rosa, Jr, MD.)*

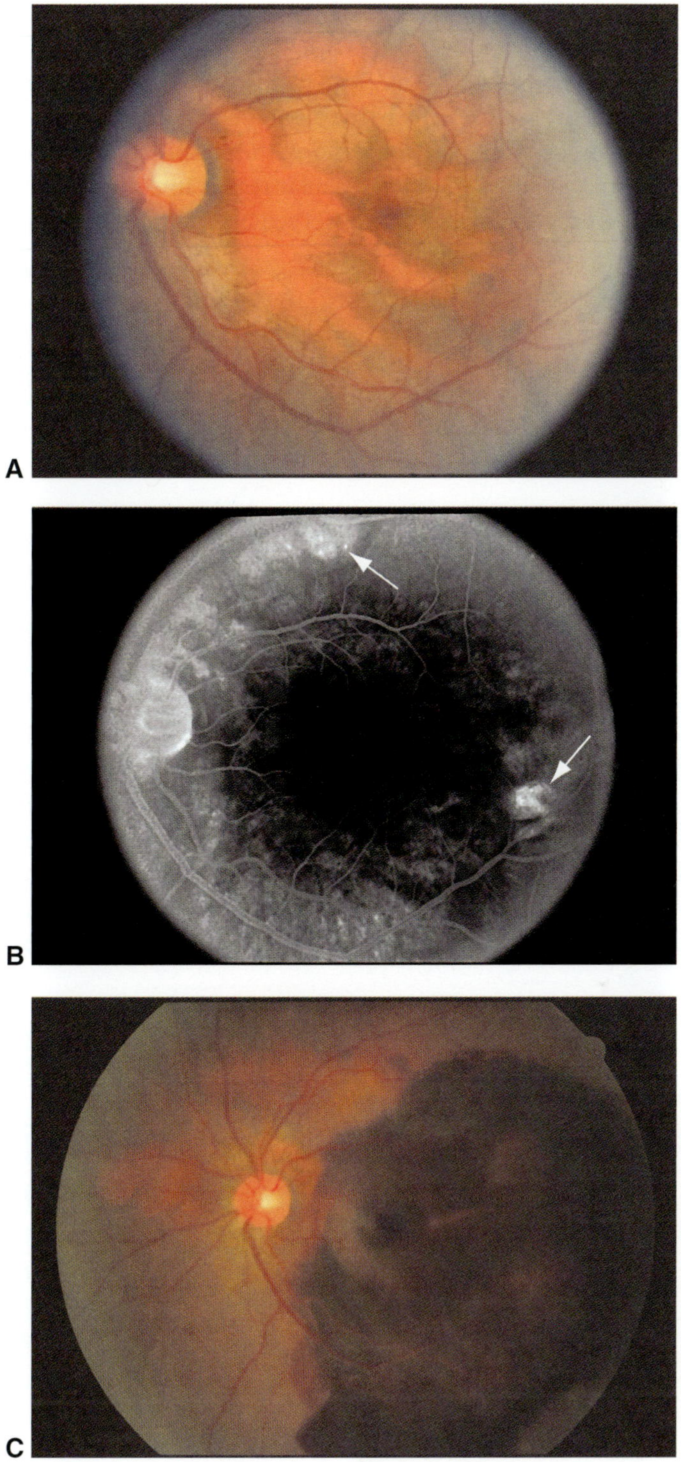

Figure 11-36 PCV. **A,** Elevated, red-orange, nodular and tubular lesions in the peripapillary and macular regions. **B,** Late fluorescein angiogram (860 seconds) shows hyperfluorescent polypoidal lesions *(arrows)* without apparent leakage. **C,** Dense subretinal hemorrhage in same patient as **A** and **B.** Note the persistent red-orange lesions in the peripapillary region. *(Courtesy of Robert H. Rosa, Jr, MD.)*

more prevalent in Asian and African American populations than in whites, accounting for up to 55% of cases of neovascular AMD in the Japanese population. PCV occurs more frequently in men than women in Asian populations; the opposite is observed in whites. The majority of PCV lesions are located in the macular region in Asian cohorts, whereas peripapillary PCV lesions are more frequently observed in American and European cohorts.

Honda S, Matsumiya W, Negi A. Polypoidal choroidal vasculopathy: clinical features and genetic predisposition. *Ophthalmologica.* 2014;231(2):59–74.

Imamura Y, Engelbert M, Iida T, Freund KB, Yannuzzi LA. Polypoidal choroidal vasculopathy: a review. *Surv Ophthalmol.* 2010;55(6):501–515.

Rosa RH Jr, Davis JL, Eifrig CW. Clinicopathologic reports, case reports, and small case series: clinicopathologic correlation of idiopathic polypoidal choroidal vasculopathy. *Arch Ophthalmol.* 2002;120(4):502–508.

Macular Dystrophies

See BCSC Section 12, *Retina and Vitreous,* for additional discussion of macular dystrophies.

Fundus flavimaculatus and Stargardt disease

Fundus flavimaculatus and Stargardt disease are thought to represent 2 ends of the spectrum of a disease process characterized by yellowish flecks at the RPE level, a generalized vermilion (reddish) color to the fundus on clinical examination, variable late RPE atrophy, a dark choroid on fluorescein angiography (Fig 11-37; see also Figs 12-7 and 12-8 in BCSC Section 12, *Retina and Vitreous*), and gradually decreasing vision. The inheritance pattern is generally autosomal recessive, but autosomal dominant forms have been reported. Several genetic mutations have been observed in patients with a Stargardt-like phenotype, including the *ABCA4, STGD4, ELOVL4,* and *PRPH2 (peripherin 2)* genes. Mutations in *ABCA4* are responsible for most cases of Stargardt disease. The *ABCA4* gene encodes a protein

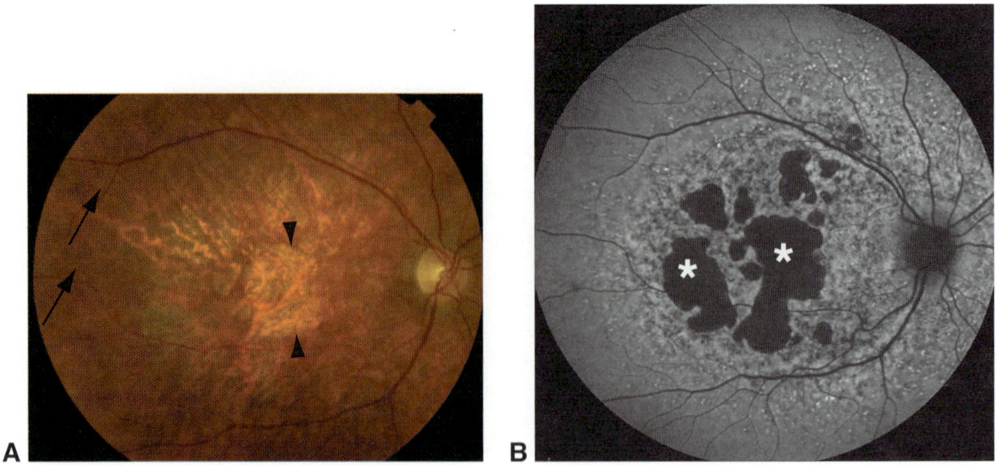

Figure 11-37 Stargardt disease. **A,** Fundus photograph shows retinal flecks *(arrows)* and focal or geographic RPE atrophy *(between arrowheads)* in the macular region. **B,** FAF imaging reveals increased FAF corresponding to retinal flecks and decreased FAF corresponding to areas of RPE atrophy *(asterisks).*

(Continued)

called RIM protein, which is a member of the ATP-binding cassette transporter family. This protein, which is expressed in the rims of rod and cone photoreceptor disc membranes, helps transport vitamin A derivatives to the RPE. The most striking feature of Stargardt disease revealed by light and electron microscopy is the marked engorgement of RPE cells

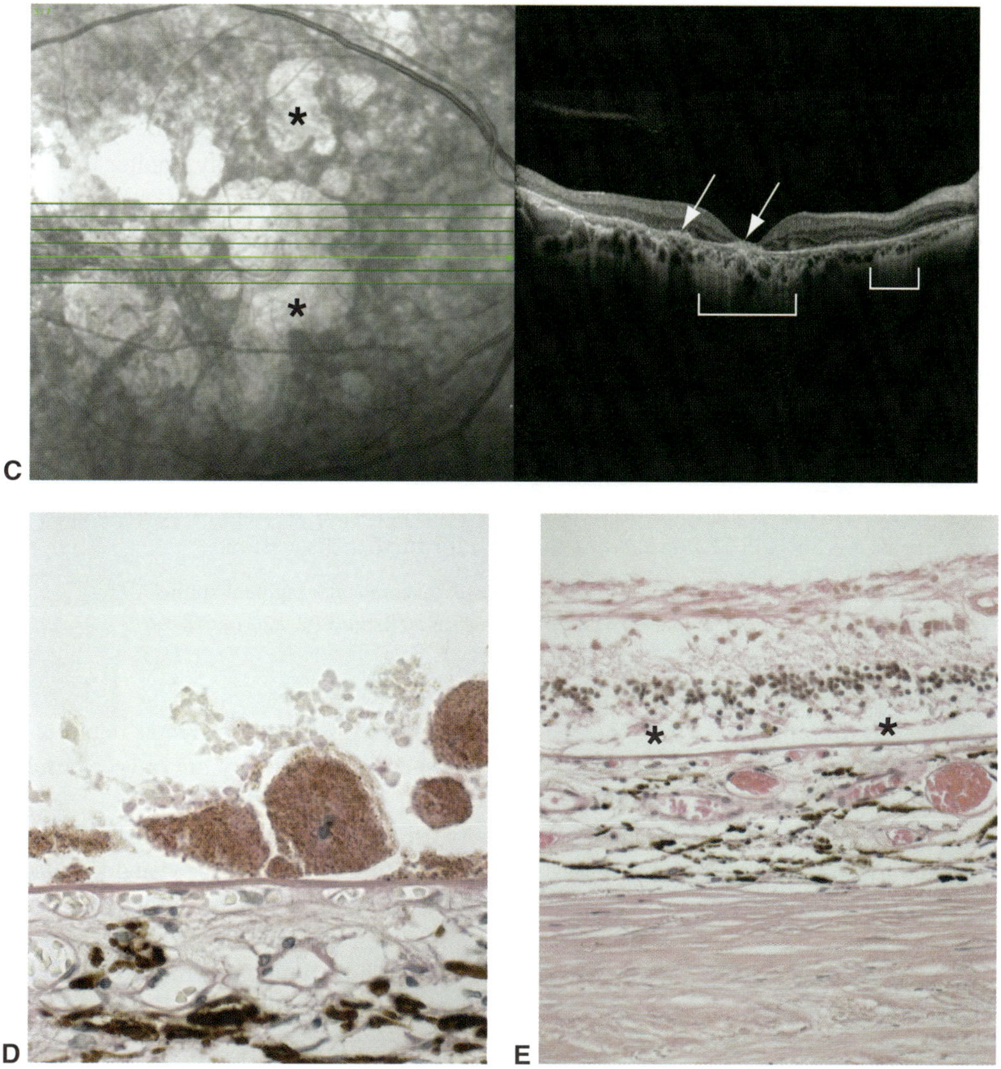

Figure 11-37 *(continued)* **C,** Near-infrared imaging (left panel) reveals increased reflectance corresponding to areas of RPE atrophy *(asterisks)*. SD-OCT (right panel) reveals hyperreflectivity at the level of the RPE (corresponding histologically with enlarged RPE cells with increased lipofuscin content) *(arrows)*, markedly thinned retina in the foveal region, and focal attenuation or loss of the photoreceptor cell layer in areas corresponding to RPE atrophy, as seen on the near-infrared image and back-shadowing on the SD-OCT image *(brackets)*. **D,** Histology with PAS stain reveals hypertrophic RPE cells with numerous PAS-positive cytoplasmic granules containing lipofuscin. This histologic finding corresponds to the retinal flecks seen clinically. **E,** In advanced stages of Stargardt disease, geographic RPE atrophy with loss of the photoreceptor cell layer *(asterisks)* may be observed (H&E stain). *(Parts A–C courtesy of Robert H. Rosa, Jr, MD; parts D and E courtesy of Sander Dubovy, MD.)*

(see Fig 11-37D; see also Fig 12-8 in BCSC Section 12, *Retina and Vitreous*) with lipofuscin-like, PAS-positive material, with apical displacement of the normal RPE melanin granules.

Pattern dystrophies

The term *pattern dystrophies* refers to a heterogeneous group of inherited macular disorders that are characterized by varying patterns of pigment deposition in the macula at the RPE level. Recognized pattern dystrophies include butterfly-shaped pattern dystrophy (BPD), adult-onset foveomacular vitelliform dystrophy (AFMVD), reticular dystrophy, and fundus pulverulentus. BPD is characterized by a butterfly-shaped, irregular, depigmented lesion at the RPE level. AFMVD is characterized by the presence of slightly elevated, symmetric, round to oval, yellow lesions at the RPE level; these lesions are typically smaller than the vitelliform lesion characteristic of Best disease (Fig 11-38). Spectral domain optical coherence tomography (SD-OCT) reveals elevation of the photoreceptor layer, with localization of the dystrophic material between the photoreceptors and RPE (see Fig 11-38C). The most common genetic mutation associated with the pattern dystrophies is in the *PRPH2 (peripherin 2)* gene. Histologic studies reveal central loss of the RPE and photoreceptor cell layer, with a moderate number of pigment-containing macrophages in the subretinal space and outer neurosensory retina (see Fig 11-38D). To either side, the RPE is distended with lipofuscin (see Fig 11-38E). Basal laminar and linear deposits may be present throughout the macular region. The pathologic finding of pigment-containing cells with lipofuscin and drusen-like material in the subretinal space correlates clinically with the vitelliform appearance. See BCSC Section 12, *Retina and Vitreous,* for further discussion.

Dubovy SR, Hairston RJ, Schatz H, et al. Adult-onset foveomacular pigment epithelial dystrophy: clinicopathologic correlation of three cases. *Retina.* 2000;20(6):638–649.

Diffuse Photoreceptor Dystrophies

Inherited dystrophies that affect the rods and cones are discussed in greater detail elsewhere in the BCSC (see BCSC Section 12, *Retina and Vitreous*). Only the most common diffuse photoreceptor dystrophy, retinitis pigmentosa, is discussed here.

Retinitis pigmentosa (RP) refers to a group of inherited retinal diseases that are characterized by photoreceptor and RPE dysfunction resulting in progressive visual field loss. The genetics of RP are complex; it can be sporadic, autosomal dominant, autosomal recessive, or X-linked. Mutations in the rhodopsin gene *(RHO)* are the most common cause of autosomal dominant RP. Ophthalmoscopic findings include pigment arranged in a bone spicule–like configuration around the retinal arterioles, arteriolar narrowing, and optic nerve head atrophy (Fig 11-39A). The disease is characterized primarily by the loss of rod photoreceptor cells via apoptosis. Cones are seldom directly affected by the identified mutations; however, they degenerate secondary to the loss of rods. The term *retinitis pigmentosa* is a misnomer, because clear evidence of inflammation is lacking. Microscopically, photoreceptor cell loss occurs, as well as RPE hyperplasia with migration into the retina around retinal vessels (Fig 11-39B). The arterioles, though narrowed clinically, show no histologic abnormality initially. Later, thickening and hyalinization of the vessel walls appear. The optic nerve may show diffuse or sectoral atrophy, with gliosis as a late change.

Ben-Arie-Weintrob Y, Berson EL, Dryja TP. Histopathologic-genotypic correlations in retinitis pigmentosa and allied diseases. *Ophthalmic Genet.* 2005;26(2):91–100.

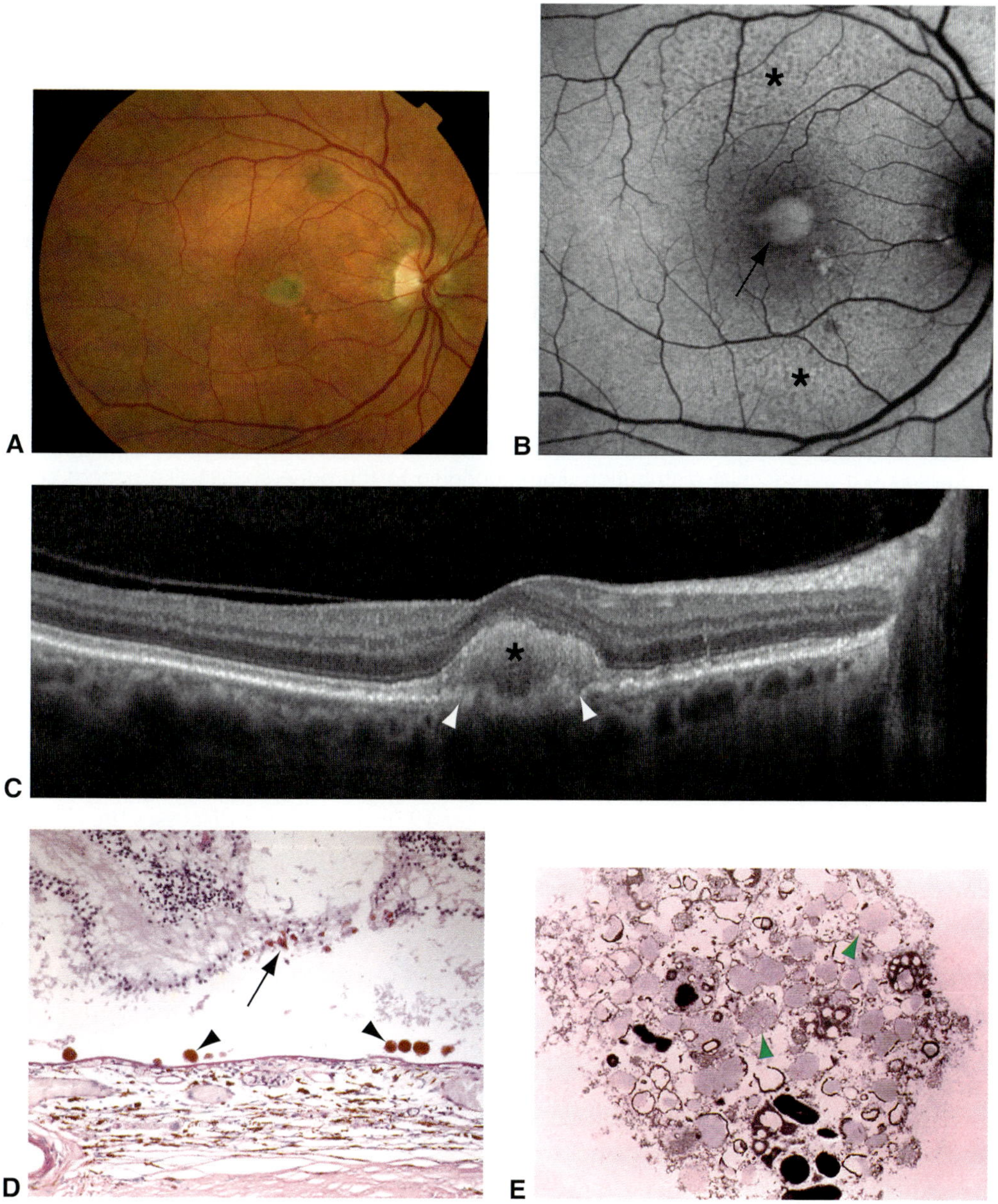

Figure 11-38 Adult-onset foveomacular vitelliform dystrophy. **A,** Yellowish, egg yolk–like lesion with focal pigment clumping and mottling in the central macula. **B,** FAF image of the same patient as shown in **A** reveals increased FAF corresponding to the vitelliform lesion *(arrow).* Note the reticular pseudodrusen, which are inconspicuous in the clinical photograph, in the superior and inferior macula *(asterisks).* **C,** SD-OCT of the same patient as shown in parts **A** and **B** reveals subfoveal hyperreflective material *(asterisk).* Note the irregular RPE elevation *(between arrowheads).* **D,** Histologic findings include pigment-containing cells in the subretinal space *(arrowheads)* and outer neurosensory retina *(arrow)* (H&E stain). **E,** Electron microscopy shows pigment-containing cells filled with lipofuscin *(arrowheads). (Parts A–C courtesy of Robert H. Rosa, Jr, MD; parts D and E courtesy of Sander Dubovy, MD.)*

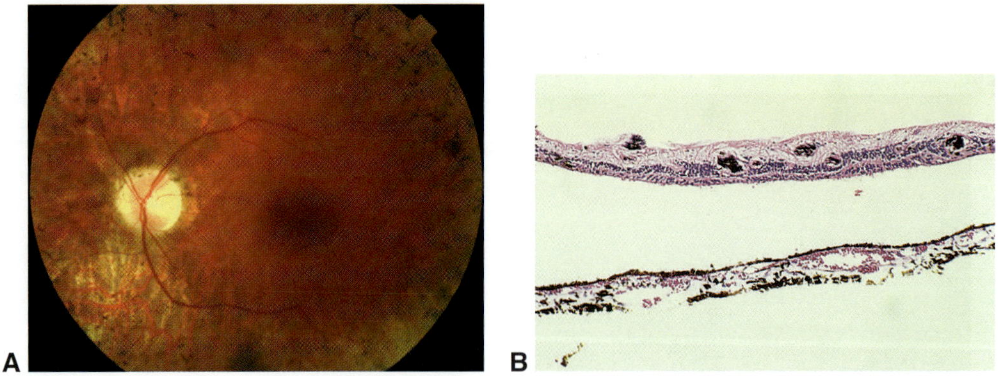

Figure 11-39 Retinitis pigmentosa. **A,** Fundus photograph shows mild optic nerve head atrophy, retinal arteriolar narrowing, focal depigmentation, and bone-spicule pigmentation in the fundus. **B,** Histologically, note the marked photoreceptor cell loss and RPE migration into the retina in a perivascular distribution, corresponding to the bone spicule–like pattern seen clinically (H&E stain). The retina is artifactitiously detached. *(Part A courtesy of Robert H. Rosa, Jr, MD.)*

Neoplasia

The tumors discussed in this section arise from tissue derived from the inner layer of the optic cup.

Retinoblastoma

Retinoblastoma is the most common primary intraocular malignancy in childhood, occurring in 1 in 14,000–20,000 live births. Chapter 19 in this volume discusses the clinical aspects of retinoblastoma. Retinoblastoma is also discussed in Chapter 25 of BCSC Section 6, *Pediatric Ophthalmology and Strabismus.*

Pathogenesis

Although retinoblastoma was once considered to be of glial origin (lesions clinically simulating retinoblastoma were formerly called *pseudogliomas*), the tumor's neuroblastic origin from the nucleated layers of the retina has been well established. Immunohistochemical studies have demonstrated that tumor cells stain positive for neuron-specific enolase, rod outer segment photoreceptor–specific S-antigen, and rhodopsin. Tumor cells also secrete an extracellular substance known as *interphotoreceptor retinoid-binding protein,* which is also a product of normal photoreceptors. Retinoblastoma tumor cells grown in a culture have been shown to express a red and a green photopigment gene, as well as cone cell α-subunits of transducin. These findings further support the concept that retinoblastoma may be a neoplasm of cone cell lineage. However, immunohistochemical and molecular studies cast some doubt on the hypothesis that a single cell type is the progenitor of retinoblastoma. The presence of small amounts of glial tissue within retinoblastoma suggests that resident glial cells may undergo reactive proliferation or become trapped within the tumor.

The *retinoblastoma gene (RB1),* localized to the long arm of chromosome 13, is deceptively named, as it does not actively cause retinoblastoma. The normal gene *suppresses* the development of retinoblastoma (and possibly other tumors, such as osteosarcoma).

Retinoblastoma develops when both homologous loci of the suppressor gene become nonfunctional, either by a deletion error or by mutation. Although 1 normal gene is sufficient to suppress the development of retinoblastoma, when 1 normal gene and 1 abnormal gene are present, the occurrence of a mutation in the normal gene may lead to loss of tumor suppression and allow retinoblastoma to develop.

Recently, it has been shown that amplification of the *MYCN* oncogene might initiate retinoblastoma in the presence of nonmutated *RB1* genes in up to 3% of unilateral retinoblastoma tumors. Genetic tests for mutations in the *RB1* gene are negative in these cases. This type of unilateral retinoblastoma is characterized by distinct histologic features (ie, undifferentiated cells with prominent and multiple nucleoli, necrosis, apoptosis, little calcification, absence of Flexner-Wintersteiner rosettes, and nuclear molding), only a few of the genomic copy number changes that are characteristic of retinoblastoma, and very early age (ie, median age of 4.5 months) at diagnosis.

Benavente CA, Dyer MA. Genetics and epigenetics of human retinoblastoma. *Annu Rev Pathol.* 2015;10:547–562.

Grossniklaus HE. Retinoblastoma. Fifty years of progress. The LXXI Edward Jackson Memorial Lecture. *Am J Ophthalmol.* 2014;158(5):875–891.

Rushlow DE, Mol BM, Kennett JY, et al. Characterisation of retinoblastomas without *RB1* mutations: genomic, gene expression, and clinical studies. *Lancet Oncol.* 2013;14(4): 327–334.

Histologic features

Histologically, retinoblastoma consists of cells with round or oval nuclei that are approximately twice the size of a lymphocyte. Nuclei are hyperchromatic and surrounded by a scant amount of cytoplasm. Mitotic activity is usually high, although frequent apoptotic cells may make this difficult to assess. As tumors expand into the vitreous or subretinal space, they frequently outgrow their blood supply, creating a characteristic pattern of necrosis with the formation of pseudorosettes (viable tumor cells surrounding a blood vessel) (Fig 11-40); calcification is a common finding in areas of necrosis (Fig 11-41). Cuffs of

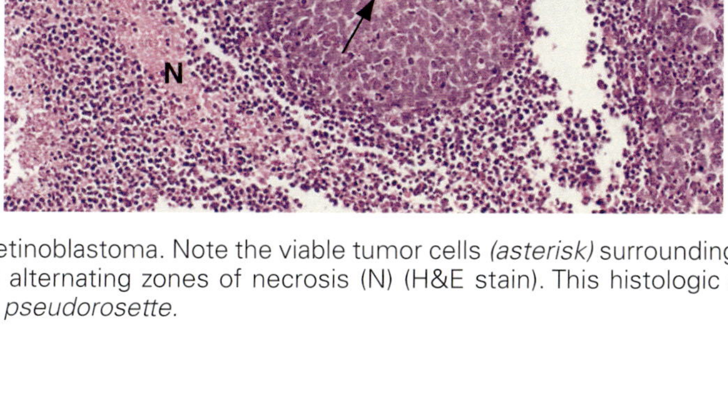

Figure 11-40 Retinoblastoma. Note the viable tumor cells *(asterisk)* surrounding a blood vessel *(arrow)* and the alternating zones of necrosis (N) (H&E stain). This histologic arrangement is referred to as a *pseudorosette.*

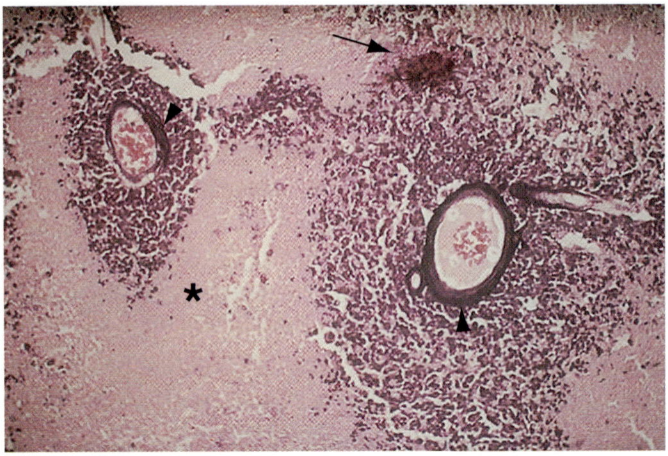

Figure 11-41 Retinoblastoma. Zones of viable tumor (usually surrounding blood vessels) alternate with zones of tumor necrosis *(asterisk)*. Calcium *(arrow)* is present in the necrotic area. The basophilic material surrounding and within the blood vessel walls *(arrowheads)* is DNA, presumably liberated from the necrotic tumor (H&E stain).

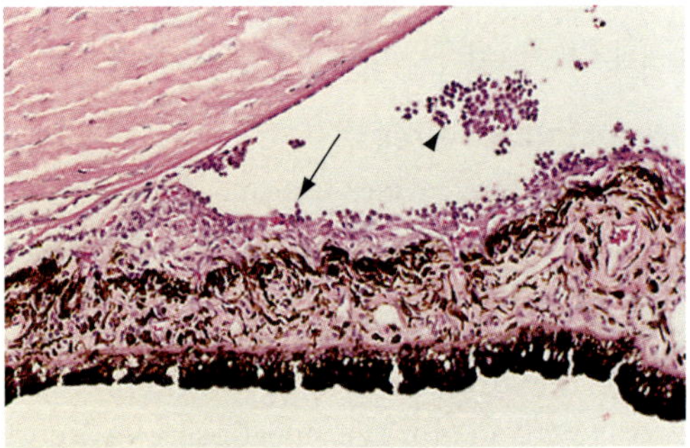

Figure 11-42 Retinoblastoma. Note the thick iris neovascular membrane *(arrow)* and free-floating tumor cells *(arrowhead)* in the anterior chamber (H&E stain).

viable cells course along blood vessels; regions of ischemic necrosis begin 90–120 μm from nutrient vessels. DNA released from necrotic cells may be detected within tumor vessels (see Fig 11-41) and within blood vessels in tissues remote from the tumor, such as the iris. Neovascularization of the iris can complicate retinoblastoma (Fig 11-42).

Cells shed from retinoblastoma tumors remain viable in the vitreous and subretinal space, and may eventually develop into seeds throughout the eye. It may be difficult to determine histologically whether multiple intraocular foci of the tumor represent multiple primary tumors, implying systemic distribution of the abnormal gene, or tumor seeds (see Chapter 19, Fig 19-7).

The formation of highly organized *Flexner-Wintersteiner rosettes* is a characteristic feature of retinoblastoma that occurs only in rare cases in other neuroblastic tumors (eg, primitive neuroectodermal tumors). Flexner-Wintersteiner rosettes are expressions of retinal differentiation. The cells of these rosettes surround a central lumen lined by a refractile structure. This refractile lining corresponds to the external limiting membrane of the retina that represents sites of attachments between photoreceptors and Müller cells.

The rosette is characterized by a single row of columnar cells with eosinophilic cytoplasm and peripherally situated nuclei in a radial arrangement (Fig 11-43A).

A rosette without features of retinal differentiation, known as the *Homer Wright rosette,* can be found in other neuroblastic tumors, such as neuroblastoma and medulloblastoma, as well as in retinoblastoma. Unlike the Flexner-Wintersteiner rosette, a Homer Wright rosette has a center that is filled with a tangle of eosinophilic cytoplasmic processes (Fig 11-43B).

Evidence of photoreceptor differentiation has also been documented for another flowerlike structure known as a *fleurette.* Fleurettes are curvilinear clusters of cells composed of rod and cone inner segments that are often attached to abortive outer segments (Fig 11-43C). The fleurette expresses a greater degree of retinal differentiation than the Flexner-Wintersteiner rosette. In a typical retinoblastoma, the undifferentiated tumor cells greatly outnumber the fleurettes and Flexner-Wintersteiner rosettes, and differentiation is not an important prognostic indicator.

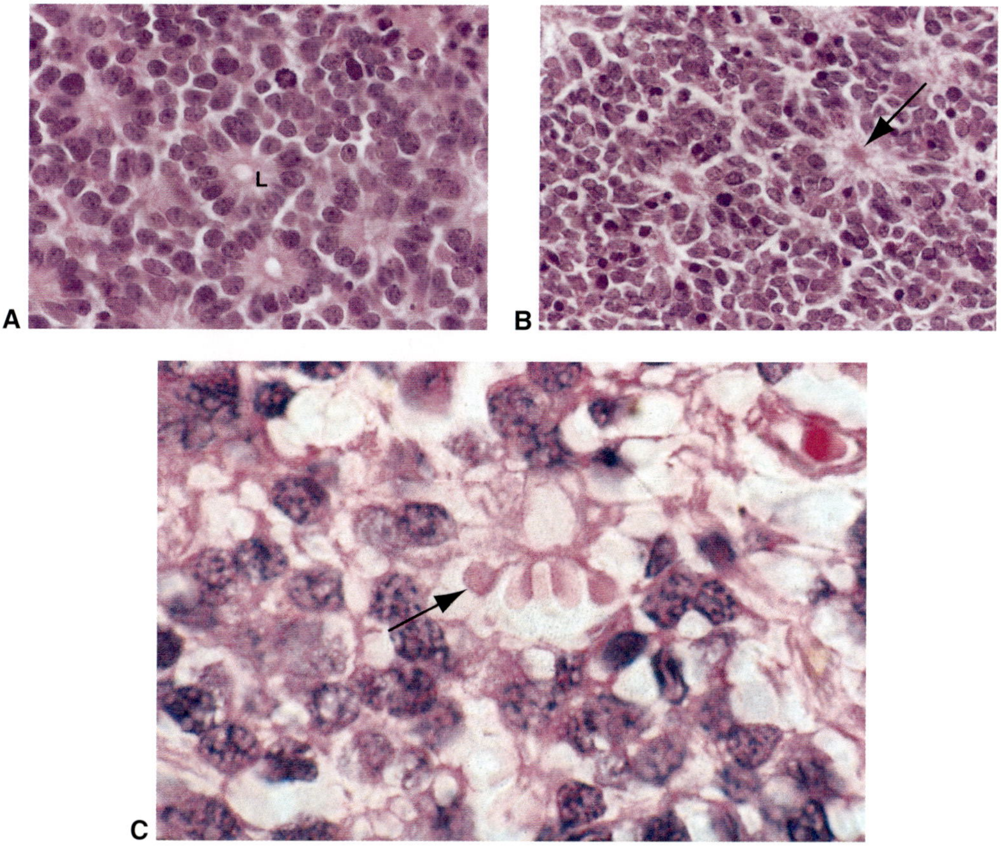

Figure 11-43 Retinoblastoma rosettes. **A,** Flexner-Wintersteiner rosettes: note the central lumen (L) (H&E stain). **B,** Homer Wright rosettes: note the neurofibrillary tangle *(arrow)* in the center of these structures (H&E stain). **C,** The fleurette *(arrow)* demonstrates bulbous cellular extensions of retinoblastoma cells that represent differentiation along the lines of photoreceptor inner segments (H&E stain).

Progression

The most common route for a retinoblastoma tumor to spread from the eye is by way of the optic nerve. Direct infiltration of the optic nerve can lead to extension into the brain. Cells that spread into the leptomeninges can gain access to the subarachnoid space, with the potential for seeding throughout the central nervous system (Fig 11-44). Invasion of the optic nerve is a poor prognostic sign (Fig 11-45). See Chapter 19 for a discussion

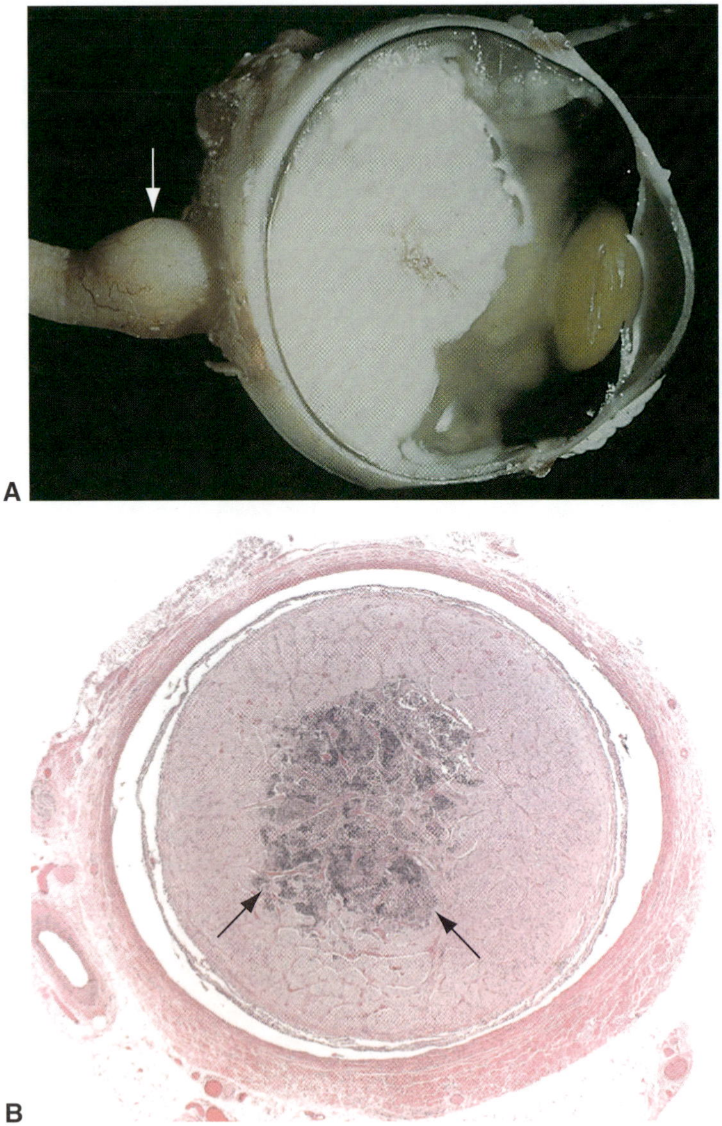

Figure 11-44 Retinoblastoma. **A,** Massive invasion of the globe posteriorly by retinoblastoma with bulbous enlargement of the optic nerve *(arrow)* caused by direct extension. **B,** A cross section of the optic nerve taken at the surgical margin of transection. Tumor *(arrows)* is present in the nerve at this point, and the prognosis is poor (H&E stain). *(Part B courtesy of Nasreen A. Syed, MD.)*

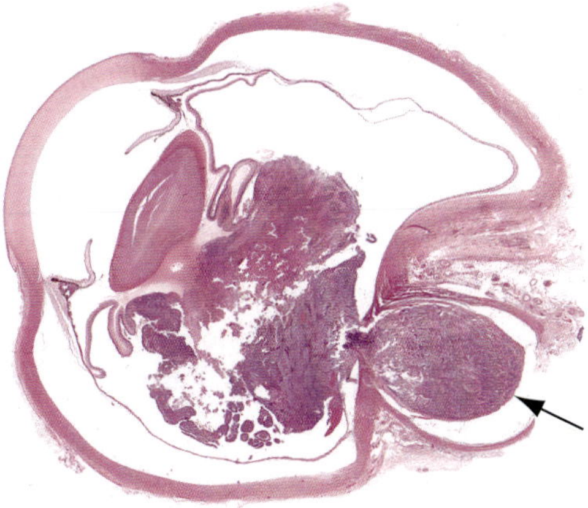

Figure 11-45 Retinoblastoma has invaded the optic nerve and extended posterior to the lamina cribrosa to the margin of resection *(arrow)* (H&E stain). This is an extremely poor prognostic sign. *(Courtesy of Nasreen A. Syed, MD.)*

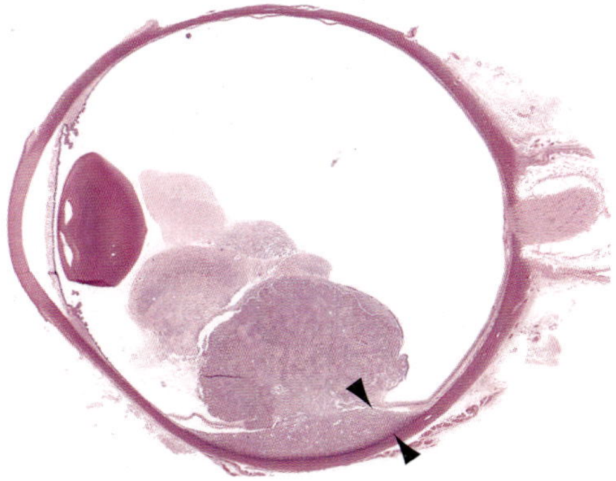

Figure 11-46 Retinoblastoma with high-risk histologic feature. Massive choroidal invasion *(between arrowheads)* (H&E stain) is defined as an invasive focus of tumor with a maximum diameter (in any dimension) measuring at least 3 mm and tumor reaching at least the inner fibers of the scleral tissue. *(Courtesy of Nasreen A. Syed, MD.)*

of prognosis. High-risk histologic features associated with metastasis and survival include optic nerve invasion (laminar, retrolaminar, or cut margin), massive choroidal invasion, extraocular extension, and extensive tumor necrosis.

Massive choroidal invasion (Fig 11-46) is commonly defined as an invasive focus of tumor with a maximum diameter (in any dimension) measuring at least 3 mm and tumor reaching at least the inner fibers of the scleral tissue. Focal choroidal invasion is defined as a tumor focus of less than 3 mm in any dimension that does not reach the sclera. Spread to regional lymph nodes may be seen when a tumor involving the anterior segment grows into the conjunctival substantia propria, especially when the trabecular meshwork is involved.

Chong EM, Coffee RE, Chintagumpala M, Hurwitz RL, Hurwitz MY, Chévez-Barrios P. Extensively necrotic retinoblastoma is associated with high-risk prognostic factors. *Arch Pathol Lab Med.* 2006;130(11):1669–1672.

Sastre X, Chantada GL, Doz F, et al.; International Retinoblastoma Staging Working Group. Proceedings of the consensus meetings from the International Retinoblastoma Staging Working Group on the pathology guidelines for the examination of enucleated eyes and evaluation of prognostic risk factors in retinoblastoma. *Arch Pathol Lab Med.* 2009;133(8): 1199–1202.

Retinocytoma

Retinocytoma is characterized histologically by numerous fleurettes admixed with individual cells that demonstrate varying degrees of photoreceptor differentiation (Fig 11-47). Retinocytoma should be differentiated from the spontaneous regression of retinoblastoma that is the end result of coagulative necrosis. See the discussion in Chapter 19.

Retinocytoma differs from retinoblastoma in the following ways:

- Retinocytoma cells have more cytoplasm and more evenly dispersed nuclear chromatin than retinoblastoma cells. Mitoses are not observed in retinocytoma.
- Although calcification may be identified in retinocytoma, necrosis is usually absent.

Medulloepithelioma

Medulloepithelioma is a congenital neuroepithelial tumor arising from primitive medullary epithelium (ie, the inner layer of the optic cup). This tumor usually occurs in the ciliary body but has also been documented in the retina and optic nerve. Clinically, medulloepithelioma may appear as a lightly pigmented or amelanotic cystic mass in the ciliary body, with erosion into the anterior chamber and iris root (see Chapter 19, Fig 19-12). Within the tumor, undifferentiated round to oval cells with little cytoplasm are organized into ribbonlike structures that have a distinct cellular polarity (Fig 11-48). Cell nuclei are

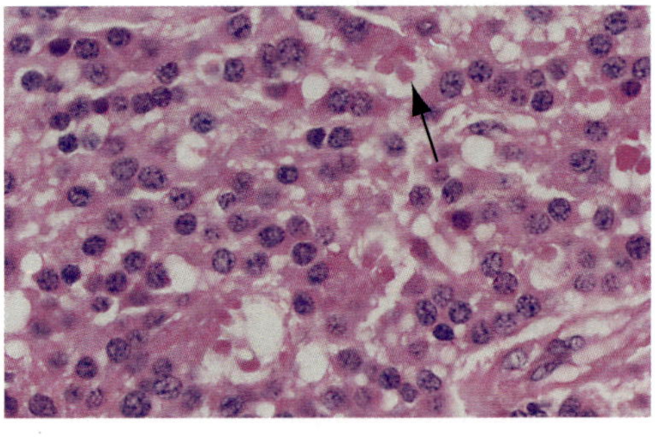

Figure 11-47 Retinocytoma. Note the exquisite degree of photoreceptor differentiation with apparent stubby inner segments *(arrow)* (H&E stain).

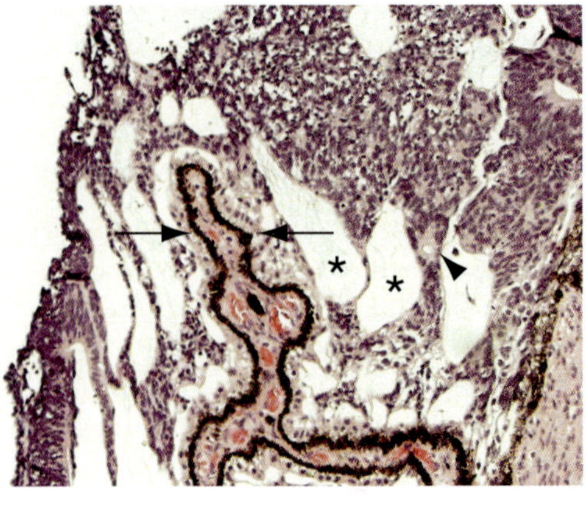

Figure 11-48 Medulloepithelioma. Histology shows a ciliary process *(between arrows)* surrounded by ribbons, cords, and small sheets of blue tumor cells with pockets of vitreous *(asterisks)* and occasional Flexner-Wintersteiner rosettes *(arrowhead)* (H&E stain). *(Courtesy of George J. Harocopos, MD.)*

stratified in 3 to 5 layers, and the entire structure is lined on one side by a thin basement membrane. One surface secretes a mucinous substance, rich in hyaluronic acid, that resembles primitive vitreous. Stratified sheets of cells are capable of forming mucinous cysts that are clinically characteristic. Homer Wright and Flexner-Wintersteiner rosettes may also be present.

Medulloepitheliomas that contain solid masses of neuroblastic cells indistinguishable from retinoblastoma are more difficult to classify. Medulloepitheliomas that have substantial numbers of undifferentiated cells with high mitotic rates and that demonstrate tissue invasion are considered malignant, although patients treated with enucleation have high survival rates, and "malignant" medulloepithelioma typically follows a relatively benign course if the tumor remains confined to the eye.

Heteroplastic tissue, such as cartilage or smooth muscle, may be found in medulloepitheliomas. Tumors composed of cells from 2 different embryonic germ layers are referred to as *teratoid medulloepitheliomas.* Malignant teratoid medulloepitheliomas demonstrate either solid areas of undifferentiated neuroblastic cells or sarcomatous transformation of heteroplastic elements. In rare cases, ciliary body medulloepithelioma presents in association with pleuropulmonary blastoma as part of a familial tumor predisposition syndrome; it may be secondary to a germline mutation in the *DICER1* gene.

Schultz KA, Yang J, Doros L, et al. *DICER1*-pleuropulmonary blastoma familial tumor predisposition syndrome: a unique constellation of neoplastic conditions. *Pathol Case Rev.* 2014;19(2):90–100.

Fuchs Adenoma

Fuchs adenoma, an acquired tumor of the nonpigmented epithelium of the ciliary body, may be associated with sectoral cataract and may simulate other iris or ciliary body neoplasms. Fuchs adenomas consist of hyperplastic, nonpigmented ciliary epithelium arranged in sheets and tubules, with alternating areas of PAS-positive basement membrane material.

Shields JA, Eagle RC Jr, Ferguson K, Shields CL. Tumors of the nonpigmented epithelium of the ciliary body: the Lorenz E. Zimmerman tribute lecture. *Retina.* 2015;35(5):957–965.

Combined Hamartoma of the Retina and RPE

A combined hamartoma of the retina and RPE is characterized clinically by the presence of a slightly elevated, variably pigmented mass that involves the RPE, peripapillary retina, optic nerve, and overlying vitreous (see Chapter 17, Fig 17-13). Frequently, a preretinal membrane that distorts the tumor's inner retinal surface is present. The lesion is often diagnosed in childhood, supporting a probable hamartomatous origin, but it is possible that the vascular changes are primary, with secondary changes in the adjacent RPE.

Histologically, the tumor is characterized by thickening of the optic nerve head and peripapillary retina, with an increased number of blood vessels (Fig 11-49). The RPE is hyperplastic and frequently migrates into the retina in a perivascular location. Vitreous condensation and fibroglial proliferation may be present on the surface of the tumor.

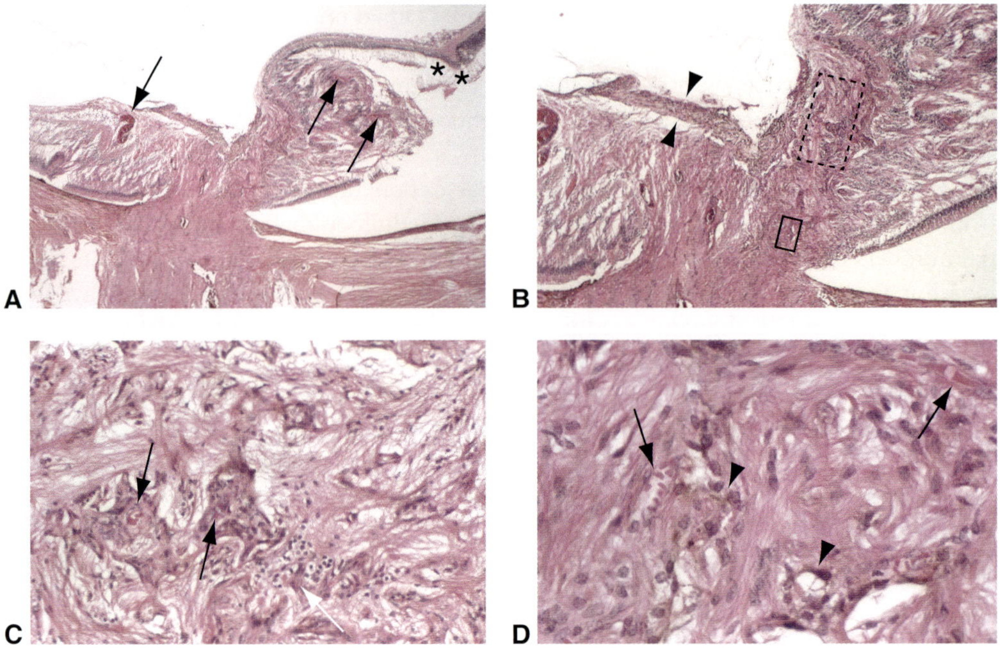

Figure 11-49 Combined hamartoma of the retina and RPE. **A,** Low-magnification photomicrograph shows thickening of the peripapillary retina, increased vascularity with variably sized blood vessels *(arrows)*, and cystic change in the outer plexiform layer *(asterisks)* (H&E stain). **B,** Thickening of the optic nerve head and peripapillary retina with an epipapillary fibroglial membrane *(between arrowheads)* (H&E stain). Box with dashed line is shown at higher magnification in part **C.** Smaller box is shown at higher magnification in part **D. C,** Hyperplastic RPE surrounding small blood vessels *(arrows)* in the peripapillary NFL (H&E stain). **D,** Small-caliber vascular channels *(arrows)* and hyperplastic RPE *(arrowheads)* in the peripapillary retina. *(Courtesy of Robert H. Rosa, Jr, MD.)*

Adenomas and Adenocarcinomas of the RPE

Neoplasia of the RPE is uncommon and is distinguished from hyperplasia of the RPE principally by the absence of a history of, or pathologic features suggesting, prior trauma or eye disease. *Adenomas* of the RPE typically retain characteristics of RPE cells, including basement membranes, cell junctions, and microvilli. *Adenocarcinomas* are distinguished from adenomas by greater anaplasia, mitotic activity, and invasion of the choroid or retina. Adenoma and adenocarcinoma of the RPE may rarely arise from CHRPE lesions. No metastases have ever been documented to occur in patients with RPE adenocarcinomas.

Shields JA, Eagle RC Jr, Shields CL, Brown GC, Lally SE. Malignant transformation of congenital hypertrophy of the retinal pigment epithelium. *Ophthalmology.* 2009;116(11): 2213–2216.

Spencer WH, ed. *Ophthalmic Pathology: An Atlas and Textbook.* 4th ed. Philadelphia: Saunders; 1997:1291–1313.

CHAPTER 12

Uveal Tract

Topography

The *iris, ciliary body,* and *choroid* constitute the uveal tract (Fig 12-1). The uveal tract is embryologically derived from mesoderm and neural crest cells. Firm attachments between the uveal tract and the sclera exist at only 3 sites: (1) the scleral spur, (2) the exit points of the vortex veins, and (3) the optic nerve.

Iris

The iris is located in front of the crystalline lens. It separates the anterior segment of the eye into 2 compartments, the anterior chamber and the posterior chamber, and forms a circular aperture (pupil) that controls the amount of light transmitted into the eye. The iris comprises 5 layers:

- anterior border layer
- stromal layer
- muscular layer
- anterior layer of pigment epithelium
- posterior layer of pigment epithelium

The anterior border layer, which represents a condensation of iris stroma and melanocytes, is coarsely ribbed with numerous crypts (Fig 12-2). The stroma contains blood vessels, nerves, melanocytes, fibrocytes, and 2 types of clump cells: macrophages containing phagocytosed pigment (type I, or clump cells of Koganei) and variants of smooth-muscle cells (type II clump cells). The vessels within the stroma have a thick collar of collagen.

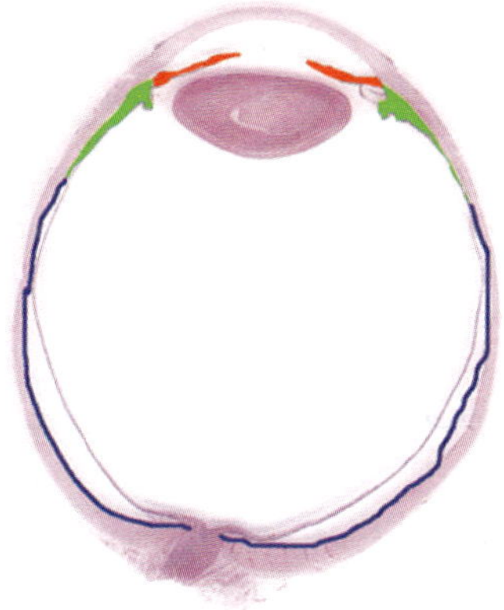

Figure 12-1 Uveal topography. The uveal tract consists of the iris *(red)*, the ciliary body *(green)*, and the choroid *(blue)*. *(Courtesy of Nasreen A. Syed, MD.)*

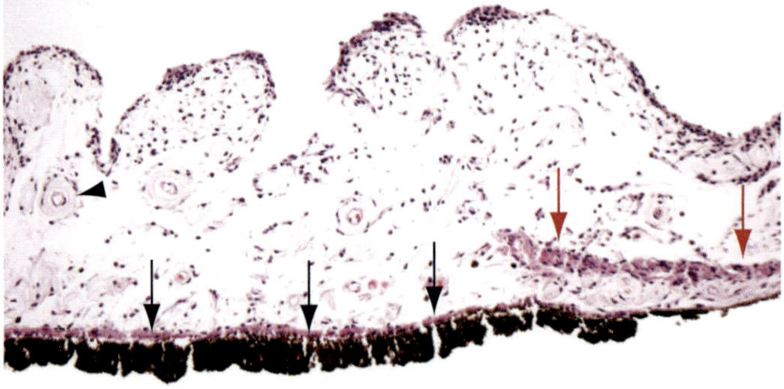

Figure 12-2 Histologic appearance of a normal iris: the anterior border layer is thrown into numerous crypts and folds. The sphincter muscle *(red arrows)* is present at the pupillary border, whereas the dilator muscle *(black arrows)* lies just anterior to the posterior pigment epithelium. Normal iris vessels demonstrate a thick collagen cuff *(arrowhead)* (hematoxylin-eosin [H&E] stain). *(Courtesy of Nasreen A. Syed, MD.)*

The muscular layer is made up of the dilator muscle and the sphincter muscle. Both are composed of smooth-muscle cells and are under autonomic control; however, the dilator muscle is part of the anterior layer of pigment epithelium. The posterior iris is lined with a double layer of cuboidal epithelium arranged in an apex-to-apex configuration. The cytoplasm of these epithelial cells is packed with melanin granules; iris color is determined by the number and size of the melanin pigment granules in the iris stromal melanocytes.

Ciliary Body

The ciliary body, which is approximately 6.0–6.5 mm wide, extends from the base of the iris and becomes continuous with the choroid at the ora serrata. The ciliary body is composed of 2 areas: the *pars plicata,* which contains the ciliary processes, and the *pars plana.*

The inner portion of the ciliary body is lined by a double layer of epithelial cells, the inner nonpigmented layer and the outer pigmented layer (Fig 12-3). The zonular fibers of the lens attach to the ciliary body in the valleys of the ciliary processes and along the pars plana. The ciliary smooth muscle comprises 3 layers of fibers: the outermost *longitudinal* layer, the middle *radial* layer, and *the innermost circular* layer. These muscle groups function as a unit during accommodation.

Choroid

The choroid is the pigmented vascular tissue that forms the middle coat of the posterior part of the eye. It extends from the ora serrata anteriorly to the optic nerve posteriorly and consists of 3 principal layers:

- lamina fusca—suprachoroidal pigmented layer with attachments to sclera
- stroma—central loose fibrovascular connective tissue with arterioles originating from the short posterior ciliary arteries
- choriocapillaris—innermost layer containing thin-walled capillaries

The choriocapillaris is the blood supply for the retinal pigment epithelium (RPE) and the outer retinal layers (Fig 12-4).

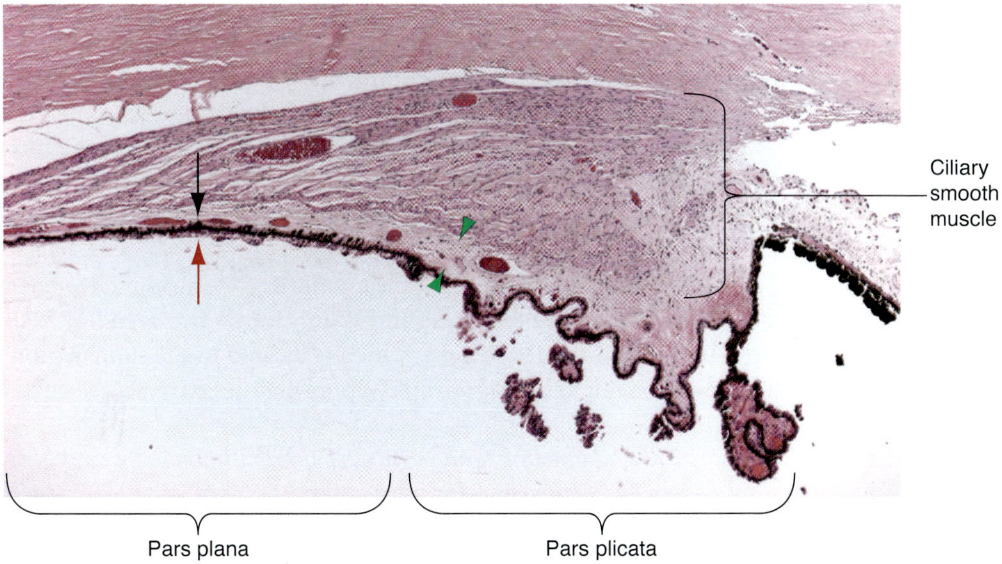

Figure 12-3 Normal ciliary body. The inner face of the ciliary body is lined with a double layer of epithelium. The inner layer is nonpigmented *(red arrow)* and the outer layer is pigmented *(black arrow).* Note the fibrovascular connective tissue interposed between the pigmented ciliary epithelium and the ciliary muscle fibers *(between green arrowheads)* (H&E stain). *(Courtesy of Nasreen A. Syed, MD.)*

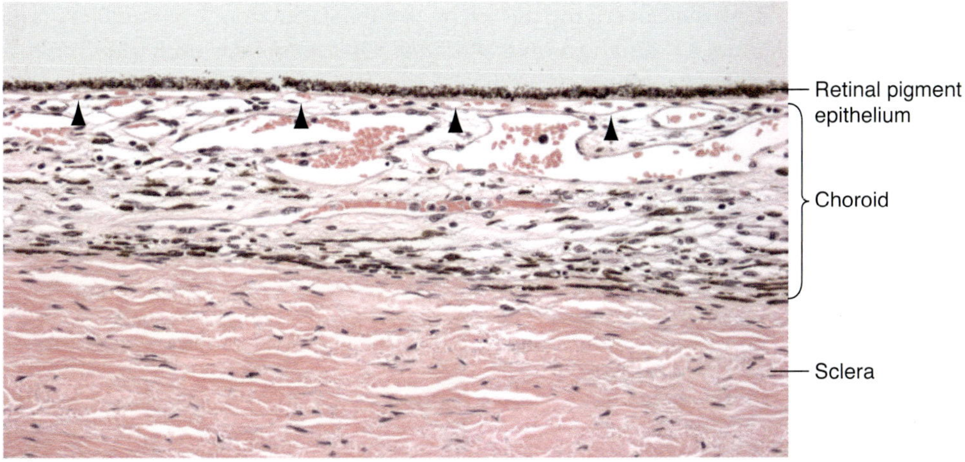

Figure 12-4 Normal choroid. The choroid is a vascular, pigmented structure present between the retinal pigment epithelium (RPE) and the sclera. The layer closest to the RPE is composed of capillaries and is known as the *choriocapillaris (arrowheads)* (H&E stain). *(Courtesy of Nasreen A. Syed, MD.)*

Congenital Anomalies

Aniridia

True aniridia, or complete absence of the iris, is rare. Most cases of aniridia are incomplete, with a narrow rim of rudimentary iris tissue present. Aniridia is usually bilateral, though sometimes asymmetric. Histologically, the rudimentary iris consists of underdeveloped ectodermal–mesodermal neural crest elements. The angle is often incompletely developed, and peripheral anterior synechiae that have an overgrowth of corneal endothelium are often present, most likely accounting for the high incidence of glaucoma associated with aniridia. Other ocular findings in aniridia include cataract, corneal pannus, and foveal hypoplasia.

Both autosomal dominant and sporadic inheritance patterns for aniridia have been described. An association between sporadic aniridia and Wilms tumor has been linked to 11p13 deletions and to mutations in the *PAX6* gene, which is located in the same region. Microcephaly, cognitive impairment, and genitourinary abnormalities have also been associated with aniridia.

See also BCSC Section 2, *Fundamentals and Principles of Ophthalmology,* and Section 6, *Pediatric Ophthalmology and Strabismus* for further discussion of aniridia.

Hingorani M, Hanson I, van Heyningen V. Aniridia. *Eur J Hum Genet.* 2012;20(10): 1011–1017.

Coloboma

A coloboma—the absence of part or all of normal ocular tissue—may affect the iris, ciliary body, choroid, or all 3 structures (Fig 12-5). Histologically, colobomas appear as an area nearly devoid of retinal and choroidal tissue. A thin layer of glial tissue (intercalary membrane) may be the only tissue overlying the sclera. See BCSC Section 2, *Fundamentals and Principles of Ophthalmology,* and Section 6, *Pediatric Ophthalmology and Strabismus,* for further discussion of uveal colobomas.

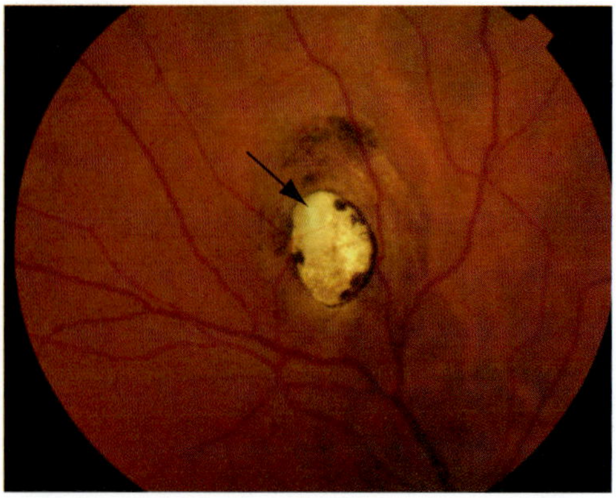

Figure 12-5 Choroidal coloboma. Note the RPE hyperplasia at the margin of the colobomatous defect and the fibroglial tissue within the coloboma *(arrow)*. *(Courtesy of Adela Castaño, COA, and Robert H. Rosa, Jr, MD.)*

Inflammations

See BCSC Section 9, *Intraocular Inflammation and Uveitis,* for further discussion of the conditions described in the following sections and an in-depth explanation of the immunologic processes involved.

Infectious

Infectious processes in the uveal tract may be restricted to that layer or part of a generalized inflammation that affects multiple or all coats of the eye. If the eye is the primary source of the infection (eg, as in posttraumatic bacterial infection), that infection is termed *exogenous.* If, however, the infection originates elsewhere in the body (eg, a ruptured diverticulum) and subsequently spreads hematogenously to involve the uveal tract, the infection is referred to as *endogenous.* A wide variety of organisms can cause infections of the uveal tract, including bacteria, fungi, viruses, and protozoa.

Histology often shows a mix of acute and chronic inflammatory cells within the choroid, ciliary body, or iris stroma. In cases of viral, fungal, or protozoal (eg, toxoplasmosis) agents, epithelioid histiocytes are typically present (granulomatous inflammation). If infection is suspected, special stains (see Chapter 3, Table 3-2) for microorganisms (tissue Gram, Gomori methenamine silver, PAS [periodic acid–Schiff], Ziehl-Neelsen) may be helpful.

Noninfectious

Sympathetic ophthalmia

Sympathetic ophthalmia is a rare bilateral granulomatous panuveitis that occurs after accidental or surgical injury to 1 eye (the *exciting,* or *inciting, eye*) followed by a latent period of weeks to years before development of uveitis in the uninjured globe (the *sympathizing eye*).

Sympathetic ophthalmia is a clinical diagnosis. The histopathologic findings are not pathognomonic. Furthermore, immunosuppressive therapy may modify the histologic findings. Histologically, a diffuse granulomatous inflammatory reaction that is composed of lymphocytes and epithelioid histiocytes containing phagocytosed melanin pigment is present within the uveal tract (Figs 12-6, 12-7). Plasma cells are usually scant, suggesting a cell-mediated response. Classically, in the early stages of the disease, the choriocapillaris is spared. Varying degrees of inflammation may be present in the anterior chamber, such as clusters of histiocytes deposited on the corneal endothelium *(mutton-fat keratic precipitates). Dalen-Fuchs nodules,* which are accumulations of epithelioid histiocytes and lymphocytes between the RPE and Bruch membrane, may be seen in some cases (see Fig 12-7). However, Dalen-Fuchs nodules may also be present in other diseases, such as Vogt-Koyanagi-Harada syndrome, and thus are not pathognomonic of sympathetic ophthalmia.

See BCSC Section 7, *Orbit, Eyelids, and Lacrimal System,* and Section 9, *Intraocular Inflammation and Uveitis,* for further discussion.

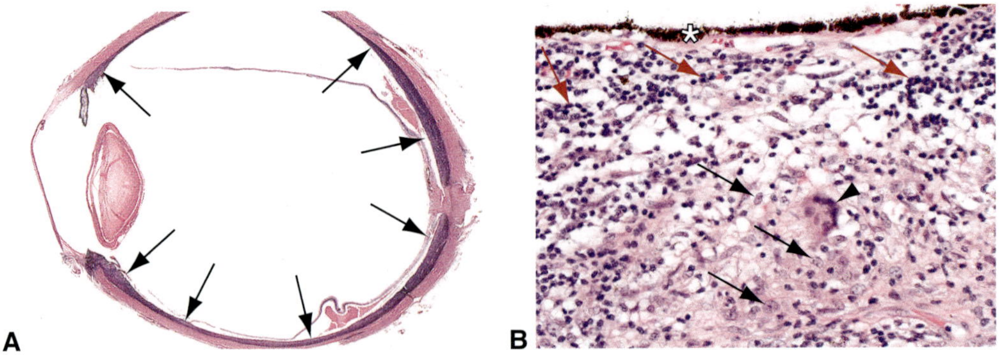

Figure 12-6 Sympathetic ophthalmia. **A,** Diffuse infiltration of the uveal tract by chronic inflammatory cells *(arrows)* (H&E stain). **B,** Higher magnification of the RPE *(asterisk)* and choroid (400×, H&E stain) shows the presence of a multinucleated giant cell *(arrowhead)* and epithelioid histiocytes *(black arrows)* and lymphocytes *(red arrows)*. Note the relative sparing of the choriocapillaris beneath the RPE. *(Part A courtesy of Hans E. Grossniklaus, MD; part B courtesy of Michele Bloomer, MD.)*

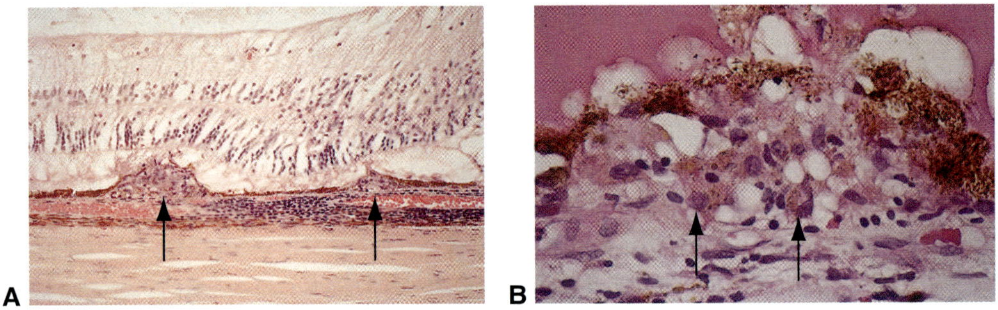

Figure 12-7 Dalen-Fuchs nodules in sympathetic ophthalmia. **A,** Focal aggregates of inflammatory cells are located between the RPE and Bruch membrane *(arrows)* (H&E stain). **B,** Higher magnification demonstrates the presence of epithelioid histiocytes containing cytoplasmic pigment *(arrows)* within the nodules (H&E stain). *(Courtesy of Hans E. Grossniklaus, MD.)*

Vogt-Koyanagi-Harada syndrome

Vogt-Koyanagi-Harada (VKH) syndrome is a rare cause of posterior or diffuse uveitis and may have both ocular and systemic manifestations. The syndrome occurs more commonly in patients with Asian or Native American ancestry and usually affects individuals between 30 and 50 years of age.

A chronic, diffuse granulomatous uveitis resembles that seen in sympathetic ophthalmia. However, in VKH, the entire choroid, including the choriocapillaris, is typically involved by the inflammatory reaction. The granulomatous inflammation may extend into the retina. Because the disease is one of exacerbation and remission, chorioretinal scarring and RPE hyperplasia and/or atrophy may also occur.

Sarcoidosis

Sarcoidosis is an inflammatory disorder that can affect nearly all systems in the body. The disease is characterized by inflammatory nodule formation in various organs and tissues.

The uveal tract is the most common site of ocular involvement. Anteriorly, inflammatory nodules of the iris may develop, either at the pupillary margin *(Koeppe nodules)* or elsewhere on the iris *(Busacca nodules).* In the posterior segment, chorioretinitis, periphlebitis, and chorioretinal nodules may be present. Periphlebitis may appear clinically as inflammatory lesions called *candlewax drippings.* Inflammatory cell infiltration may cause the optic nerve to become edematous.

Histologically, the classic sarcoid nodule is composed of non-necrotizing (noncaseating) granulomas. These granulomas are collections of epithelioid histiocytes, sometimes accompanied by multinucleated giant cells, surrounded by a cuff of lymphocytes (Fig 12-8). In the uvea, the inflammatory infiltrate may show a more diffuse distribution of lymphocytes and epithelioid histiocytes (granulomatous inflammation). The multinucleated giant cells may demonstrate *asteroid bodies* (star-shaped, acidophilic bodies) and/or *Schaumann bodies* (spherical, basophilic, calcified bodies). Neither asteroid nor Schaumann bodies are pathognomonic for sarcoidosis.

Behçet disease

Behçet disease is an occlusive systemic vasculitis that can cause nongranulomatous necrotizing inflammation in the uveal tract. See BCSC Section 9, *Intraocular Inflammation and Uveitis,* for further discussion.

Juvenile xanthogranuloma

Juvenile xanthogranuloma (JXG) is an uncommon inflammatory condition that occurs in children. The skin and uvea are commonly affected areas; in the uveal tract, lesions may present as a solid mass, mimicking a neoplastic process. Histologically, the characteristic appearance of the lesions includes the presence of lipid-laden histiocytes, Touton giant cells, lymphocytes, and occasional eosinophils (Fig 12-9). The lesions are often vascularized, and the blood vessels tend to be fragile, resulting in intralesional hemorrhage. Iris JXG lesions may cause a spontaneous hyphema.

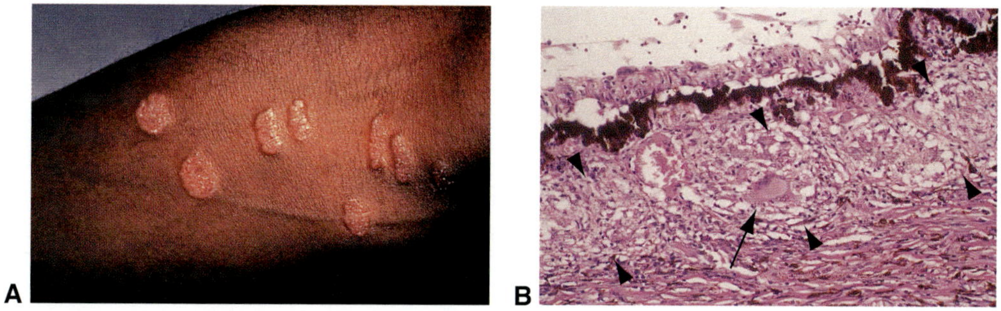

Figure 12-8 Sarcoidosis. **A,** Gross appearance of multiple discrete nodules on the skin of the upper extremity. **B,** Histology of sarcoid nodule showing epithelioid histiocytes *(between arrowheads)* and multinucleated giant cells *(arrow)* (H&E stain). *(Part A courtesy of Curtis E. Margo, MD; part B courtesy of Hans E. Grossniklaus, MD.)*

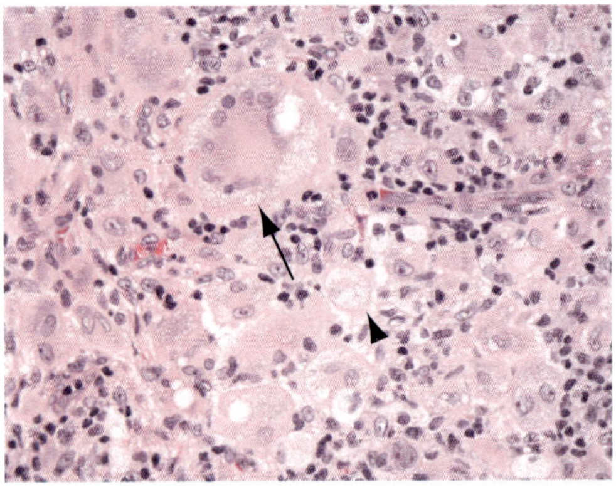

Figure 12-9 Juvenile xanthogranuloma. Touton giant cells *(arrow)* with ring of nuclei, inner eosinophilic cytoplasm, and outer vacuolated or foamy cytoplasm; foamy histiocytes *(arrowhead)*; and lymphocytes are admixed (H&E stain). *(Courtesy of Nasreen A. Syed, MD.)*

Degenerations

Rubeosis Iridis

Rubeosis iridis, or neovascularization of the iris (see Chapter 11, Fig 11-27), is commonly found in surgically enucleated blind eyes. It may be associated with a wide variety of conditions (see BCSC Section 10, *Glaucoma,* Table 5-4). Histologically, the new vessels tend to lack supporting tissue and do not possess the thick fibrous cuff that encircles normal iris vessels. The new vessels grow on the anterior surface of the iris and may extend into the angle. The neovascular membrane has a fibrous component consisting of myofibroblasts, which contract and eventually lead to angle closure due to formation of peripheral anterior synechiae. Neovascularization of the angle often results in *neovascular glaucoma,* a secondary glaucoma. Membrane contraction may also lead to *ectropion uveae,* an anterior displacement or dragging of the posterior iris pigment epithelial layer onto the anterior iris surface at the pupillary border. The anterior surface of the iris often becomes flattened. In advanced cases, atrophy of the dilator muscle, attenuation of the pigment epithelium, and stromal fibrosis may occur (Fig 12-10).

Hyalinization of the Ciliary Body

Over time, the ciliary body processes become hyalinized and fibrosed, losing stromal cellularity; occasionally, dystrophic calcification develops (Fig 12-11). The thin, delicate processes become blunted and attenuated, and the stroma becomes more eosinophilic. This process is a normal age-related change to the ciliary body and is not considered pathologic, although it does contribute functionally to the development of presbyopia.

Choroidal Neovascularization

Choroidal neovascularization is discussed at length in Chapter 11 and in BCSC Section 12, *Retina and Vitreous.*

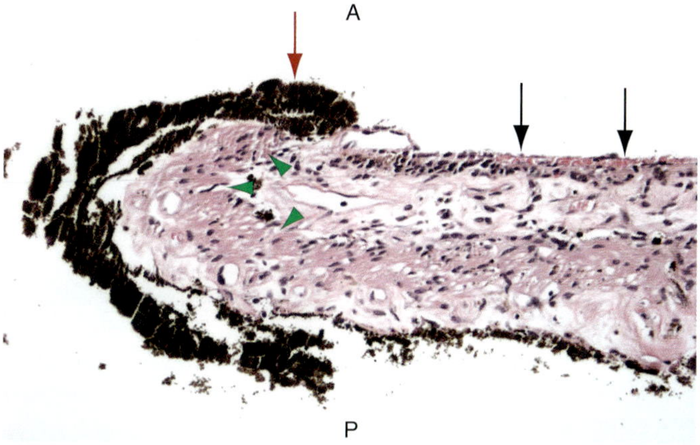

Figure 12-10 Iris neovascularization (rubeosis iridis). Small blood vessels sprout from existing iris vasculature, typically on the surface of the iris *(black arrows)*. Note the flat anterior surface of the iris (A = anterior, P = posterior). The contractile component of the neovascular membrane may result in dragging of the iris pigment epithelium *(red arrow)* and sphincter muscle *(green arrowheads)* anteriorly at the pupillary margin, in turn resulting in *ectropion uveae* (H&E stain). *(Courtesy of Nasreen A. Syed, MD.)*

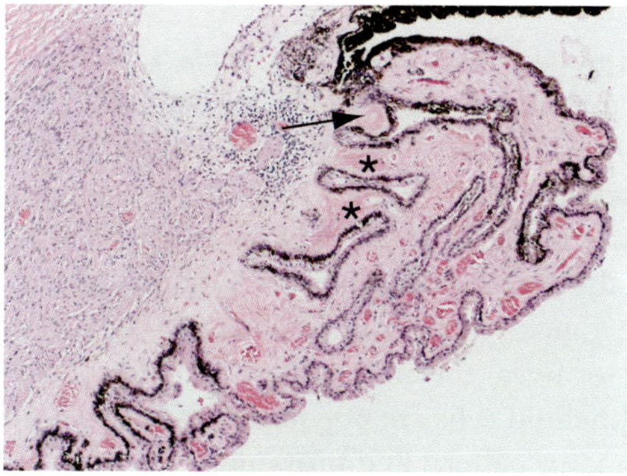

Figure 12-11 Age-related changes in the ciliary body include sclerotic vessels *(arrow)* and hyalinization *(asterisks)* (100×, H&E stain). *(Courtesy of Michele Bloomer, MD.)*

Neoplasia

Uveal neoplasms are also discussed in detail in Chapters 17, 18, and 20. The discussion of uveal neoplasms in this chapter focuses primarily on histopathology.

Iris

Nevus

An *iris nevus* is a localized proliferation of melanocytic cells that generally appears as a darkly pigmented lesion of the iris stroma with minimal distortion of the iris architecture (see Chapter 17, Fig 17-1). An iris nevus appears histologically as an accumulation of branching dendritic cells or spindle cells, usually with melanin granules in the cytoplasm.

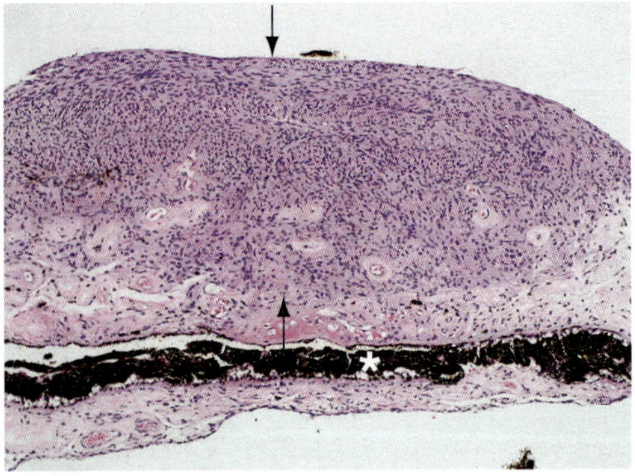

Figure 12-12 Iris nevus (100×, H&E stain). Spindle-shaped nevus cells *(arrows)* form a plaque on the surface of the iris and extend down into the iris stroma just anterior to the posterior pigmented epithelium *(asterisk)*. *(Courtesy of Michele Bloomer, MD.)*

The nuclei of these cells are typically oblong or ovoid with a bland appearance and indistinct nucleoli. Less commonly, epithelioid nevus cells may be observed. A variety of growth patterns and cytologic appearances is possible, but cellular atypia and significant mitotic activity are not present. The nevus cells aggregate within the stroma and sometimes also appear in a plaquelike distribution on the surface of the iris (Fig 12-12). Occasionally, nevus cells may extend into the adjacent angle structures.

Melanoma

Melanomas arising in the iris tend to follow a nonaggressive clinical course, in contrast to posterior (ciliochoroidal) melanomas. The majority of iris melanomas develop in the inferior sectors of the iris (see Chapter 17, Fig 17-3). The lesions can be quite vascularized and may occasionally cause spontaneous hyphema.

Iris melanomas can be composed of spindle melanoma cells, epithelioid melanoma cells, or a combination of these. Histologically, spindle cells possess plump, spindle-shaped nuclei that have a coarse, granular appearance and prominent nucleoli. These cells are the equivalent of spindle-B cells in posterior uveal melanoma (see the "Melanoma" section under Choroid and Ciliary Body). Epithelioid cells are polyhedral in shape, with large, round nuclei that have a clumped chromatin pattern and prominent eosinophilic nucleoli. Both types of cells tend to have a high nuclear-to-cytoplasmic ratio. The cytoplasm of melanoma cells can range from amelanotic to heavily pigmented. Typically, iris melanomas grow as a solid mass in the stroma, sometimes covered by a surface plaque. Occasionally, they may demonstrate satellite lesions or a diffuse growth pattern that replaces normal stroma (Fig 12-13). The modified Callender classification for posterior melanomas (see the "Melanoma" section) is not applicable to iris melanomas in terms of prognostic significance. Iris melanomas are classified by a separate staging system, which is based on infiltration of adjacent structures and the presence or absence of coexisting glaucoma.

Although iris melanomas may grow in a locally aggressive fashion, they rarely metastasize. One exception occurs when melanomas grow to diffusely involve the entire iris stroma. The melanoma may invade into the anterior chamber angle and extend posteriorly to involve the ciliary body.

Edge S, Byrd DR, Compton CC, Fritz AG, Greene FL, Trotti A, eds. *AJCC Cancer Staging Manual.* 7th ed. New York: Springer; 2010.

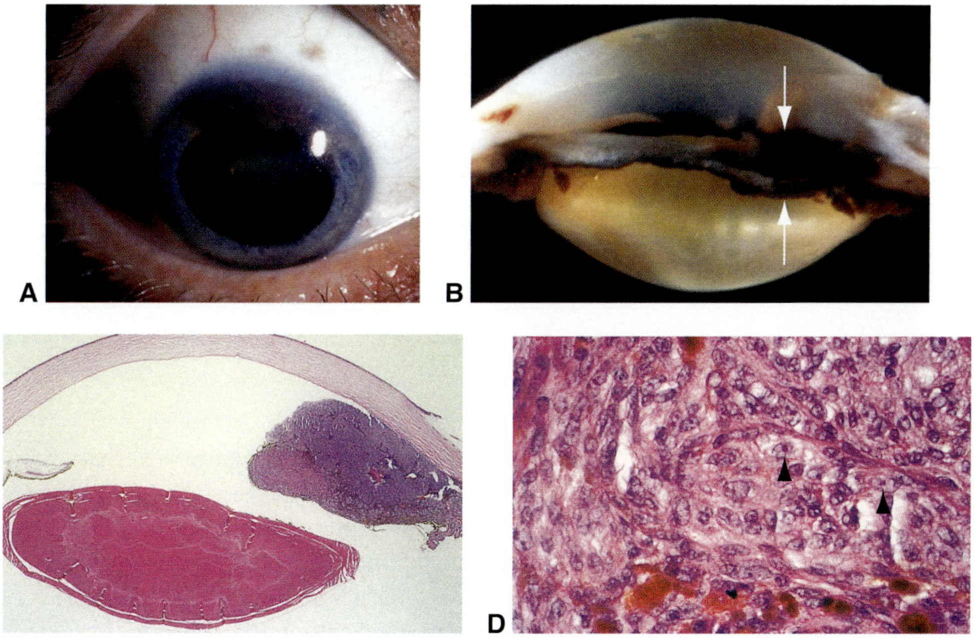

Figure 12-13 Iris melanoma. **A,** Clinical appearance. The pigmented tumor is seen between 10:30 and 2:00. **B,** Gross appearance of pigmented iris mass *(between arrows)*. **C,** Low magnification shows the iris melanoma completely replacing the normal iris stroma, extending into the anterior chamber, touching the posterior cornea, and occluding the angle (H&E stain). **D,** Histologic examination shows numerous plump epithelioid melanoma cells containing prominent nucleoli *(arrowheads)* (H&E stain). *(Courtesy of Hans E. Grossniklaus, MD.)*

Choroid and Ciliary Body

Nevus

Most uveal tract nevi (>90%) develop in the choroid (see Chapter 17, Fig 17-2). Nevus cells are divided into one of the following 4 types:

- *plump polyhedral:* abundant cytoplasm is filled with pigment and has a small, round to oval nucleus with bland appearance
- *slender spindle* (Fig 12-14): cytoplasm contains scant pigment and a small, dark, elongated nucleus
- *plump fusiform dendritic:* morphology is intermediate between plump polyhedral and slender spindle
- *balloon cells:* abundant, foamy cytoplasm lacks pigment and has a bland nucleus

Depending on the size and location of the nevus, it may exert nonspecific effects on adjacent ocular tissues. The associated choriocapillaris may become compressed or obliterated, and drusen may form overlying the nevus. Less commonly, the nevus may be associated with localized serous detachments of the overlying RPE or neurosensory retina; in addition, secondary choroidal neovascularization may develop.

Most choroidal nevi remain stationary over long periods of observation. However, the presence of nevus cells that are associated with some melanomas supplies evidence that melanomas may arise from choroidal nevi.

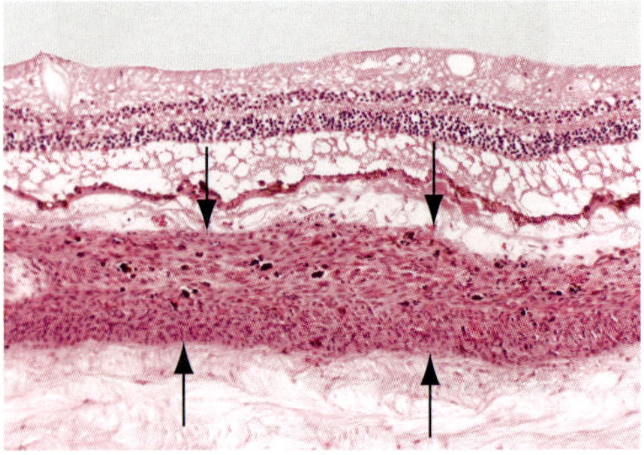

Figure 12-14 Spindle-cell choroidal nevus *(between arrows)* is composed of slender, spindle-shaped cells with thin, homogeneous nuclei (H&E stain). *(Courtesy of Nasreen A. Syed, MD.)*

Melanocytoma

Melanocytoma is a specific type of uveal tract nevus (magnocellular nevus) that warrants separate consideration. These jet-black lesions may occur anywhere in the uveal tract, but they appear most commonly in the peripapillary region (see Chapter 15, Fig 15-12B).

Histologically, a melanocytoma is composed of plump polyhedral cells with small nuclei and abundant cytoplasm. Because the nevus cells are so heavily pigmented, it is usually necessary to obtain bleached sections to accurately study the cytologic features (see Chapter 15, Fig 15-12C, D). Areas of cystic degeneration or necrosis may be observed.

Melanoma

The most common primary intraocular malignancy in adults is melanoma arising from the ciliary body and choroid. When this type of tumor grows to a significant size, it may extend beyond its site of origin (ie, from the choroid to the ciliary body and vice versa). Ciliary body and choroidal melanomas exhibit similar features and may be referred to collectively as posterior uveal melanomas, which have similar histologic features and prognostic implications.

Histologically, posterior uveal melanomas are composed of spindle cells and/or epithelioid cells (Figs 12-15, 12-16, 12-17). Less commonly, balloon cells similar to those seen in nevi may be present. Spindle cell melanomas consist primarily of spindle-B melanoma cells. They may also contain spindle-A cells; however, a tumor consisting entirely of spindle-A cells is considered a nevus. The cytoplasmic melanin content in melanoma cells

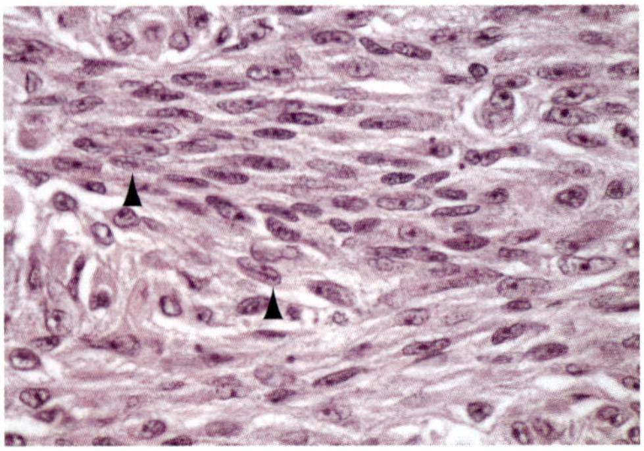

Figure 12-15 Spindle-A cells have slender, elongated nuclei with small nucleoli. A central stripe may be present down the long axis of the nucleus *(arrowheads)* (H&E stain). *(Courtesy of Nasreen A. Syed, MD.)*

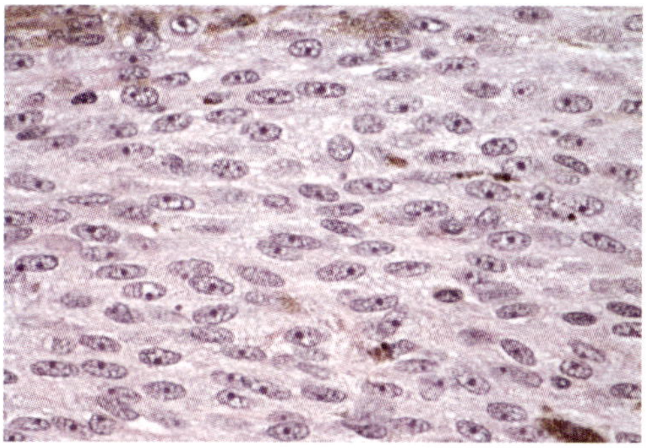

Figure 12-16 Compared with spindle-A cells, spindle-B cells demonstrate a higher nuclear-to-cytoplasmic ratio, more coarsely granular chromatin, and plumper, large nuclei. Nucleoli are prominent, and mitoses are present, though not in large numbers (H&E stain). Tumors composed of a mix of spindle-A and spindle-B cells are designated *spindle cell melanomas.* *(Courtesy of Nasreen A. Syed, MD.)*

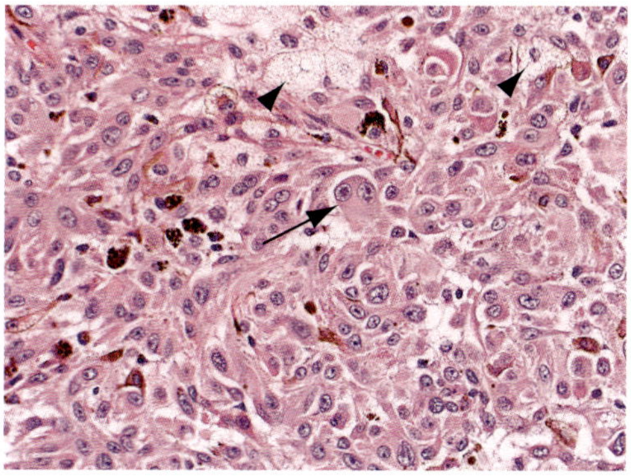

Figure 12-17 Epithelioid melanoma cells (400×, H&E). These cells resemble epithelium because of abundant eosinophilic cytoplasm and enlarged round to oval-shaped nuclei. Epithelioid melanoma cells often lack cohesiveness and demonstrate marked pleomorphism, including the formation of multinucleated tumor cells *(arrow).* Nuclei have a conspicuous nuclear membrane, very coarse chromatin, and large nucleoli. Note the balloon cells *(arrowheads).* *(Courtesy of Michele Bloomer, MD.)*

can vary considerably. The mitotic rate in melanomas tends to be low, and these tumors may exhibit variable amounts of necrosis.

Melanomas typically start as dome-shaped lesions and, as they grow and break through Bruch membrane, they acquire a mushroom or collar-button shape (Fig 12-18). Less commonly, choroidal lesions may grow in a diffuse pattern, replacing normal choroid without achieving significant height (Fig 12-19). In the ciliary body, the equivalent of the diffuse pattern is the *ring melanoma,* in which the tumor extends for the entire circumference of the ciliary body (Fig 12-20).

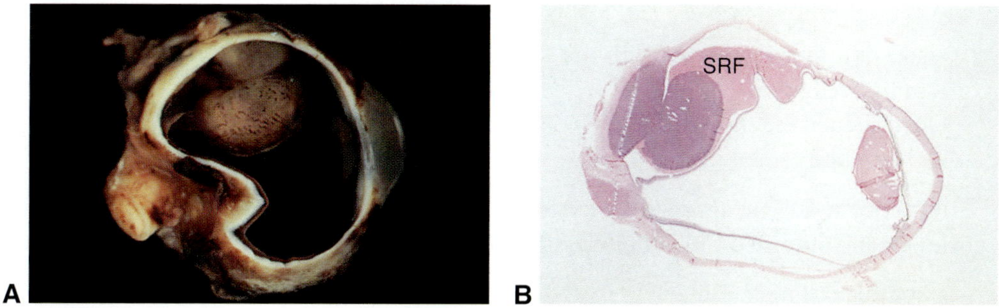

Figure 12-18 Choroidal melanoma with rupture through Bruch membrane. **A,** Gross appearance. **B,** Microscopic appearance. Note the subretinal fluid (SRF) adjacent to the tumor (H&E stain).

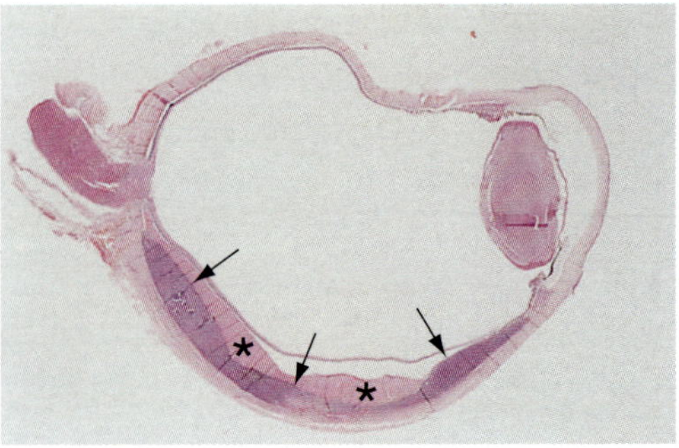

Figure 12-19 Some melanomas grow in a diffuse placoid fashion, replacing normal choroid, without achieving significant height *(arrows)*. Note the eosinophilic proteinaceous material *(asterisks)* interposed between the retina and the tumor, corresponding to exudative retinal detachment overlying the tumor (H&E stain).

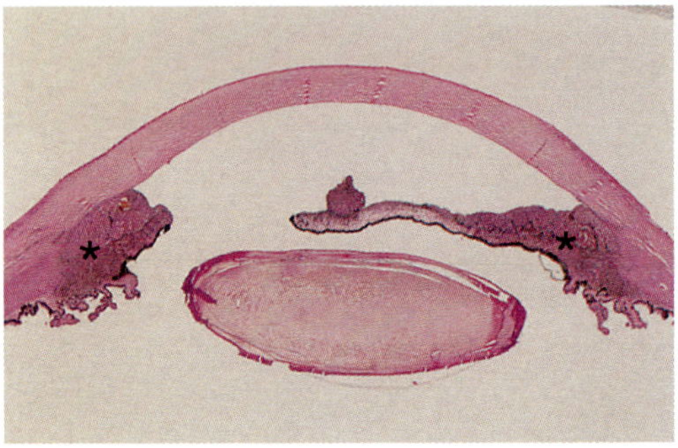

Figure 12-20 By definition, a ring melanoma *(asterisks)* follows the major arterial circle of the iris circumferentially around the eye (H&E stain).

Choroidal melanomas may also cause serous detachments of the overlying and adjacent retina, with subsequent degenerative changes in the outer segments of the photoreceptors (see Figs 12-18B, 12-19). Melanomas may extend through scleral emissary canals to gain access to the episcleral surface and the orbit (Fig 12-21). Less commonly, aggressive melanomas may directly invade the underlying sclera or overlying retina (Fig 12-22). Direct invasion of the anterior chamber or mechanical blockage due to forward iris displacement may lead to secondary glaucoma (Fig 12-23). In addition, tumor necrosis may lead to the dispersal of melanin pigment, which can then enter the anterior chamber and angle, causing a type of secondary glaucoma called *melanomalytic glaucoma* (see Chapter 7, Fig 7-12).

Several factors, which can be identified via pathologic examination, have been significantly correlated with survival in patients with posterior uveal melanomas. The most important histologic variables associated with survival are

- size of tumor in contact with the sclera
- tumor cell type
- extraocular extension
- ciliary body involvement

Posterior uveal melanomas are cytologically classified into one of the following categories via the modified Callender classification:

- spindle cell melanoma
- epithelioid melanoma
- mixed-cell type (mixture of spindle and epithelioid cells)

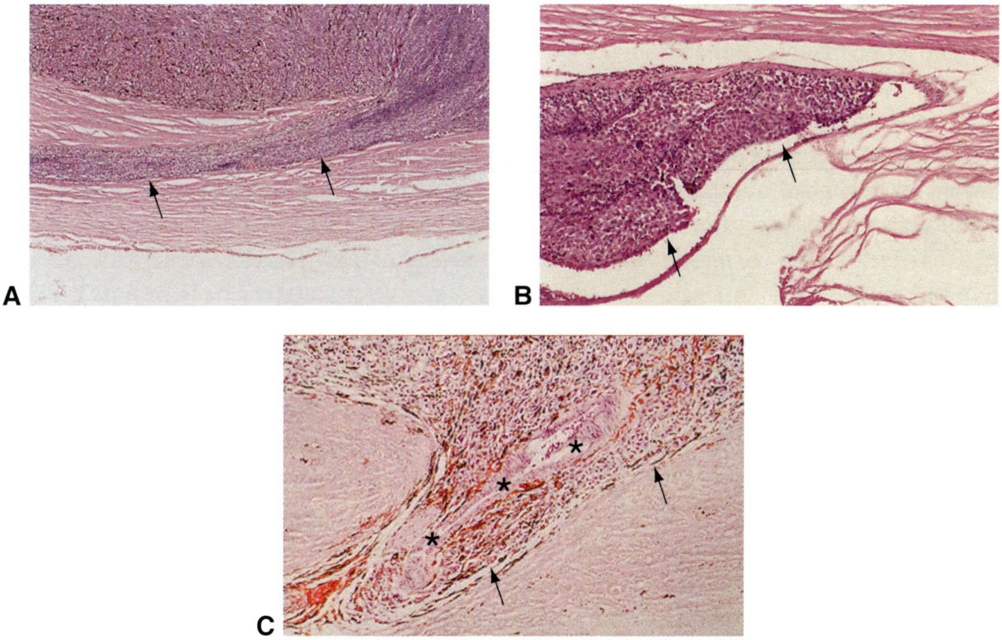

Figure 12-21 Scleral canal and vortex vein invasion by melanoma. **A,** Note the melanoma cells tracking along scleral emissary canals *(arrows)* (H&E stain). **B,** Melanoma is found within the vortex vein *(arrows)* (H&E stain). **C,** Some melanomas *(arrows)* track along the outer sheaths of posterior ciliary vessels *(asterisks)* and nerves (H&E stain).

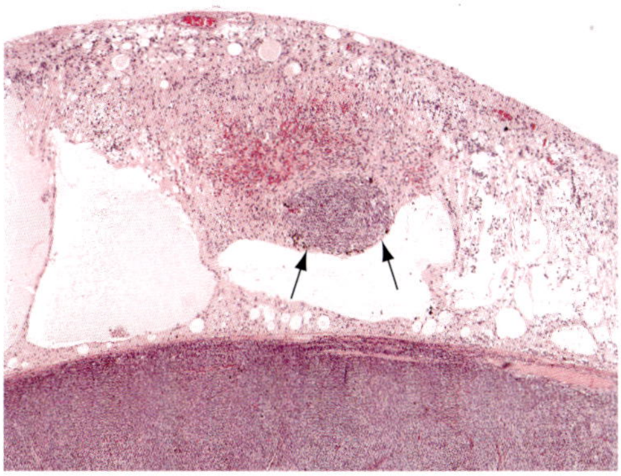

Figure 12-22 Invasion of neurosensory retina by melanoma *(arrows).* Note the atrophy of overlying outer retina, cystoid edema, and intraretinal hemorrhage (H&E stain). *(Courtesy of Nasreen A. Syed, MD.)*

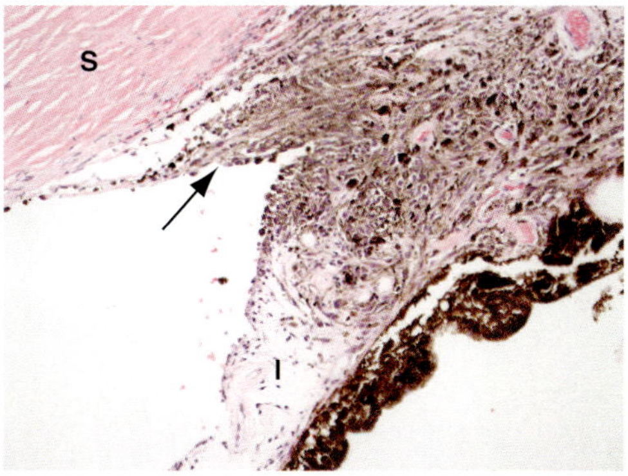

Figure 12-23 Ciliary body melanoma invading the angle (100×, H&E). Pigmented melanoma cells from a ciliary body melanoma extend anteriorly into the trabecular meshwork *(arrow).* S = Sclera, I = Iris. *(Courtesy of Michele Bloomer, MD.)*

Spindle cell melanoma has the best prognosis, and epithelioid melanoma the worst. Melanomas of mixed-cell type have an intermediate prognosis. Some authors have suggested that survival following enucleation in mixed-cell melanomas decreases with increasing proportions of epithelioid cells. In rare cases, a melanoma undergoes extensive necrosis, and precludes classification. Completely necrotic melanomas assume the same prognosis as mixed-cell melanomas.

The modified Callender classification has some disadvantages. First, there is continuing controversy about the minimum number of epithelioid cells needed for a melanoma to be classified as mixed-cell type. Second, the classification is difficult to reproduce, even among experienced ophthalmic pathologists, because the cytologic features of the melanoma cells reflect a continuous spectrum.

The *mean of the 10 largest melanoma cell nucleoli (MLN)* correlates well with mortality after enucleation. Intrinsic tumor extravascular matrix patterns have prognostic significance. Tumors containing more complex extravascular matrix patterns such as closed loops or networks (3 back-to-back loops) are associated with an increased incidence of subsequent metastases (Fig 12-24). Tumor infiltrating macrophages, some of which are pigmented, are universally found; their number relates to tumor prognostication.

Microvascular density shows an association with increased incidence of subsequent metastases that is the same, if not higher, than MLN and extravascular matrix patterns, and is relevant given that the mode of metastasis is overwhelmingly hematogenous.

Other factors associated with an increased mortality rate include extrascleral extension, anterior or juxtapapillary location of the tumor, and the presence of tumor-infiltrating lymphocytes. Invasion through Bruch membrane does not affect survival rates.

Metastases almost invariably result from the hematogenous spread of melanoma to the liver; more than 95% of tumor-related deaths have liver involvement. In as many as one-third of tumor-related deaths, the liver is the sole site of metastasis.

Some types of posterior uveal melanomas show biologic behavior that cannot be predicted according to the criteria just discussed. Survival rates of patients with diffuse ciliary body melanomas (ring melanoma) are particularly poor. These relatively flat tumors, which are almost always of mixed-cell type, may grow circumferentially without becoming significantly elevated. Diffuse choroidal melanomas have a similarly poor prognosis.

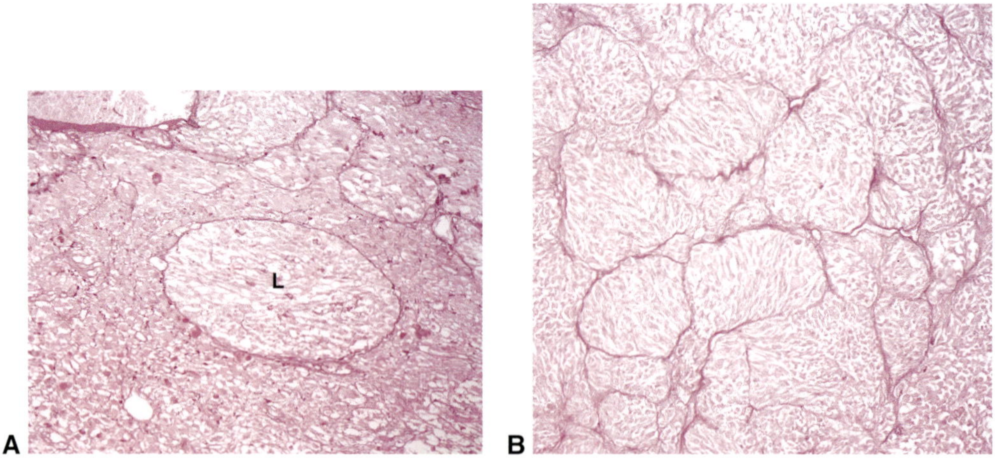

Figure 12-24 Extravascular matrix patterns in uveal melanoma. **A,** Closed loop (L) (PAS stain). **B,** Network (3 or more back-to-back loops) (PAS stain). *(Courtesy of Nasreen A. Syed, MD.)*

Cytogenetic studies of posterior uveal melanoma have shown that mutually exclusive mutations in *GNAQ* and *GNA11* are an initiating event in the development of uveal melanomas and nevi. Approximately half of uveal melanomas demonstrate monosomy of chromosome 3. A smaller proportion demonstrates gain or loss of a chromosome in chromosomes 1, 6, or 8. Monosomy 3 and trisomy 8 are associated with increased mortality. Gene expression profiling provides prognostic classification of uveal melanomas. The test, which requires a small amount of fresh or paraffin-embedded tissue, classifies these tumors as either Class 1a (low metastatic potential), Class 1b (intermediate metastatic potential), or Class 2 (high metastatic potential). Mutation of *BAP1* is thought to be a later event that confers metastatic potential. More recently, mutations in *SF3B1* and *EIF1AX* have been found to be associated with a better prognosis in uveal melanoma.

See Chapter 17 for further discussion of posterior uveal melanomas.

Coupland SE, Lake SL, Zeschnigk M, Damato BE. Molecular pathology of uveal melanoma. *Eye (Lond).* 2013;27(2):230–242.

Harbour JW, Chao DL. A molecular revolution in uveal melanoma: implications for patient care and targeted therapy. *Ophthalmology.* 2014;121(6):1281–1288.

Metastatic Tumors

Metastatic lesions are the most common intraocular tumors in adults. These lesions most often involve the choroid, but can affect any ocular structure. Unlike primary uveal melanoma, metastatic lesions are often multiple and may be bilateral. Although these lesions typically assume a flattened growth pattern, rare cases of collar-button or mushroom-shaped lesions have been reported. Although tumors from many different primary sites have been reported, the most common primary tumors metastasizing to the eye are breast carcinoma in women and lung carcinoma in men (Fig 12-25). Histologically, metastatic tumors may recapitulate the appearance of the primary lesion, or they may appear less differentiated. Special histochemical and immunohistochemical stains can be helpful in diagnosing metastatic lesions, determining the origin of the primary tumor and in some cases guiding therapy for that tumor. The importance of a careful clinical history cannot be overemphasized. See Chapter 20 for further discussion of metastatic tumors.

Other Uveal Tumors

Hemangioma

Hemangiomas of the choroid occur in 2 specific forms: circumscribed (ie, localized) and diffuse. *Circumscribed* choroidal hemangioma typically occurs in patients without systemic disorders; *diffuse* choroidal hemangioma is generally seen in patients with Sturge-Weber syndrome (encephalofacial angiomatosis).

Histologically, both diffuse and circumscribed hemangiomas show accumulations of variably sized vessels within the choroid (Fig 12-26). The lesions may appear as predominantly capillary hemangiomas, cavernous hemangiomas, or a mix of the two. There may be compressed melanocytes, hyperplastic RPE, and fibrous tissue proliferation in the adjacent and overlying choroid. See also Chapter 18 (particularly Figs 18-1 and 18-2) in this volume and BCSC Section 12, *Retina and Vitreous* (particularly Fig 9-6).

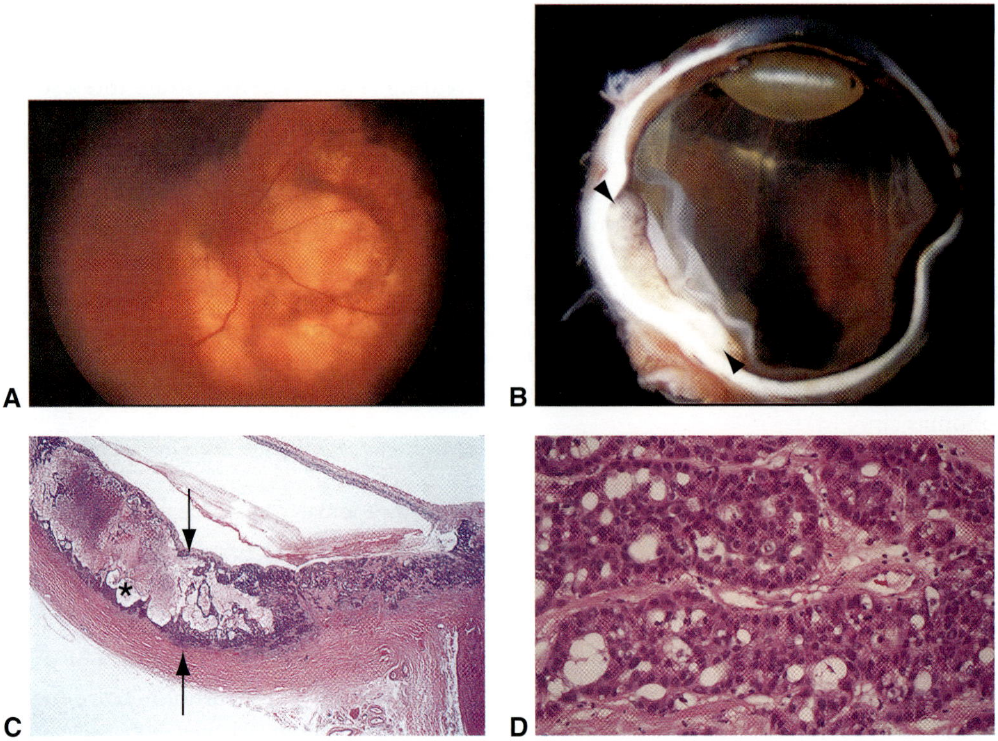

Figure 12-25 Choroidal metastasis. **A,** Clinical appearance of a metastatic lesion from a primary lung tumor. **B,** Gross appearance of lesion *(between arrowheads).* **C,** Choroidal metastasis from lung adenocarcinoma; histology shows adenocarcinoma *(between arrows)* with mucin production *(asterisk)* (H&E stain). Note overlying retinal detachment. **D,** Higher magnification depicts a well-differentiated adenocarcinoma with distinct glandular appearance (H&E stain). *(Courtesy of Hans E. Grossniklaus, MD.)*

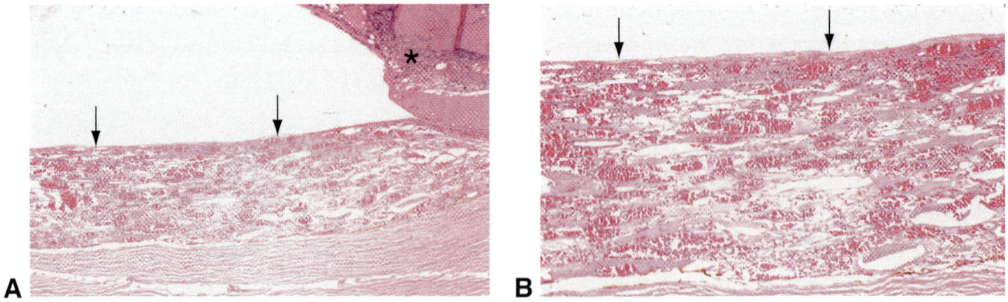

Figure 12-26 Choroidal hemangioma with a large number of thin-walled, variably sized vessels within the choroid. **A,** Low-magnification view shows exudative retinal detachment overlying the lesion *(asterisk)* (H&E stain). *Arrows* designate Bruch membrane. **B,** Higher magnification (H&E stain); *arrows* designate Bruch membrane. *(Courtesy of Nasreen A. Syed, MD.)*

Choroidal osteoma

Choroidal osteomas are benign bony tumors that typically arise from the juxtapapillary choroid; they are seen in adolescent to young adult patients, more commonly in females. The characteristic lesion appears yellow to orange and has well-defined margins (see Chapter 17, Fig 17-11D). Histologically, the tumor is composed of compact bone and is located in the peripapillary choroid. The intratrabecular spaces are filled with a loose connective tissue that contains large and small blood vessels, vacuolated mesenchymal cells, and scattered mast cells. The bony trabeculae contain osteocytes, cement lines, and occasional osteoclasts. See Chapter 17 for further discussion.

Lymphoid proliferation

The choroid may be the site of lymphoid proliferation, either as a primary ocular process or in association with systemic lymphoproliferative disease.

Primary choroidal lymphomas (previously known as *uveal lymphoid hyperplasia or infiltration*) are mostly low-grade, B-cell tumors similar to extranodal marginal zone lymphomas elsewhere. High-grade choroidal lymphomas (Fig 12-27) are usually secondary to systemic disease or an extension of vitreoretinal lymphoma. The classification of lymphomas is further discussed in Chapter 14.

Coupland SE, Damato B. Understanding intraocular lymphomas. *Clin Experiment Ophthalmol.* 2008;36(6):564–578.

Neural sheath tumors

Neurilemomas (schwannomas) and neurofibromas are rare tumors found in the uveal tract. Multiple neurofibromas may occur in the ciliary body, iris, and choroid in patients with neurofibromatosis 1 (Fig 12-28).

Leiomyoma

Neoplasms arising from the smooth muscle of the ciliary body have been reported in rare instances. When they occur, they may be clinically confused with amelanotic melanoma or neurofibroma. Histologically, these tumors consist of a proliferation of tightly packed slender spindle cells lacking pigment. Immunohistochemical stains may be useful in diagnosing leiomyomas, because leiomyomas express smooth muscle–related antigens. Under light and transmission electron microscopy, these tumors sometimes exhibit both myogenic and neurogenic features. In such cases, the tumors are called *mesectodermal leiomyoma.*

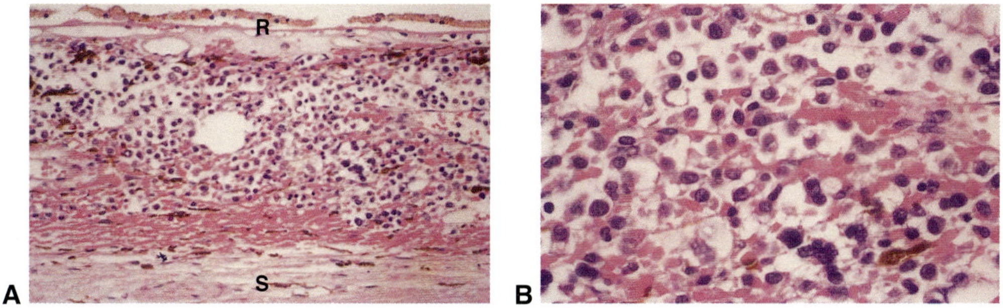

Figure 12-27 Choroidal lymphoma. **A,** Diffuse expansion of choroid by lymphoma (H&E stain). R = RPE, S = sclera. **B,** Higher magnification depicts atypical lymphocytes (H&E stain). *(Courtesy of Hans E. Grossniklaus, MD.)*

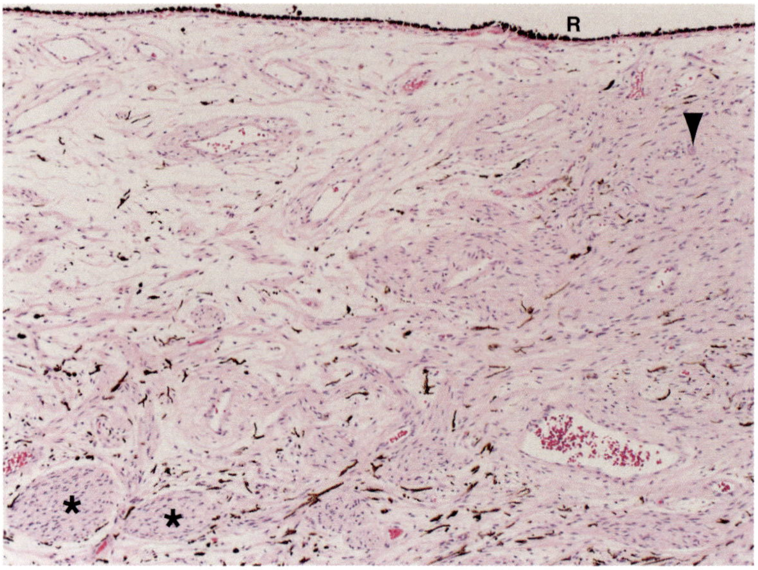

Figure 12-28 Choroidal neurofibromatosis (H&E). The choroid is diffusely infiltrated by spindle-shaped cells, occasional ganglion cells *(arrowhead),* and enlarged choroidal nerves *(asterisks).* R = RPE. *(Courtesy of Michele Bloomer, MD.)*

CHAPTER 13

Eyelids

Topography

The eyelids extend from the eyebrow superiorly to the cheek inferiorly and can be subdivided into orbital and tarsal components. At the level of the tarsus, the eyelid consists of 4 main histologic layers, from anterior to posterior:

- skin
- orbicularis oculi muscle
- tarsus
- palpebral conjunctiva

A surgical plane of dissection may be made through an incision along an isolated section of pretarsal orbicularis muscle (Riolan muscle), indicated by the gray line of the eyelid margin. This functionally divides the eyelid into anterior and posterior lamellae (Fig 13-1). See also BCSC Section 7, *Orbit, Eyelids, and Lacrimal System.*

The skin of the eyelids is thinner than that of most other body sites. It consists of an epidermis of keratinized stratified squamous epithelium, which contains melanocytes and antigen-presenting Langerhans cells, and a dermis of loose collagenous connective tissue, which contains the following:

- cilia and associated sebaceous glands (of Zeis)
- apocrine sweat glands (of Moll)
- eccrine sweat glands
- pilosebaceous units

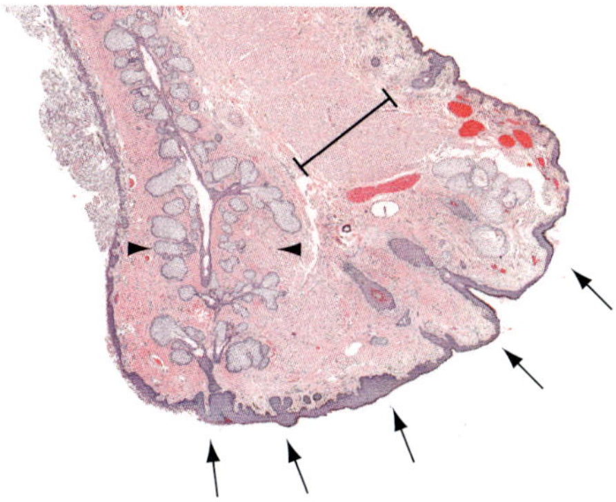

Figure 13-1 Cross section of a normal eyelid. Proceeding from left (posterior) to right (anterior) are the palpebral conjunctiva; the tarsus, containing the meibomian glands *(between arrowheads);* the orbicularis oculi *(bracket);* and the dermis, underlying the epidermis. *Arrows* point to the eyelid margin. *(Courtesy of Heather Potter, MD.)*

Eyelid glands secrete their products in various ways. Apocrine sweat glands secrete sweat by decapitating the apical part of the cell. Eccrine and lacrimal glands secrete sweat without losing any part of the cell. Sebaceous glands are holocrine glands, meaning they lose the entire cell as they secrete.

Two muscles elevate the eyelid: the *levator palpebrae superioris* (a skeletal muscle), of which only the aponeurotic portion is present in the eyelid, and the *Müller muscle* (a smooth muscle). The *orbicularis oculi* (a striated skeletal muscle) closes the eyelid. The *tarsal plate,* a thick plaque of dense, fibrous connective tissue, contains the sebaceous meibomian glands. Also present near the upper border of the superior tarsal plate (and less so along the lower border of the inferior tarsal plate) are the accessory lacrimal glands of Wolfring; the accessory lacrimal glands of Krause are located in the conjunctival fornices. The *palpebral conjunctiva* adheres tightly to the posterior surface of the tarsus.

The following are some common dermatopathological terms that also relate to ophthalmology:

- *acanthosis:* increased thickness (hyperplasia) of the stratum malpighii (consisting of the strata basale and spinosum) of the epidermis
- *hyperkeratosis:* increased thickness of the stratum corneum of the epidermis
- *parakeratosis:* retention of nuclei within the stratum corneum
- *papillomatosis:* formation of fingerlike upward projections of epidermis lining fibrovascular cores
- *dyskeratosis:* premature keratinization of the individual cells within the stratum malpighii
- *acantholysis:* loss of cohesion (dissolution of intercellular bridges) between adjacent epithelial cells

Congenital Anomalies

For additional discussion of the congenital anomalies listed in this chapter, see also BCSC Section 7, *Orbit, Eyelids, and Lacrimal System.*

Distichiasis

Distichiasis is the aberrant formation of cilia within the tarsus that causes them to exit the eyelid margin through the orifices of the meibomian glands. The pathogenesis of distichiasis is thought to be an anomalous formation within the tarsus of a complete pilosebaceous unit rather than the normal sebaceous (meibomian) gland. Histologically, hair follicles can be seen within the tarsal plate. The tarsus may be rudimentary, and the glands of Moll are often hypertrophic. See BCSC Section 6, *Pediatric Ophthalmology and Strabismus,* and Section 8, *External Disease and Cornea,* for additional discussion.

Phakomatous Choristoma

A rare congenital tumor, phakomatous choristoma (Zimmerman tumor), is formed from the aberrant location of lens epithelium within the inferonasal portion of the lower eyelid. These cells may undergo cytoplasmic enlargement, identical to the "bladder" cell in a cataractous lens. Basement membrane material that exhibits positive periodic

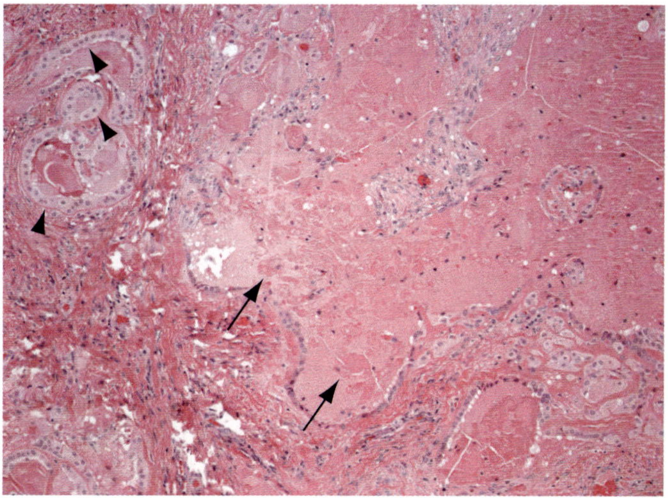

Figure 13-2 Phakomatous choristoma of the eyelid. The dermis displays a disorganized proliferation of lens epithelium *(arrowheads)* and occasional "bladder" cells *(arrows)*. Note the large amount of eosinophilic material, which represents lens nuclear and cortical proteins. *(Courtesy of Nasreen A. Syed, MD.)*

acid–Schiff staining is produced, recapitulating the lens capsule (Fig 13-2). The nodule formed is usually present at birth and enlarges slowly. Complete excision is the usual treatment.

Congenital Dermoid Cyst

Congenital dermoid cysts are not uncommon in the lateral brow of the eyelid. However, they are more traditionally regarded as orbital lesions and are therefore discussed in Chapter 14 of this volume.

Inflammations

Infectious

Depending on the causative agent, eyelid infections may produce disease that is localized (eg, hordeolum), multicentric (eg, papillomas), or diffuse (eg, cellulitis). Routes of infection include primary inoculation through a bite or wound, direct spread from a contiguous site such as a paranasal sinus infection, or hematogenous dissemination from a remote site. Infectious agents may be

- bacterial, such as *Staphylococcus aureus* in hordeolum and infectious blepharitis
- viral, such as poxvirus in molluscum contagiosum
- fungal, such as blastomycosis, coccidioidomycosis, or aspergillosis

Hordeolum

Also known as a *stye,* hordeolum is a primary, acute, self-limited inflammatory process typically involving the glands of Zeis and, less often, the meibomian glands. A small abscess, or focal collection of neutrophils and necrotic debris (ie, pus), forms at the site of infection. Lesions may drain spontaneously or require surgical drainage.

Cellulitis

The diffuse spread of acute inflammatory cells through tissue planes is known as *cellulitis. Preseptal cellulitis* involves the tissues of the eyelid anterior to the orbital septum, which is the fibrous membrane that connects the borders of the tarsal plates to the bony orbital rim. Cellulitis is most often secondary to bacterial infection of the paranasal sinuses. Histologic examination reveals neutrophilic infiltration of the soft tissues, accompanied by interstitial edema and, occasionally, necrosis (Fig 13-3). See BCSC Section 7, *Orbit, Eyelids, and Lacrimal System,* for further information.

Viral infections

Human papillomavirus may infect the skin of the eyelids, typically manifesting as *verruca vulgaris,* commonly known as a *wart.* Clinically, it is usually an elevated papillary lesion. Histologically, the lesions exhibit a papillary growth pattern and demonstrate hyperkeratosis and acanthosis (Fig 13-4A). Infected cells may demonstrate cytoplasmic clearing (koilocytosis) (Fig 13-4B). A mixed inflammatory cell infiltrate is typically present in the superficial dermis.

In *molluscum contagiosum,* which is caused by a member of the poxvirus family, dome-shaped, waxy epidermal nodules with central umbilication form. If present on the eyelid margin, the nodules may cause a secondary follicular conjunctivitis (Fig 13-5). Histologically, the lesions are distinctive; they are described in the legend for Figure 13-6.

Noninfectious

Chalazion

A chalazion is a chronic, often painless nodule of the eyelid that develops when the lipid secretions of the meibomian glands or, less often, the glands of Zeis are discharged into the surrounding tissues, inciting a lipogranulomatous reaction (Fig 13-7).

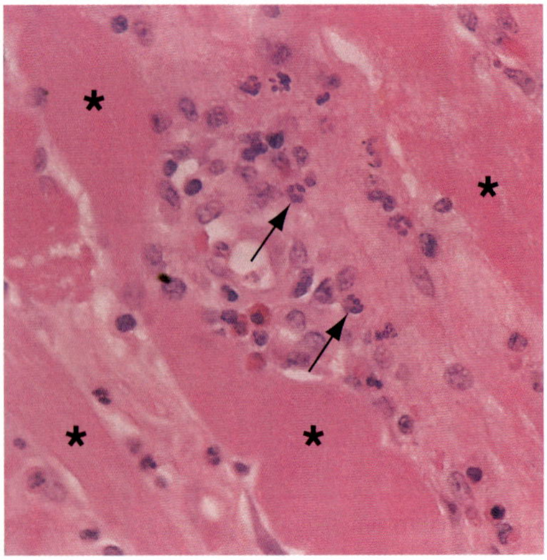

Figure 13-3 Biopsy of a preseptal cellulitis of the eyelid. Neutrophils *(arrows)* dissect between the skeletal muscle fibers *(asterisks)* of the orbicularis.

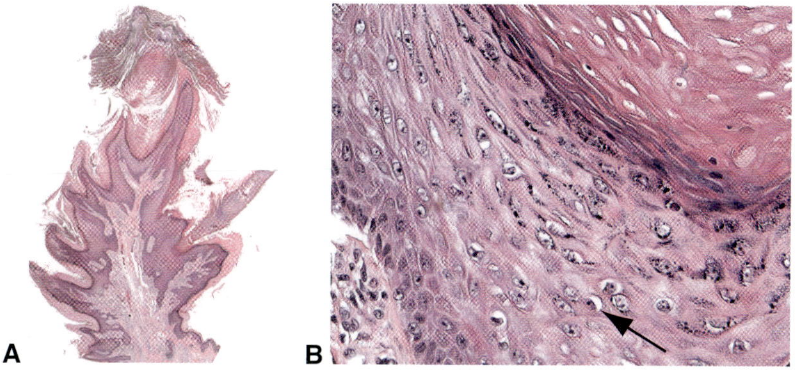

Figure 13-4 Verruca vulgaris. **A,** Verruca vulgaris is a form of infection of the eyelid with human papillomavirus (HPV). The lesion has a papillary growth pattern with fingerlike projections. **B,** Occasional koilocytes with nuclear contraction and cytoplasmic clearing are present *(arrow).* *(Courtesy of Nasreen A. Syed, MD.)*

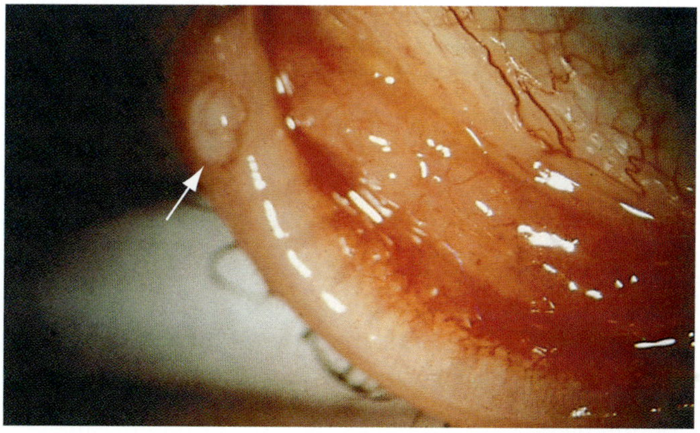

Figure 13-5 Molluscum contagiosum involving the eyelid margin *(arrow).* Note the associated follicular conjunctivitis.

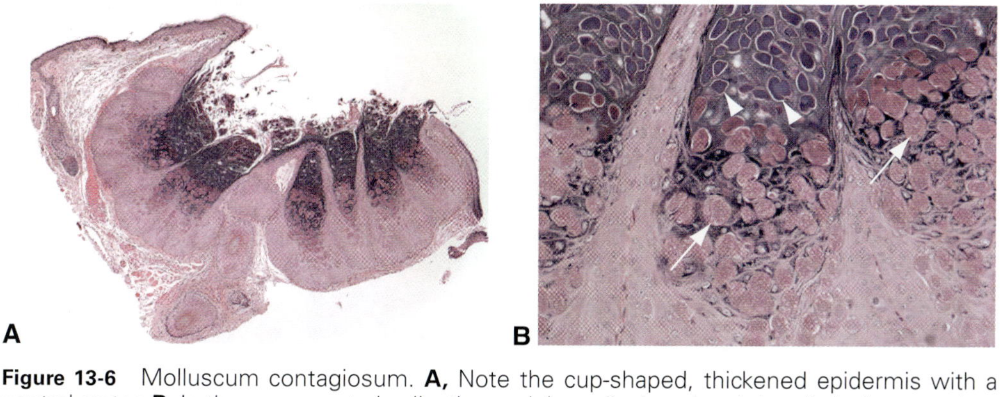

Figure 13-6 Molluscum contagiosum. **A,** Note the cup-shaped, thickened epidermis with a central crater. **B,** In the more central cells, the nuclei are displaced peripherally by large eosinophilic viral inclusions known as molluscum bodies *(arrows).* The molluscum bodies become more basophilic near the surface of the epithelium *(arrowheads).* *(Courtesy of Nasreen A. Syed, MD.)*

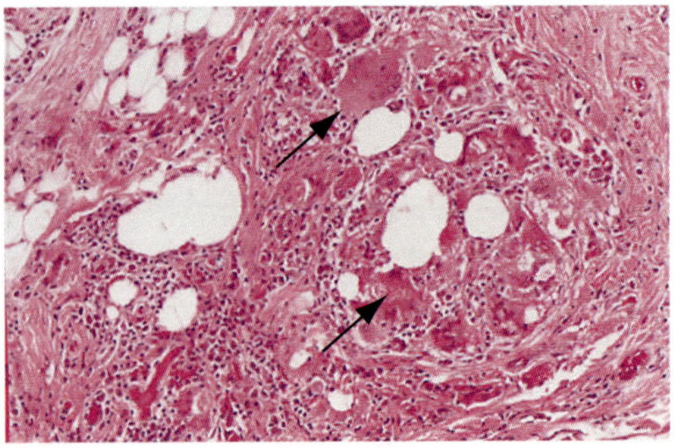

Figure 13-7 Chalazion. Granulomatous inflammation consisting of epithelioid histiocytes and multinucleated giant cells *(arrows)* surrounds clear spaces (lipogranuloma). Because the lipid is dissolved by solvents during routine tissue processing, optically clear ("lipid dropout") spaces remain. Lymphocytes, plasma cells, and neutrophils are also often present.

Degenerations

Xanthelasma

Xanthelasma consists of single or multiple soft yellow plaques occurring in the medial canthal region of the eyelids. Associated hyperlipoproteinemic states, particularly hyperlipoproteinemia types II and III, are present in 30%–40% of patients with xanthelasma. These eyelid xanthomas consist of collections of histiocytes with foamy, lipid-laden cytoplasm distributed diffusely and often around blood vessels within the dermis (Fig 13-8). Associated inflammation is minimal.

Amyloidosis

The term *amyloid* refers to a heterogeneous group of extracellular proteins that exhibit birefringence and dichroism under polarized light when stained with Congo red (see Chapter 5 and Fig 5-13). These features result from the 3-dimensional configuration of the proteins into a β-pleated sheet. Proteins that may form amyloid deposits include

- immunoglobulin light chain fragments (AL amyloid) in plasma cell dyscrasias
- transthyretin mutations in familial amyloid polyneuropathy types I and II
- gelsolin mutations in familial amyloidosis—Finnish type, also known as gelsolin amyloidosis or Meretoja syndrome

A 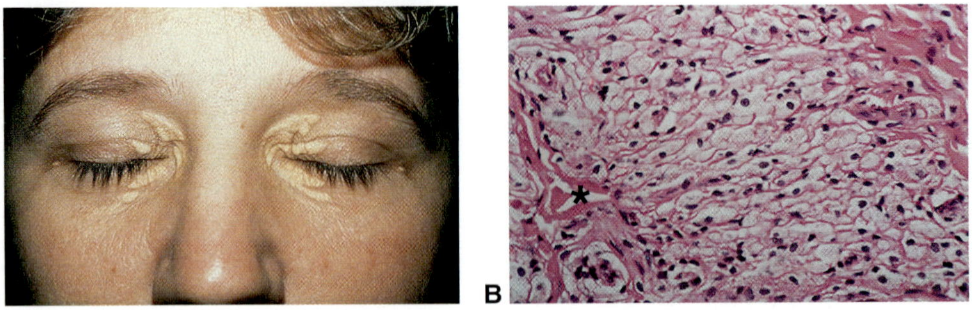 B

Figure 13-8 Xanthelasma. **A,** Patient with prominent xanthelasma. Note the yellow papules on the medial aspect of the upper and lower eyelids. **B,** Note the foam cells (filled with lipid) surrounding a venule *(asterisk)*. *(Part A from* External Disease and Cornea: A Multimedia Collection. *San Francisco: American Academy of Ophthalmology; 1994:slide 10.)*

Amyloid deposits in the skin are usually multiple, bilateral, symmetric, waxy yellow-white nodules. The deposition of amyloid within blood vessel walls in the skin causes increased vascular fragility and often results in intradermal hemorrhages, accounting for the purpura seen clinically (Fig 13-9). On routine histologic sections, amyloid appears as an amorphous, eosinophilic extracellular deposit. Stains useful in demonstrating amyloid deposits include Congo red, crystal violet, and thioflavin T (see Figure 10-12). Electron microscopy reveals that the deposits are composed of randomly oriented extracellular fibrils measuring 7–10 nm in diameter.

Amyloid deposits within the skin of the eyelid are highly indicative of a systemic disease process, either primary or secondary, whereas deposits elsewhere in the ocular adnexa are more likely to represent a localized disease process. Other systemic diseases with eyelid manifestations are listed in Table 13-1.

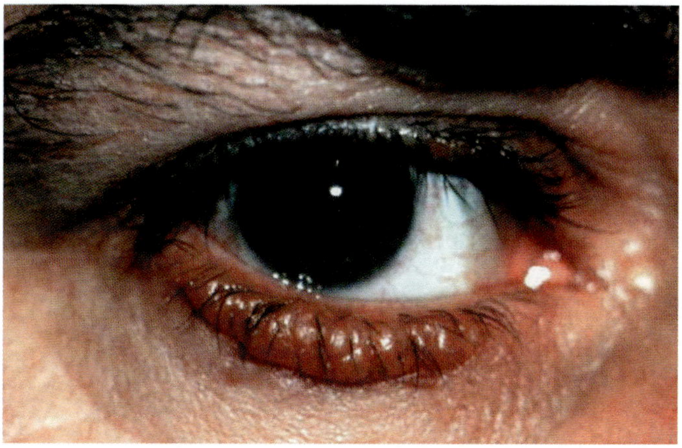

Figure 13-9 Cutaneous amyloid in a patient with multiple myeloma. Note the waxy elevation and the associated purpura of the lower eyelid. *(Courtesy of John B. Holds, MD.)*

Table 13-1 Eyelid Manifestations of Systemic Diseases

Systemic Condition	Eyelid Manifestations
Amyloidosis	Waxy papules, ptosis, purpura
Carney complex	Myxoma
Dermatomyositis	Edema, erythema
Erdheim-Chester disease	Xanthelasma, xanthogranuloma
Fraser syndrome	Cryptophthalmos
Granulomatosis with polyangiitis (formerly Wegener granulomatosis)	Edema, ptosis, lower eyelid retraction
Hyperlipoproteinemia	Xanthelasma
Polyarteritis nodosa	Focal infarct
Relapsing polychondritis	Papules
Sarcoidosis	Papules
Scleroderma	Reduced mobility, taut skin
Systemic lupus erythematosus	Telangiectasias, edema
Treacher Collins syndrome	Lower eyelid coloboma

Modified from Wiggs JL, Jakobiec FA. Eyelid manifestations of systemic disease. In: Albert DM, Jakobiec FA, eds. *Principles and Practice of Ophthalmology.* Philadelphia: Saunders; 1994:1859.

Cysts

Epidermoid Cysts

Epidermoid cysts, also known as *epidermal inclusion cysts,* are common in the eyelids. They may arise spontaneously or as a result of the entrapment of epidermis beneath the skin surface following surgery or trauma. Epidermoid cysts are lined with keratinized stratified squamous epithelium and contain keratin (Fig 13-10).

Ductal Cysts

The eyelid contains the ducts of numerous structures, including the lacrimal gland and the apocrine and eccrine sweat glands. Cysts may develop in any of these ducts. Ducts are typically lined with a double layer of cuboidal epithelium, as are ductal cysts. The lumen of the cyst typically appears empty histologically. A cyst arising from the duct of the lacrimal gland is called *dacryops.* Cysts arising from sweat ducts are referred to as either *apocrine* or *eccrine hidrocystomas* (Fig 13-11).

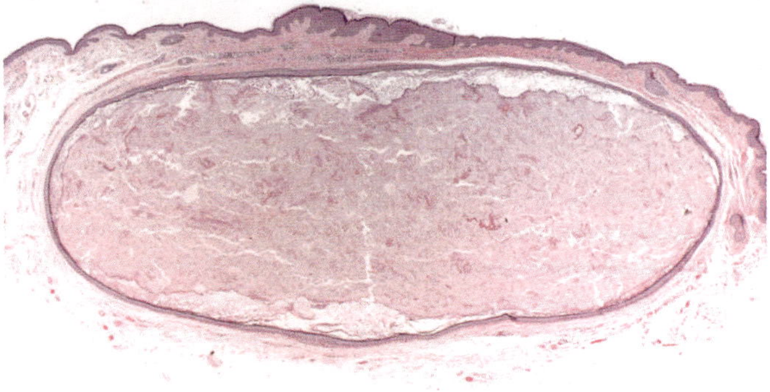

Figure 13-10 Epidermal inclusion cyst in the dermis. The cyst lining resembles epidermis, and the lumen contains keratin. *(Courtesy of Nasreen A. Syed, MD.)*

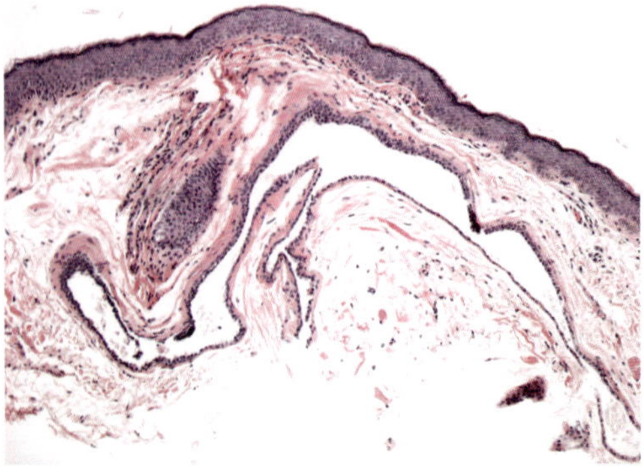

Figure 13-11 An apocrine hidrocystoma is typically lined by a double layer of epithelium (ie, an inner low cuboidal layer and an outer flattened myoepithelial layer). Epithelial cells may demonstrate decapitation secretion. *(Courtesy of Nasreen A. Syed, MD.)*

Neoplasia

Epidermal Neoplasms

Seborrheic keratosis

Seborrheic keratosis, a common benign epithelial proliferation, typically occurs in middle age. Clinically, it is a well-circumscribed, oval, dome-shaped to verrucoid "stuck-on" papule, varying from pink to dark brown in color. Histologically, although several architectural patterns are possible, all of them demonstrate hyperkeratosis, acanthosis, and some degree of papillomatosis. The acanthosis is a result of the proliferation of either polygonal or basaloid squamous cells without dysplasia.

Pseudohorn cysts, which are concentrically laminated collections of surface keratin within the acanthotic epithelium, are a characteristic finding in most types of seborrheic keratosis (Fig 13-12). Irritated seborrheic keratosis, also termed *inverted follicular keratosis,* shows nonkeratinized squamous epithelial whorling, or squamous "eddies," instead of pseudohorn cysts (Fig 13-13). Sudden onset of multiple seborrheic keratoses is known as the *Leser-Trélat sign* and is associated with malignancy, usually a gastrointestinal adenocarcinoma; these keratoses may in fact represent evolving acanthosis nigricans. Table 13-2 lists other systemic malignant tumors with cutaneous manifestations.

Keratoacanthoma

Keratoacanthoma is a rapidly growing epithelial proliferation with a potential for spontaneous involution. Strong evidence supports the idea that keratoacanthomas are a variant of a well-differentiated squamous cell carcinoma. These dome-shaped nodules, which have keratin-filled central craters, may attain a considerable size, up to 2.5 cm in diameter, within a matter of weeks to months (Fig 13-14). The natural history is typically spontaneous involution over several months, resulting in a slightly depressed scar.

Histologically, keratoacanthomas show a cup-shaped invagination of well-differentiated squamous cells that form irregularly configured nests and strands and incite a chronic inflammatory host response. The proliferating epithelial cells undermine the adjacent

A B

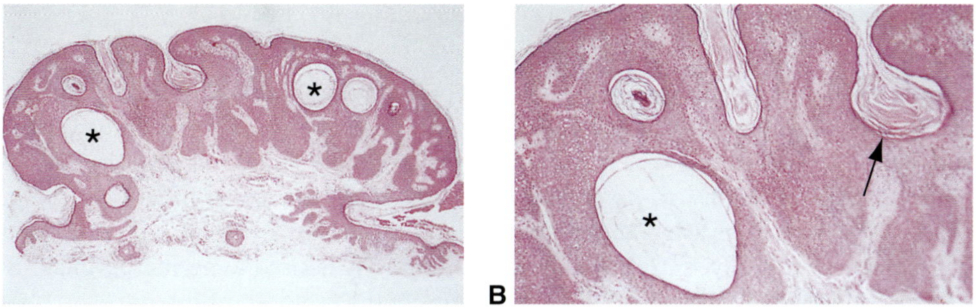

Figure 13-12 Seborrheic keratosis. **A,** The epidermis is acanthotic with a papillary configuration. Note the keratin-filled cysts *(asterisks).* **B,** When serial histologic sections are studied, pseudohorn cysts *(asterisk)* within the epidermis represent crevices or infoldings of epidermis *(arrow). (Courtesy of Hans E. Grossniklaus, MD.)*

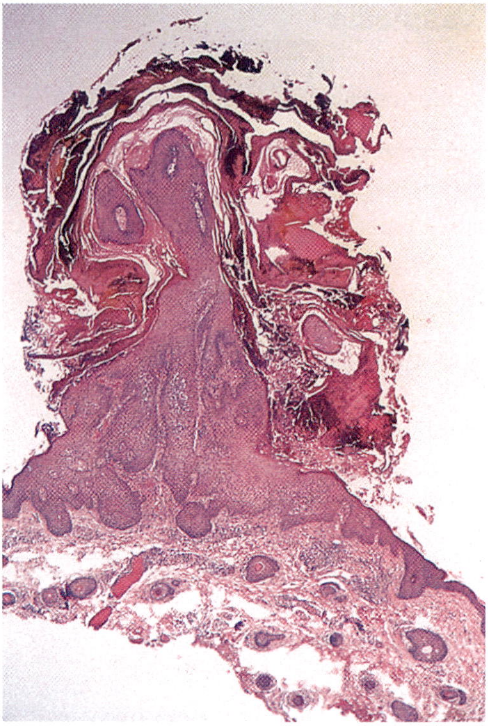

Figure 13-13 Irritated seborrheic keratosis, which is also known as *inverted follicular keratosis.* Clinically, this lesion appeared as a cutaneous horn.

Table 13-2 Neoplastic Eyelid Manifestations of Malignant Syndromes

Syndrome	Eyelid Manifestations
Basal cell nevus syndrome (medulloblastoma, fibrosarcoma)	Multiple basal cell carcinomas
Cowden disease (breast carcinoma; fibrous hamartomas of breast, thyroid, gastrointestinal tract)	Multiple trichilemmomas
Muir-Torre syndrome (visceral carcinoma, usually colon)	Keratoacanthoma, sebaceous neoplasm (adenoma, carcinoma)

Modified from Wiggs JL, Jakobiec FA. Eyelid manifestations of systemic disease. In: Albert DM, Jakobiec FA, eds. *Principles and Practice of Ophthalmology.* Philadelphia: Saunders; 1994:1859.

normal epidermis. At the deep aspect of the proliferating nodules, mitotic activity and nuclear atypia may occur, making it difficult to differentiate between keratoacanthoma and squamous cell carcinoma. Many dermatopathologists and ophthalmic pathologists prefer to call this lesion *well-differentiated squamous cell carcinoma* because of the possibility of perineural invasion and metastasis.

If treated surgically, the lesion should be completely excised to permit optimal histologic examination of the lateral and deep margins of the tumor–host interface.

Actinic keratosis

Actinic keratoses are precancerous squamous lesions that appear, clinically in middle age, as erythematous, scaly macules or papules on sun-exposed skin, particularly on the face and the dorsal surfaces of the hands. Actinic keratoses range from a few millimeters to

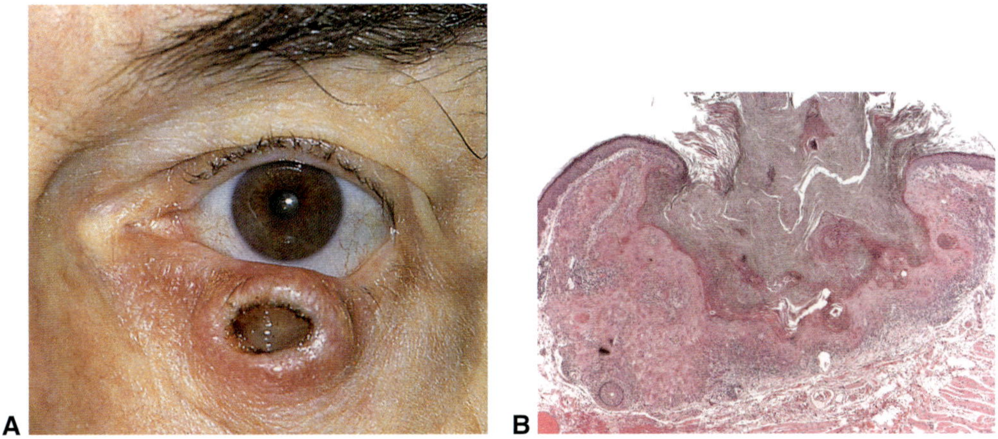

Figure 13-14 Keratoacanthoma. **A,** Clinical appearance. Note the cuplike configuration. In this case, the central crater was originally filled with keratin. **B,** Low-magnification histologic section illustrating the central keratin crater and the downward (invasive) growth pattern. *(Part B courtesy of Nasreen A. Syed, MD.)*

1 cm. Hyperkeratotic types of these lesions may form a cutaneous horn, and hyperpigmented types may clinically simulate lentigo maligna. Squamous cell carcinoma may develop from preexisting actinic keratosis. However, when squamous cell carcinoma arises in actinic keratosis, the risk of subsequent metastatic dissemination is very low (0.5%–3.0%).

Histologically, there are 5 subtypes, which range from hypertrophic to atrophic. All types demonstrate changes in the epidermis with hyperkeratosis and parakeratosis. Cellular atypia (nuclear hyperchromasia and pleomorphism and an increased nuclear-to-cytoplasmic ratio) is present and ranges from mild (involving only the basal epithelial layers) to frank carcinoma in situ (full-thickness involvement of the epidermis). Dyskeratosis (premature individual cell keratinization) and mitotic figures above the basal epithelial layer are often found (Fig 13-15). The underlying dermis shows solar elastosis (elastotic

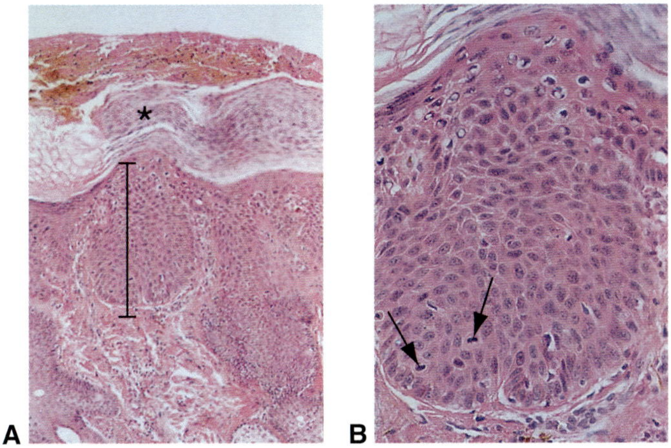

Figure 13-15 Actinic keratosis. **A,** Note the epidermal acanthosis *(bracket),* disorganization within the epidermis (dysplasia), parakeratosis *(asterisk),* and inflammation within the dermis. **B,** At higher magnification, note the epidermal dysplasia and mitotic figures *(arrows).*

degeneration of collagen) (Fig 13-16), which manifests as fragmentation, clumping, and loss of eosinophilia of dermal collagen. A chronic inflammatory cell infiltrate is usually seen in the superficial dermis. Histologic examination of the base of the lesion is necessary to determine whether stromal invasion indicative of squamous cell carcinoma is present.

Carcinoma

Basal cell carcinoma Basal cell carcinoma (BCC), the most common malignant neoplasm of the eyelids, accounts for more than 90% of all malignant eyelid tumors. Although exposure to sunlight is the main risk factor, genetic factors can play a role in familial syndromes. The lower eyelid is more commonly involved than the upper eyelid, with the medial canthus being the second most common site of involvement. Tumors in the medial canthal area are more likely to be deeply invasive and to involve the orbit. Nodular BCC (the most common type) is a slow-growing, slightly elevated lesion with ulceration and pearly, raised, rolled edges (Fig 13-17). The morpheaform, or sclerosing, variant of BCC is a flat or slightly depressed, pale yellow, indurated plaque; this type is

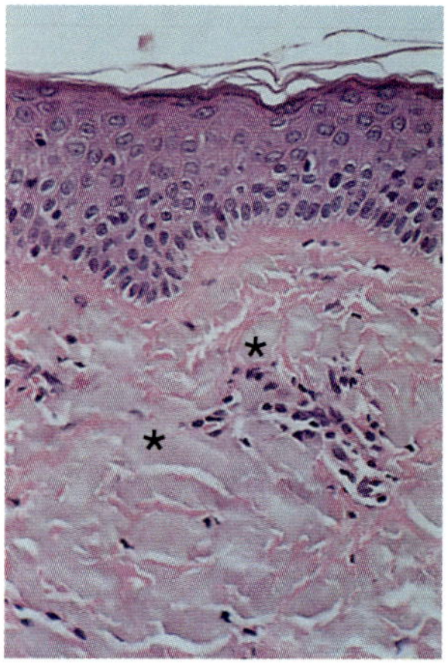

Figure 13-16 Solar elastosis. The collagen of the dermis appears bluish *(asterisks)* in this hematoxylin-eosin (H&E) stain, instead of pink. This is a histologic sign of ultraviolet light–induced damage.

A 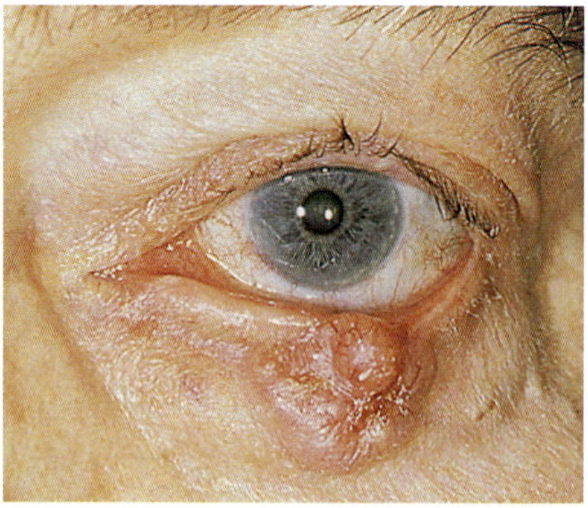 B 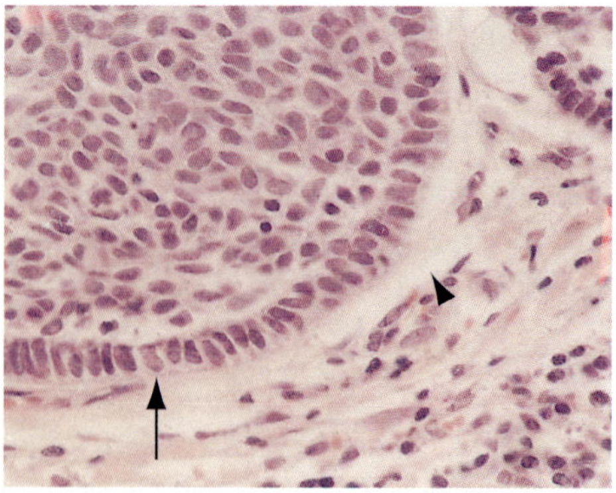

Figure 13-17 Basal cell carcinoma. **A,** Clinical appearance of the nodular type. **B,** Histologic appearance. Note the characteristic palisading of the cells around the outer edge of the tumor *(arrow)* and the artifactitious separation (due to tissue processing) between the nests of tumor cells and the dermis (retraction artifact, *arrowhead*).

often infiltrative, and its extent is difficult to determine clinically. A small percentage of BCCs are pigmented or multicentric.

As the name implies, BCCs originate from the stratum basale, or stratum germinativum, of the epidermis and the outer root sheath of the hair follicle and occur only in hair-bearing tissue. Tumor cells are characterized by relatively bland, monomorphous nuclei and a high nuclear-to-cytoplasmic ratio. BCC forms cohesive islands with nuclear palisading of the peripheral cell layer. BCCs may exhibit a variety of histologic patterns, including keratotic (hair follicle), squamous (metatypical), sebaceous, adenoid, and eccrine (syringoid) differentiation. In the morphea (sclerosing) variant, thin cords and strands of tumor cells are set in a fibrotic stroma (Fig 13-18).

The treatment of choice is complete excision, and surgical margin control is required. Typically, margin control is achieved with frozen sections or Mohs micrographic surgery. Morbidity in BCCs is almost always the result of local spread; metastasis is extremely unusual.

Squamous cell carcinoma Although *squamous cell carcinoma (SCC)* may occur in the eyelids, it is far less common than BCC. Like BCCs, most SCCs arise in solar-damaged skin, so the lower eyelid is more frequently involved than the upper. However, SCC is more likely to involve the upper eyelid than is BCC. The clinical appearance of SCC is diverse, ranging from ulcers to plaques to fungating or nodular growths. Accordingly, the clinical differential diagnosis is long; an accurate diagnosis requires pathologic examination of excised tissue.

Histologic examination shows atypical squamous cells that form nests and strands, extend beyond the epidermal basement membrane, infiltrate the dermis, and incite a fibrotic tissue reaction (Fig 13-19). Tumor cells may be well differentiated (forming keratin and easily recognizable as squamous), moderately differentiated, or poorly differentiated (requiring ancillary studies to confirm the nature of the neoplasm). When the diagnosis is in question, the pathologist should look for the presence of intercellular bridges between tumor cells. Perineural and lymphatic invasion may be present and should be reported when identified microscopically. To treat this tumor adequately, frozen section (conventional or Mohs micrographic surgery) or permanent section margin control is required. Regional lymph node metastasis may occur in patients with SCC of the eyelid.

Chévez-Barrios P. Frozen section diagnosis and indications in ophthalmic pathology. *Arch Pathol Lab Med.* 2005;129(12):1626–1634.

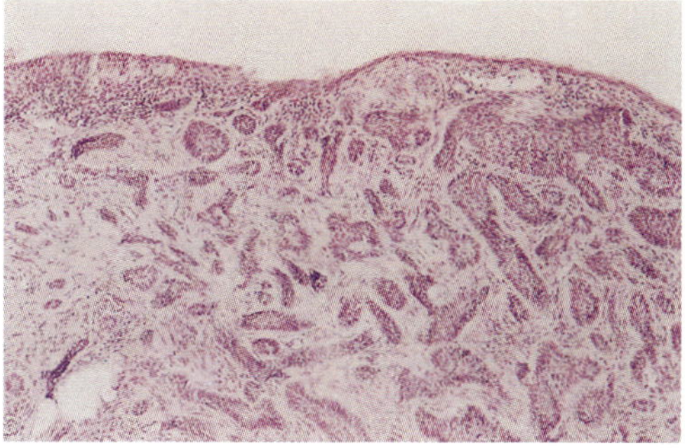

Figure 13-18 Basal cell carcinoma, morphea-form (sclerosing) type. Thin strands and cords of tumor cells are seen in a fibrotic (desmoplastic) dermis.

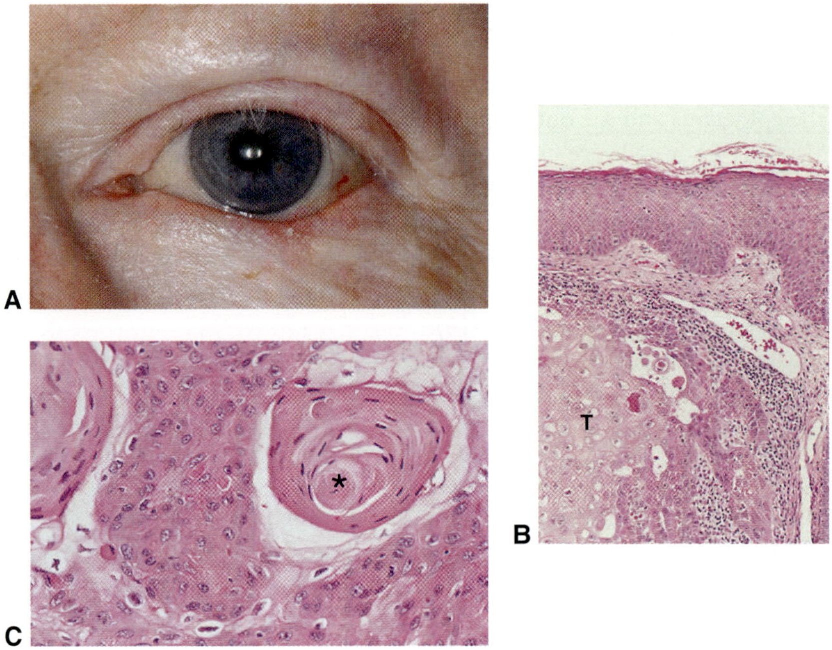

Figure 13-19 Squamous cell carcinoma. **A,** Clinical appearance. Note the focal loss of lashes and scaly appearance of the lower eyelid. **B,** Note the tumor cells (T) invading the dermis. **C,** A keratin pearl *(asterisk)* is present in this well-differentiated squamous cell carcinoma. *(Part A courtesy of Keith D. Carter, MD.)*

Dermal Neoplasms

Capillary hemangiomas are common in the eyelids of children. They usually appear at or shortly after birth as a bright red lesion, grow over weeks to months, and involute by school age. Intervention is reserved for lesions that affect vision because of ptosis or astigmatism, promoting amblyopia.

The histologic appearance depends on the stage of evolution of the hemangioma. Early lesions may be very cellular, with solid nests of plump endothelial cells and correspondingly little vascular luminal formation. Established lesions typically show well-developed, flattened, endothelium-lined capillary channels in a lobular configuration (Fig 13-20). Involuting lesions demonstrate increased fibrosis and hyalinization of capillary walls with luminal occlusion.

Neoplasms and Proliferations of the Dermal Appendages

Syringoma

Syringoma, a common benign lesion of the lower eyelid, typically manifests as multiple, tiny, flesh-colored papules. Syringomas result from a malformation of the eccrine sweat gland ducts. Histologically, syringomas consist of multiple comma-shaped or round ductules lined with a double layer of epithelium and containing a central lumen, often with secretory material (Fig 13-21).

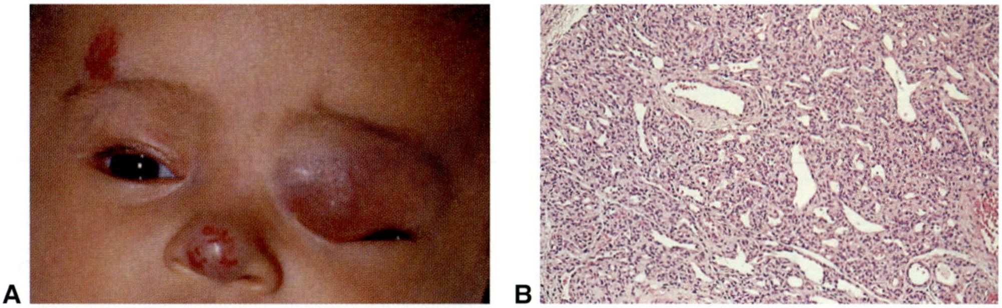

Figure 13-20 Capillary hemangioma. **A,** Infant with multiple capillary hemangiomas. **B,** Note the small capillary-sized vessels and the proliferation of benign endothelial cells. *(Part A courtesy of Sander Dubovy, MD.)*

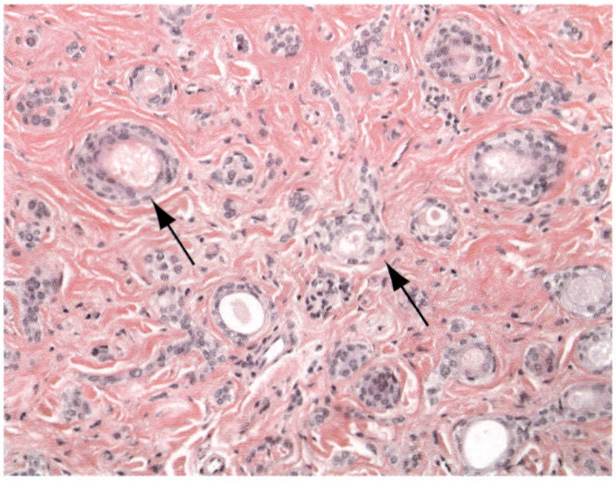

Figure 13-21 Syringoma. Note the round and comma-shaped epithelial-lined ductules *(arrows). (Courtesy of Nasreen A. Syed, MD.)*

Sebaceous hyperplasia

Sebaceous hyperplasia is an uncommon benign lesion of the eyelid and face. Clinically, it appears as a small, yellow papule. Histologically, it is typically a single enlarged sebaceous gland with numerous lobules attached to a single central duct (Fig 13-22).

Sebaceous adenoma

Sebaceous adenoma is a rare benign lesion of the eyelid that typically manifests as a yellow, circumscribed nodule. Histologically, it is composed of multiple sebaceous lobules that are irregularly shaped and incompletely differentiated (Fig 13-23). The possibility of Muir-Torre syndrome should be considered when sebaceous adenoma is diagnosed (see Table 13-2).

Sebaceous carcinoma

Sebaceous carcinoma most commonly involves the upper eyelid of elderly persons. It may originate in the meibomian glands of the tarsus, the glands of Zeis in the skin of the eyelid, or the sebaceous glands of the caruncle. Clinically, the diagnosis is often missed or delayed because of this lesion's propensity to mimic a chalazion or chronic unilateral blepharoconjunctivitis (Fig 13-24).

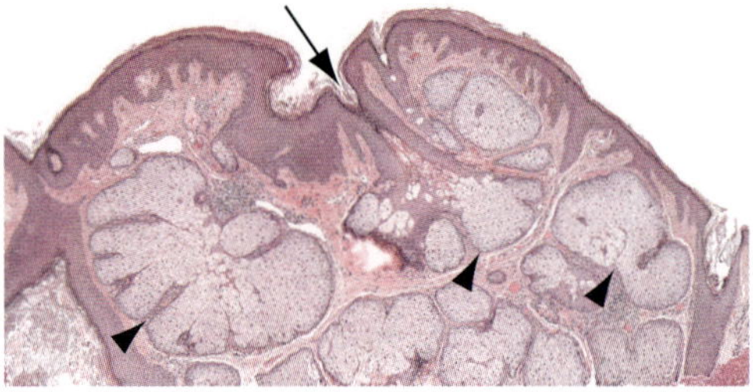

Figure 13-22 Sebaceous hyperplasia. Numerous sebaceous lobules *(arrowheads)* surround a hair follicle *(arrow)*. *(Courtesy of Nasreen A. Syed, MD.)*

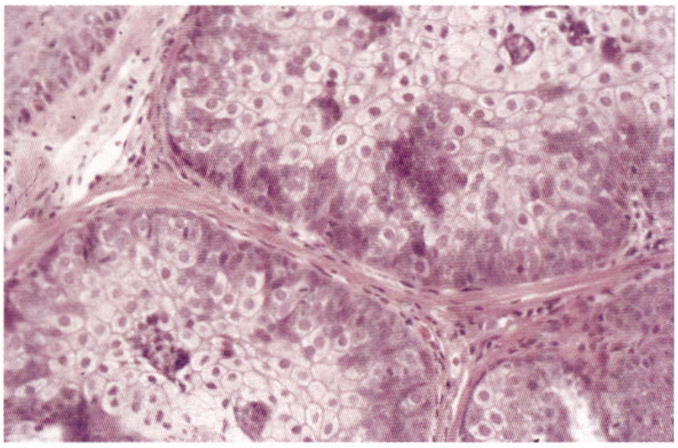

Figure 13-23 Sebaceous adenoma. Sebaceous lobules demonstrate focal proliferations of basophilic (blue) sebocytes. This lesion is most commonly associated with Muir-Torre syndrome. *(Courtesy of Nasreen A. Syed, MD.)*

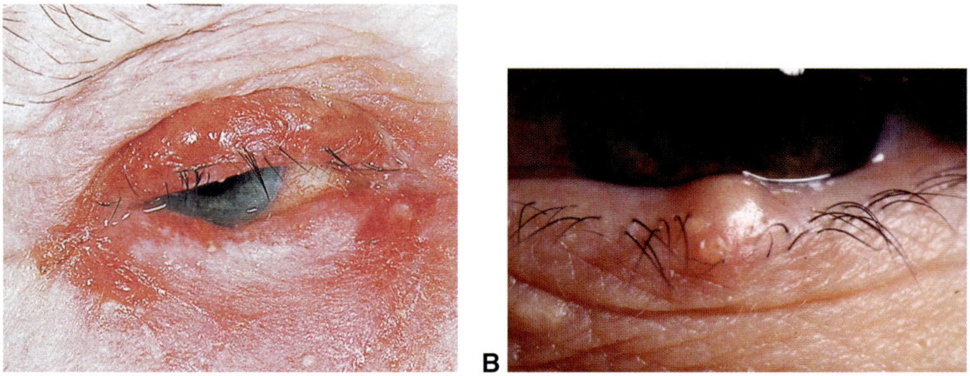

Figure 13-24 Sebaceous carcinoma, clinical appearance. **A,** Note the eyelid erythema suggesting blepharitis, in addition to the loss of eyelashes and the irregular eyelid thickening. **B,** This lesion mimics a chalazion of the lower eyelid. Focal lash loss is present. *(Part B courtesy of Roberta E. Gausas, MD.)*

Histologically, well-differentiated sebaceous carcinomas are readily identified by the microvesicular foamy nature of the tumor cell cytoplasm (Fig 13-25A). Moderately differentiated tumors may show some sebaceous features. Poorly differentiated tumors, however, may be difficult to distinguish from other, more common malignant epithelial tumors. Special stains, such as oil red O or Sudan black B, can be used to diagnose sebaceous carcinomas, because they reveal lipid within the cytoplasm of tumor cells. Tissue staining for lipids should be performed on frozen or cryostat sections, because the lipid constituents are often removed during paraffin processing. When sebaceous carcinoma is suspected clinically, the pathologist should be alerted so that tissue handling allows for any special stains needed.

A primary characteristic of sebaceous carcinoma is *pagetoid spread,* the dissemination of both individual tumor cells and clusters of tumor cells within the epidermis or conjunctival epithelium (Fig 13-25B). Another characteristic is the complete replacement

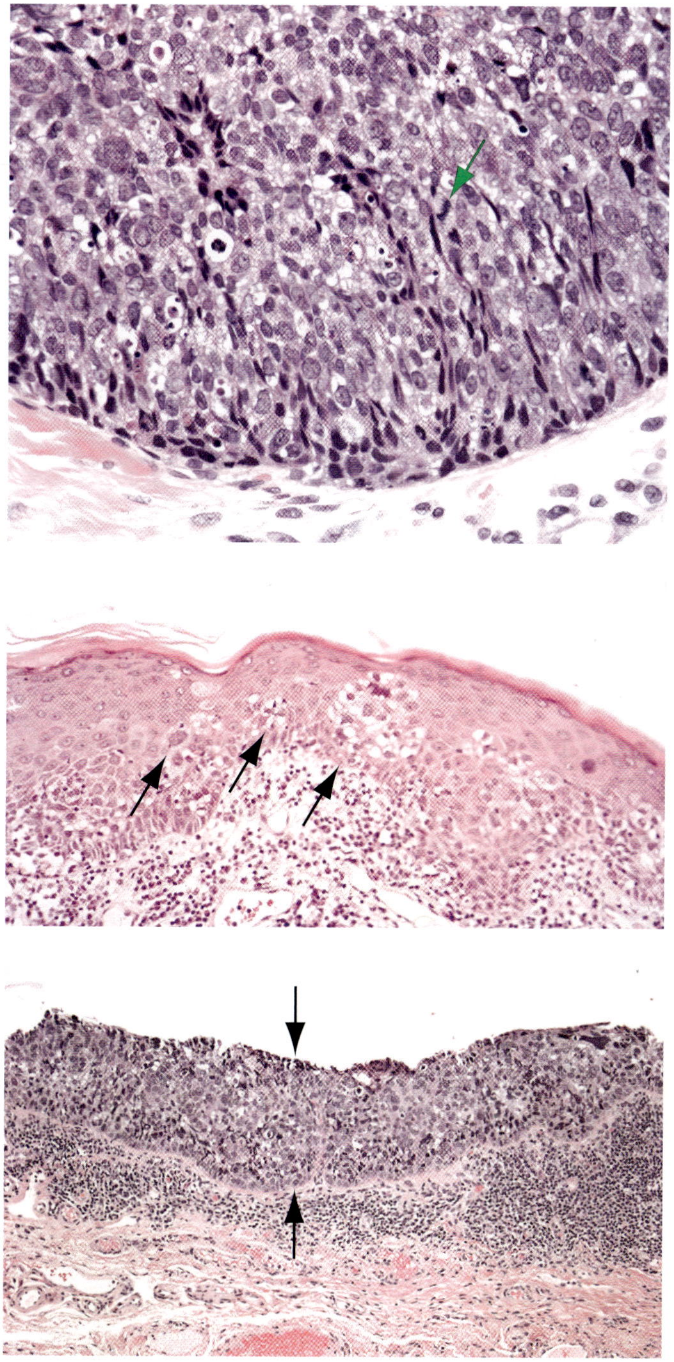

Figure 13-25 Sebaceous carcinoma, histologic appearance. **A,** Tumor cells often have hyperchromatic, pleomorphic nuclei. The cytoplasm frequently has a foamy or vacuolated appearance. Note the mitotic figure *(arrow)*. **B,** Pagetoid invasion of epidermis by individual tumor cells and small clusters of tumor cells *(arrows)*. These areas are subtle and may be difficult to identify. **C,** Sebaceous carcinoma in situ, with complete replacement of normal conjunctival epithelium by tumor cells *(between arrows)*. *(Courtesy of Nasreen A. Syed, MD.)*

of conjunctival epithelium by tumor cells, or *sebaceous carcinoma in situ* (Fig 13-25C). A rare variant of sebaceous carcinoma involves only the epidermis and conjunctiva without demonstrable invasive tumor.

Treatment recommendations include wide local excision of nodular lesions. Large or deeply invasive tumors may require exenteration. Because it can be difficult to identify intraepithelial spread, permanent margins are often more reliable than frozen section control of surgical margins or Mohs micrographic surgery. Preoperative mapping via routine processing of multiple biopsies may afford a more accurate assessment of the extent of spread of the carcinoma. Survival rates for sebaceous carcinoma are worse than those for SCC, but they have improved in recent years as a result of increased awareness, earlier detection, more accurate diagnosis, and more appropriate treatment. Metastases first involve regional lymph nodes; sentinel lymph node biopsy can therefore be helpful in tumor staging.

Melanocytic Neoplasms

Melanocytic nevus

Melanocytic nevi are benign proliferations of melanocytes that commonly occur on the eyelids. Melanocytic nevi may be visible at birth or shortly after birth (congenital nevi) or become apparent in adolescence or adulthood; congenital nevi tend to be larger than those appearing in later years. Nevi greater than 20 cm in diameter are called *giant congenital melanocytic nevi.* The risk for development of melanoma in congenital nevi is proportional to the size of the nevus; close follow-up and/or excision of congenital nevi is warranted. Congenital nevi of the eyelid may develop in utero before the separation of the upper and lower eyelids, resulting in a "kissing" nevus (Fig 13-26). Nevi in adults often appear as dome-shaped lesions on the eyelid margin. Other forms of rare nevi can occur on the eyelid, including blue nevi, Spitz nevi, and dysplastic nevi.

Histologically, most nevi are composed of nevus cells, specialized melanocytes that have a round rather than dendritic shape and tend to cluster together in nests. The cytoplasm of the nevus cell contains a variable amount of melanosomes. Other characteristics of these cells include growth within and around adnexal structures, vessel walls, and the perineurium and extension into the deep reticular dermis or subcutaneous tissue. When a combination of round and spindle-shaped cells is seen in a lesion, the term *combined nevus* is used.

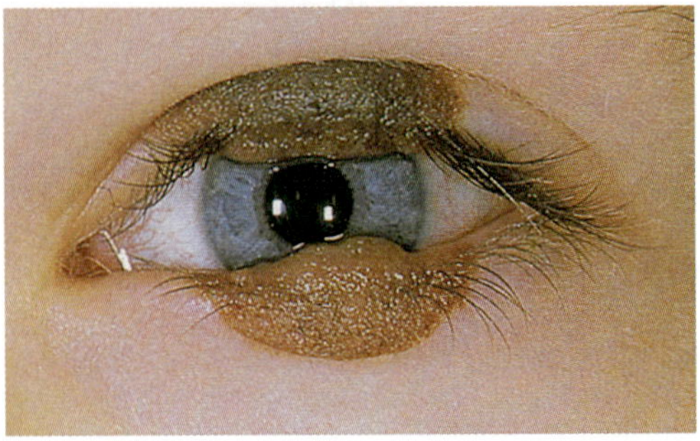

Figure 13-26 Congenital split, or "kissing," nevus of the eyelid.

Nevi typically begin as macular (flat) lesions and evolve with age. When histologic examination reveals nests of melanocytes along the dermal–epidermal junction, these lesions are termed *junctional nevi* (Fig 13-27). Clinically, a junctional nevus is indistinguishable from an ephelis, or freckle, but in the latter, the basal layer of epidermal cells contains the pigment. Typically in adolescence, the junctional nests of nevus cells begin to migrate into the superficial dermis, and the nevus becomes increasingly elevated. At this stage, the nevus may also increase in pigmentation. When both junctional and intradermal components are present, the histologic classification becomes *compound nevus* (Fig 13-28). Finally, sometime in adulthood, the junctional component disappears, leaving only nevus cells within the dermis, and the classification accordingly becomes *intradermal or dermal nevus* (Fig 13-29).

The cytomorphology of the nevus cells also evolves: the cells in the superficial portion of the nevus are polygonal, or epithelioid, in shape (type A nevus cells). Within the

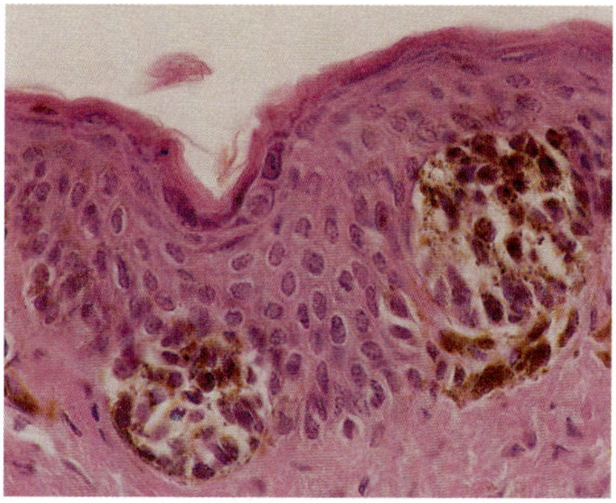

Figure 13-27 Junctional nevus. Nests of nevus cells are seen at the dermal–epidermal junction.

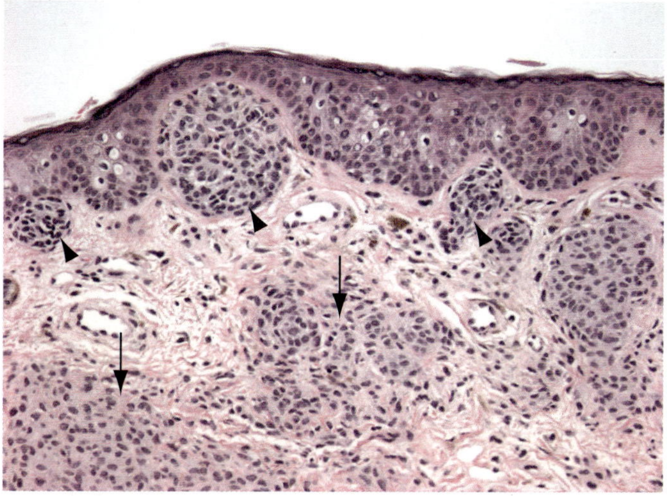

Figure 13-28 Compound nevus. Nests of nevus cells are present in the dermis *(arrows)* as well as at the dermal–epidermal junction *(arrowheads)*. *(Courtesy of Nasreen A. Syed, MD.)*

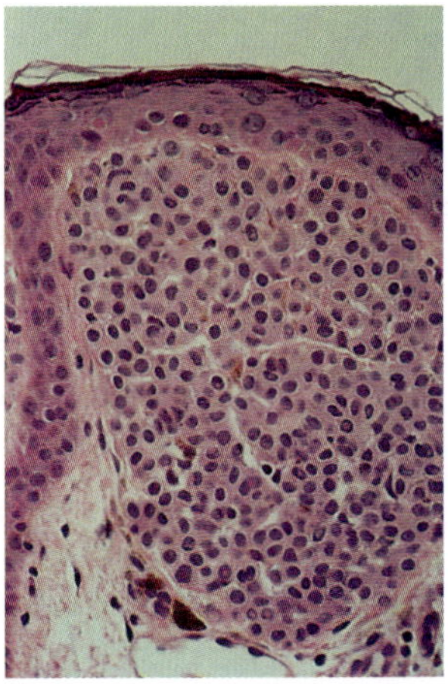

Figure 13-29 Intradermal nevus. The nests of nevus cells are confined to the dermis.

midportion, the cells become smaller, have less cytoplasm, and resemble lymphocytes (type B nevus cells). At the deepest levels, the nevus cells appear similar to Schwann cells of peripheral nerves with a spindle configuration (type C nevus cells). Recognition of this "maturation" is useful for classifying melanocytic neoplasms as benign. Multinucleated giant melanocytes and interspersed adipose tissue are common in older nevi.

Melanoma

Cutaneous melanoma occurs rarely on the eyelids. It may be associated with a preexisting nevus, develop de novo, or extend from a tumor elsewhere on the face. Clinical features that suggest malignancy are the same as those for dysplastic nevi; in addition, melanoma is heralded by a vertical (perpendicular to the skin surface) growth phase. There are 3 main histologic subtypes of melanoma that occur on the eyelids (Fig 13-30):

- lentigo maligna
- superficial spreading
- nodular

Lentigo maligna melanoma, which develops on the face of elderly individuals, has a long preinvasive phase and is the most common type occurring on the eyelids. *Superficial spreading melanoma* is the most common type of cutaneous melanoma; it demonstrates a radial (intraepidermal) growth pattern that extends beyond the invasive component. *Nodular melanoma* has a significant vertical growth phase that results in a raised or indurated mass.

The characteristic histologic features of melanoma include pagetoid intraepidermal spread of atypical melanocytic nests and single cells, nuclear abnormalities (as previously listed), lack of maturation in the deeper portions of the mass, and atypical mitotic figures. A bandlike lymphocytic host response along the base of the mass is more common in melanoma than in benign proliferations. Prognosis is correlated with tumor thickness (Breslow thickness) in stage I (localized) disease. Metastases, when they occur, typically involve regional lymph nodes first.

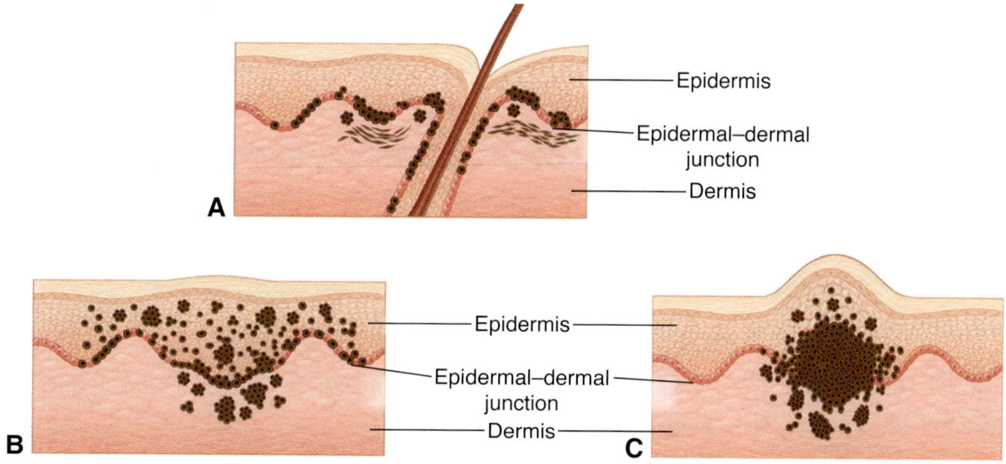

Figure 13-30 Schematic illustration of cutaneous melanoma types. **A,** Lentigo maligna melanoma. Atypical melanocytes (brown cells) proliferate predominantly in the basal layers of the epidermis in a linear or nested pattern, similar to primary acquired melanosis with atypia of the conjunctiva. Note the tendency of the melanocytes to involve the outer sheaths of the hair shafts. The invasive component is seen as brown cells (spindle and epithelioid) in the superficial dermis. **B,** In superficial spreading melanoma, tumor cell nests are present in all levels of the epidermis, often in a pagetoid fashion, with cells or clusters of cells scattered among epithelial cells. Lentigo maligna and superficial spreading melanomas spread horizontally (radial growth) through the skin, staying close to the dermal–epidermal junction. **C,** Nodular melanoma has a narrow intraepidermal component and more prominent vertical growth within the dermis; it is therefore more deeply invasive than the other types. *(Modified with permission from Spencer WH, ed.* Ophthalmic Pathology: An Atlas and Textbook. *Vol 4. Philadelphia: Saunders; 1996:2270. Illustration by Christine Gralapp.)*

CHAPTER 14

Orbit

Topography

Bony Orbit and Soft Tissues

Seven bones form the boundaries of the orbit (see Figs 1-1 through 1-3 in BCSC Section 7, *Orbit, Eyelids, and Lacrimal System*). They are the ethmoidal, frontal, lacrimal, maxillary, palatine, sphenoid, and zygomatic bones.

The orbital cavity contains the globe, lacrimal gland, muscles, tendons, fat, fasciae, vessels, nerves, ciliary ganglion, and cartilaginous trochlea. Inflammatory and neoplastic processes that increase the volume of the orbital contents lead to *proptosis* (protrusion) of the globe and/or *displacement* (deviation) from the horizontal or vertical position. The degree and direction of ocular displacement help to localize the position of the mass.

The *lacrimal gland* is situated anteriorly in the superotemporal quadrant of the orbit. The gland is divided into orbital and palpebral lobes by the aponeurosis of the levator palpebrae superioris muscle. The lacrimal gland acini are composed of low cuboidal epithelium. The ducts, which lie within the fibrovascular stroma, are lined by low cuboidal epithelium and a second outer layer of low, flat myoepithelial cells. See BCSC Section 2, *Fundamentals and Principles of Ophthalmology*, and Section 7, *Orbit, Eyelids, and Lacrimal System*, for additional discussion.

Congenital Anomalies

Cysts

Although some cysts are congenital, there are also acquired cysts. The major categories of orbital cysts include cysts of the surface epithelium, teratomatous cysts, neural cysts, secondary cysts (mucoceles), inflammatory cysts (parasitic), and noncystic lesions with a cystic component.

Congenital dermoid cysts are believed to develop as embryonic epithelial nests that become entrapped during embryogenesis. Most manifest in childhood as a mass in the lateral brow. Cyst rupture may produce a marked granulomatous reaction. Histologically, a dermoid cyst is lined by keratinized stratified squamous epithelium and contains keratin, sebum, and hair. By definition, its walls contain dermal elements, including sebaceous glands, hair follicles, and sweat glands (Fig 14-1). If the cyst wall does not have adnexal

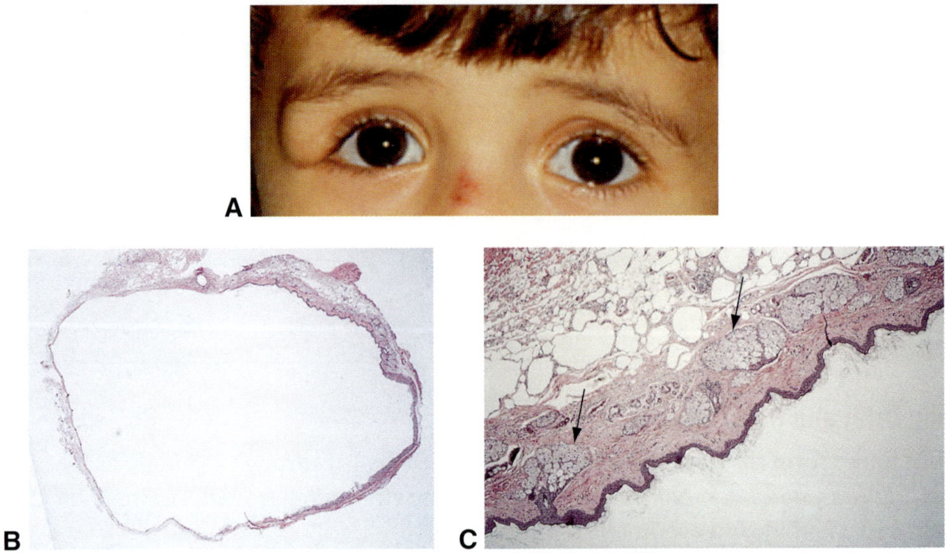

Figure 14-1 Cysts. **A,** Clinical appearance of dermoid cyst of the right orbit. Note the typical superotemporal location. **B,** Low-magnification photomicrograph reveals a cyst lined by keratinized stratified squamous epithelium. **C,** The wall of the cyst contains sebaceous glands *(arrows)* and adnexal structures. *(Part A courtesy of Sander Dubovy, MD; parts B and C courtesy of Hans E. Grossniklaus, MD.)*

structures, the term *simple epithelial (epidermoid) cyst* is applied. Simple epithelial cysts may also be lined by respiratory, conjunctival, or apocrine epithelium.

Inflammations

Orbital inflammation may be idiopathic or secondary to a systemic inflammatory disease (eg, Graves disease), a retained foreign body, or infectious disease. Orbital inflammation includes diffuse inflammation of multiple tissues (eg, sclerosing orbititis, diffuse anterior inflammation) and preferential involvement of specific orbital structures (eg, orbital myositis, optic perineuritis). Conditions masquerading as orbital inflammation include congenital orbital mass lesions and orbital neoplastic disease, such as lymphoma and rhabdomyosarcoma.

Noninfectious

Nonspecific orbital inflammation

Nonspecific orbital inflammation (NSOI) refers to a space-occupying inflammatory disorder that simulates a neoplasm (thus, it is sometimes known as *orbital pseudotumor*) but has no recognizable cause. This disorder accounts for approximately 5% of orbital lesions. Clinically, patients have an abrupt onset and usually report pain. The condition may affect children as well as adults. The inflammatory response may be diffuse or compartmentalized. When localized to an extraocular muscle, the condition is called *orbital myositis* (Fig 14-2); when localized to the lacrimal gland, it is called *dacryoadenitis.*

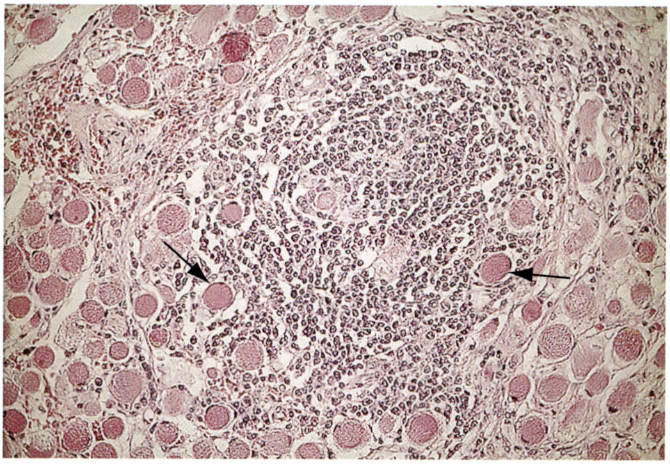

Figure 14-2 Nonspecific orbital inflammation (NSOI). NSOI can affect any orbital structure. In myositis, the skeletal muscle fibers *(arrows)* are surrounded by a dense infiltrate of chronic inflammatory cells. Unlike thyroid eye disease, in myositis the muscle tendons are involved.

In the early stages of NSOI, inflammation predominates, with a polymorphous inflammatory response (eosinophils, neutrophils, plasma cells, lymphocytes, and macrophages) that is often perivascular and that frequently infiltrates muscle and fat, producing fat necrosis. In later stages, fibrosis is the predominant feature, often with interspersed lymphoid follicles bearing germinal centers. The fibrosis may replace orbital fat and encase extraocular muscles and the optic nerve (Fig 14-3). Immunophenotypic and molecular genetic analyses can differentiate NSOI from lymphoid tumors based on whether the proliferation of lymphocytes is polyclonal (NSOI) or monoclonal (lymphoma). CD20 and CD25 receptors have been found in cases of NSOI and may provide the basis for future treatments. Immunoglobulin G4 (IgG4)–positive plasmacytic infiltrates have recently become a marker for a sclerosing variant of fibroinflammatory diseases. The nature of the pathologic findings dictates the recommended treatment. See also BCSC Section 7, *Orbit, Eyelids, and Lacrimal System.*

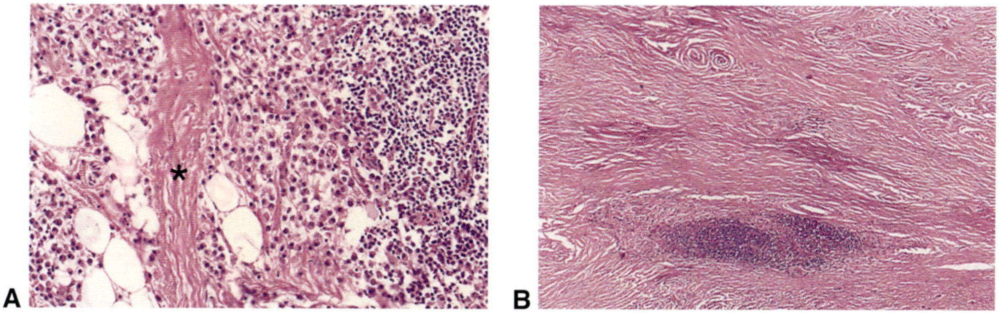

Figure 14-3 NSOI. **A,** Note the mixture of inflammatory cells, mostly lymphocytes (small, blue) and plasma cells (larger, with pink cytoplasm), and the bundle of collagen *(asterisk)* running through the orbital fat. **B,** Diffuse fibrosis dominates the histologic picture of this fibrosing orbititis, representing a later stage of the condition in **A.**

Wallace ZS, Khosroshahi A, Jakobiec FA, et al. IgG4-related systemic disease as a cause of "idiopathic" orbital inflammation, including orbital myositis, and trigeminal nerve involvement. *Surv Ophthalmol.* 2012;57(1):26–33.

Thyroid eye disease

Thyroid eye disease (TED) (also known as *Graves disease, thyroid ophthalmopathy, thyroid-associated orbitopathy,* and *Basedow disease*) is related to thyroid dysfunction and is the most common cause of unilateral or bilateral proptosis (exophthalmos) in adults. Signs and symptoms of TED are related to inflammation of the orbital connective tissue, inflammation and fibrosis of the extraocular muscles, and adipogenesis. The muscles appear firm and white, and the tendons are usually not involved. A cellular infiltrate of mononuclear inflammatory cells (eg, lymphocytes, plasma cells, mast cells) and fibroblasts involves the interstitial tissues of the extraocular muscles, most commonly the inferior and medial rectus muscles (Fig 14-4). The fibroblasts synthesize hyaluronan and other glycosaminoglycans.

Because orbital fibrocytes (considered precursor cells of fibroblasts) are derived from the neural crest and are pluripotent, the enhanced signaling promotes adipocyte differentiation and adipogenesis. For more discussion of the molecular process of TED development, see BCSC Section 1, *Update on General Medicine,* and Section 7, *Orbit, Eyelids, and Lacrimal System.*

As a result of the increased bulk within the orbit, the optic nerve may be compromised at the orbital apex, and optic nerve head swelling may result. Late stages of TED are associated with progressive fibrosis that results in restriction of ocular movement and severe eyelid retraction with resultant exposure keratitis.

Shan SJ, Douglas RS. The pathophysiology of thyroid eye disease. *J Neuroophthalmol.* 2014; 34(2):177–185.

Infectious

Bacterial infections

The causes of bacterial infections of the orbit include bacteremia, trauma, retained surgical hardware, and, most commonly, spread from an adjacent sinus infection. Infection may involve a variety of organisms, including *Haemophilus influenzae, Streptococcus, Staphylococcus aureus, Clostridium, Bacteroides, Klebsiella,* and *Proteus.* Histologically, acute inflammation, necrosis, and abscess formation may be present. Tuberculosis, which rarely involves the orbit, produces a necrotizing granulomatous reaction.

Fungal and parasitic infections

Rhinocerebral or rhino-orbito-cerebral zygomycosis (mucormycosis) (Fig 14-5A) usually occurs in patients with poorly controlled diabetes mellitus (especially those with ketoacidosis), solid malignant neoplasms, or extensive burns; in patients undergoing treatment with corticosteroid agents; or in patients with neutropenia related to hematologic malignant neoplasms. It usually represents spread from an adjacent sinus infection. Histologically, inflammation (acute and chronic) is present in a background of necrosis and is often granulomatous. Broad, nonseptate hyphae may be identified with hematoxylin-eosin,

A

B

C

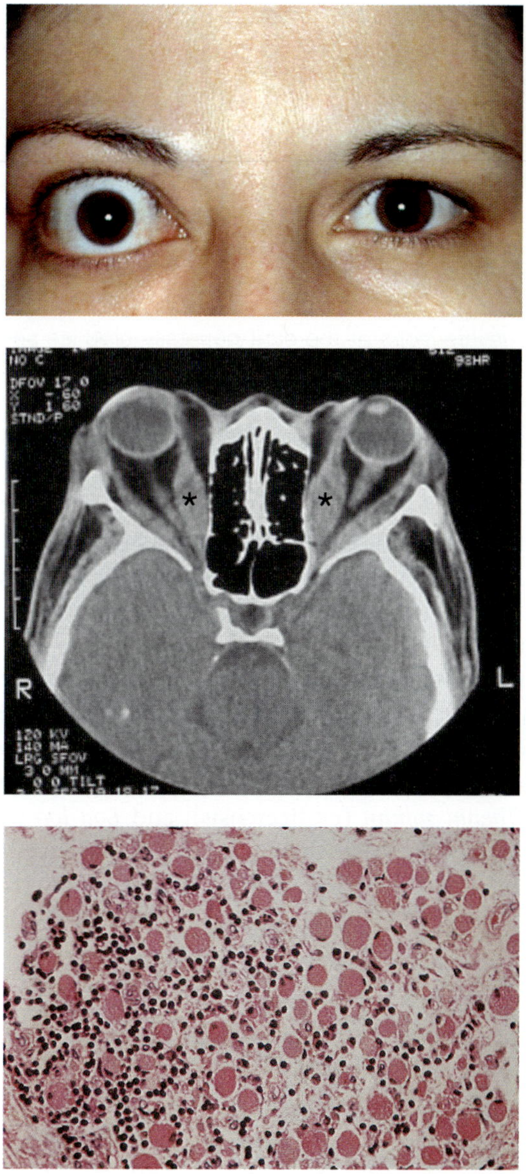

Figure 14-4 Thyroid eye disease. **A,** Clinical appearance demonstrating asymmetric proptosis and eyelid retraction, most prominent on the right. **B,** Computed tomography (CT) scan (axial view) shows fusiform enlargement of the extraocular muscles *(asterisks)* with sparing of the muscle tendons. **C,** The muscle bundles of the extraocular muscle are separated by fluid, accompanied by an infiltrate of mononuclear inflammatory cells. *(Parts A and B courtesy of Sander Dubovy, MD.)*

periodic acid–Schiff (PAS), and Gomori methenamine silver (GMS) stains. These fungi can invade blood vessel walls and produce a thrombosing vasculitis and necrosis. Diagnosis is achieved by biopsy of necrotic-appearing tissues (eschar) in the nasopharynx.

Aspergillus infection of the orbit from the adjacent sinuses may occur in immunocompromised or otherwise healthy individuals. With its slowly progressive and insidious

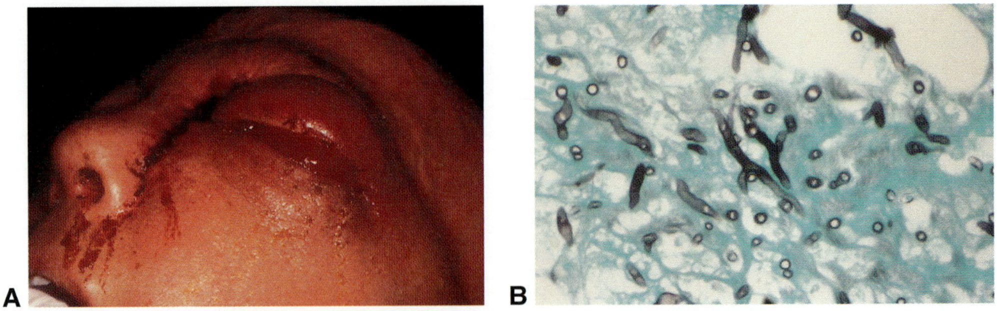

Figure 14-5 *Aspergillus* infections of the orbit generally produce severe, insidious orbital inflammation. **A,** Clinical appearance, which is similar to the clinical presentation of patients with mucormycosis. **B,** Microscopic section shows branching fungal hyphae on silver stains. *(Courtesy of Hans E. Grossniklaus, MD.)*

symptoms, sino-orbital aspergillosis often goes unrecognized, producing a sclerosing granulomatous disease. *Aspergillus* is often difficult to culture but may be observed in tissue as septate hyphae with 45° angle branching (Fig 14-5). Despite aggressive surgical therapy and adjunct therapy with antifungal agents, if extension into the brain occurs, orbital infections due to *Aspergillus* may be fatal.

Allergic fungal sinusitis is a form of noninvasive fungal disease resulting from an IgE-mediated hypersensitivity reaction in atopic individuals. It is caused by several species of fungi. The disease may extend into the orbit and intracranially in some instances.

Parasitic infections of the orbit are rare. They may be produced by *Echinococcus* (orbital hydatid cyst), *Taenia solium* (cysticercosis), and *Loa loa* (ocular filariasis). These infections are seen mostly in patients who come from, or have traveled to, areas where the infections are endemic. Enzyme-linked immunosorbent assay (ELISA) for serum antibodies may aid diagnosis. See BCSC Section 7, *Orbit, Eyelids, and Lacrimal System.*

Degenerations

Amyloid

Amyloid deposition in the orbit occurs in primary systemic amyloidosis. When it involves the extraocular muscles and nerves, it can cause ophthalmoplegia and ptosis. See Chapters 5, 6, 10, and 13 in this volume and BCSC Section 8, *External Disease and Cornea.*

Neoplasia

Neoplasms of the orbit may be primary or secondary (extensions from adjacent structures or metastatic disease). Secondary tumors are slightly more common than primary tumors. (See the section Secondary Tumors later in this chapter.) Children and adults are affected by different varieties of orbital tumors. Vascular and lymphoid tumors are the primary orbital lesions most often encountered in adults, and congenital tumors are the primary orbital lesions most often encountered in children.

In children, approximately 90% of orbital tumors are benign. Benign cystic lesions (dermoid or simple epithelial cysts) represent 50% of orbital lesions in childhood. Rhabdomyosarcoma is the most common orbital malignant tumor in childhood; it represents 3% of all orbital masses. The orbit may be involved secondarily in cases of retinoblastoma, neuroblastoma, and leukemia/lymphoma. See BCSC Section 7, *Orbit, Eyelids, and Lacrimal System,* for additional discussion.

Lacrimal Sac Neoplasia

Lacrimal sac neoplasms are rare. In one study of patients undergoing dacryocystorhinostomy (DCR) for chronic nasolacrimal duct obstruction, neoplasm was the cause in only 5% of cases. Most lacrimal sac tumors are papillomatous neoplasms that arise in the epithelial lining, but a wide variety have been reported.

Anderson NG, Wojno TH, Grossniklaus HE. Clinicopathologic findings from lacrimal sac biopsy specimens obtained during dacryocystorhinostomy. *Ophthal Plast Reconstr Surg.* 2003;19(3):173–176.

Lacrimal Gland Neoplasia

Because the lacrimal gland is a modified salivary gland, epithelial lacrimal gland tumors are classified according to the World Health Organization (WHO) epithelial salivary gland classification system. The most common types of epithelial lacrimal gland tumors are pleomorphic adenoma, adenocarcinoma (carcinoma ex pleomorphic adenoma), and adenoid cystic carcinoma.

Weis E, Rootman J, Joly TJ, et al. Epithelial lacrimal gland tumors: pathologic classification and current understanding. *Arch Ophthalmol.* 2009;127(8):1016–1028.

Pleomorphic adenoma

The most common epithelial tumor of the lacrimal gland is pleomorphic adenoma (benign mixed tumor). The tumor is pseudoencapsulated and grows slowly by expansion. This progressive expansive growth may excavate the bone of the lacrimal fossa. Tumor growth stimulates the periosteum to deposit a thin layer of new bone (ie, cortication). The adjacent orbital bone is not eroded. Typically, the patient experiences no pain. This tumor is slightly more common in men than in women, and the median age at presentation is 35 years.

Histologically, pleomorphic adenoma has a fibrous pseudocapsule and comprises a mixture of ductal-derived epithelial and stromal elements. The epithelial component may form nests or tubules lined by 2 layers of cells, the outermost layer blending imperceptibly with the stroma (Fig 14-6). The stroma may appear myxoid and may contain heterologous elements, including cartilage and bone. Immunohistochemistry reflects the epithelial and myoepithelial components, both derived from epithelium. The tumor typically tests positive for keratin and epithelial membrane antigen in the ductal areas and positive for keratin, actin, myosin, fibronectin, and S-100 protein in the myoepithelial areas.

Chromosomal translocations are recognized in pleomorphic adenomas. Transformation into a malignant mixed tumor may take place in a long-standing or incompletely excised pleomorphic adenoma, with relatively rapid growth after a period of relative

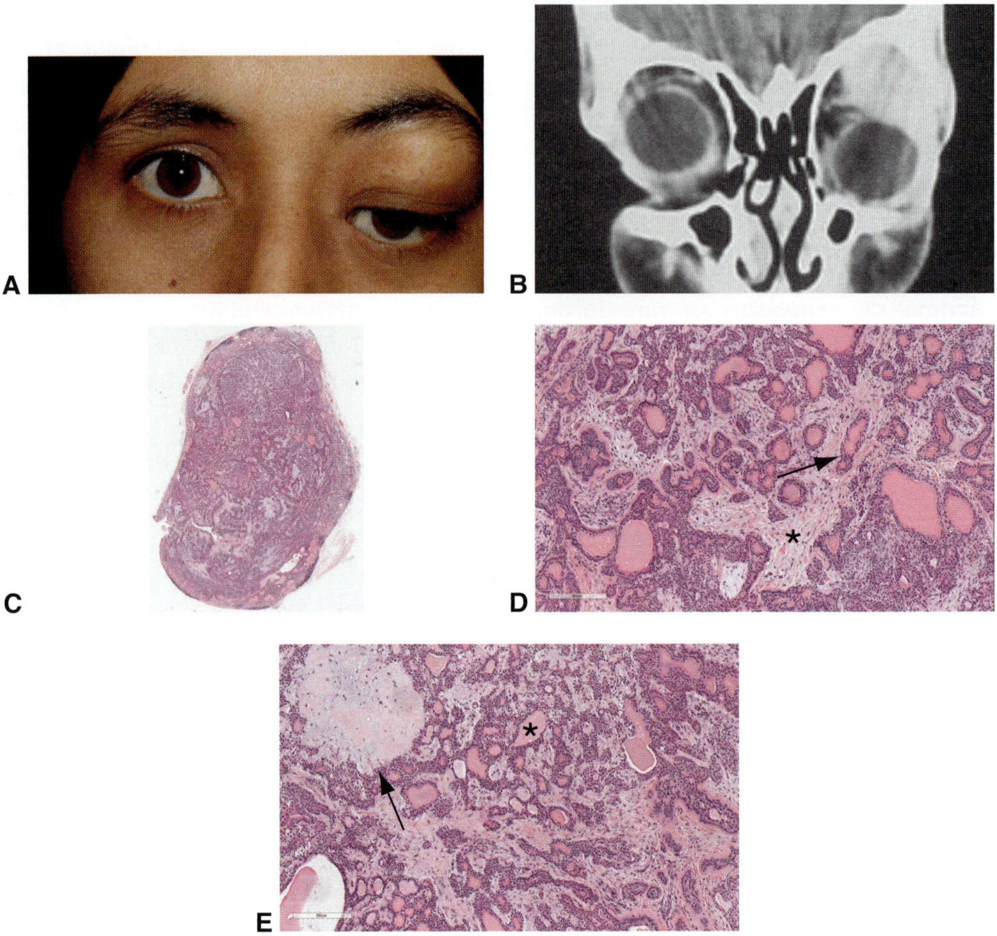

Figure 14-6 Pleomorphic adenoma (benign mixed tumor) of the lacrimal gland. **A,** Clinical appearance. A superotemporal orbital mass is present, causing proptosis and downward displacement of the left globe. **B,** CT scan (coronal view) demonstrating left orbit tumor. **C,** Low-magnification photomicrograph shows the circumscribed nature of this pleomorphic adenoma. **D,** Note both the neoplastic epithelial elements *(arrow)* and the fibromyxoid stroma *(asterisk)*. **E,** Well-differentiated glandular structures with lumina *(asterisk)*. The outer myoepithelial layer can become metaplastic to form other mesenchymal tissue (eg, adipose, cartilage *[arrow]*). *(Parts A and B courtesy of Sander Dubovy, MD; parts C–E courtesy of Heather Potter, MD.)*

quiescence. Carcinomas, including adenocarcinoma (carcinoma ex pleomorphic adenoma) and adenoid cystic carcinoma, may also develop in recurrent pleomorphic adenomas.

Adenoid cystic carcinoma

Adenoid cystic carcinoma (ACC) can develop in a pleomorphic adenoma or de novo in the lacrimal gland. The tumor is slightly more common in women than in men, and the median age at presentation is about 40 years. Unlike pleomorphic adenoma, ACC has no pseudocapsule; it tends to cause bone destruction and invade orbital nerves, accounting for the pain that is frequently reported on presentation. The gross appearance is grayish white, firm, and nodular. Histologic examination may reveal a variety of patterns, including the cribriform (Swiss cheese) pattern, which is the most common (Fig 14-7). Other histologic patterns include basaloid (solid), comedocarcinoma, sclerosing, and tubular (ductal). Presence of a basaloid pattern has been associated with a worse prognosis (5-year survival rate of 20%) when compared with absence of a basaloid component (5-year survival rate of 70%). Immunohistochemistry is typically positive for S-100 protein, keratin, and actin, with areas of epithelial and myoepithelial differentiation. There is a positive correlation between prognosis and protein expression of Bcl-2 and BAX. Expression of p53 is associated with a poor prognosis. Exenteration is one of the currently accepted treatments for this tumor, but some advocate globe-sparing intra-arterial chemotherapy.

Ahmad SM, Esmaeli B, Williams M, et al. American Joint Committee on Cancer classification predicts outcome of patients with lacrimal gland adenoid cystic carcinoma. *Ophthalmology.* 2009;116(6):1210–1215.

von Holstein SL, Coupland SE, Briscoe D, Le Tourneau C, Heegaard S. Epithelial tumours of the lacrimal gland: a clinical, histopathological, surgical and oncological survey. *Acta Ophthalmol.* 2013;91(3):195–206.

Lymphoproliferative Lesions

Most classifications of lymphoid lesions have been based on lymph node architecture; therefore such nodal classifications have been difficult to apply to extranodal lymphoid lesions. In the ocular adnexa, the diagnosis of lymphoma involves identifying a monoclonal population of cells. Because there are no lymph nodes in the orbit, it is problematic to classify these lesions according to the criteria used for lymph nodes. The development of classification schemes for lymphomas is, thus, an ongoing and controversial process. In general, lymphoproliferative lesions are divided into reactive lymphoid hyperplasia (RLH), atypical lymphoid hyperplasia (ALH), and ocular adnexal lymphoma (OAL). OAL is subtyped according to the *WHO Classification of Tumours of Haematopoietic and Lymphoid Tissues.* Many lymphoid masses in the orbit that had previously been classified as reactive or atypical hyperplasia would now be considered neoplasia.

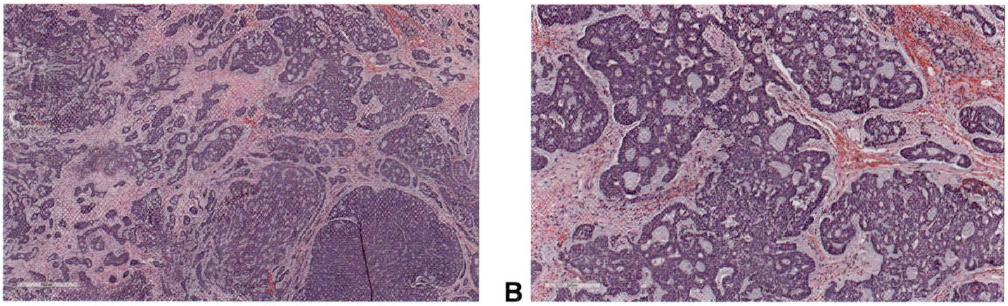

A B

Figure 14-7 Adenoid cystic carcinoma of the lacrimal gland. **A,** Low-magnification photomicrograph showing numerous invasive tumor lobules (H&E stain). **B,** Note the characteristic cribriform ("Swiss cheese") appearance. *(Courtesy of Heather Potter, MD.)*

Unlike patients with NSOI, those with orbital lymphoproliferative lesions present with gradual, painless progression of proptosis. Bilateral disease may occur; when it does, it heightens suspicion for systemic disease. Every patient with an orbital lymphoproliferative lesion should be staged in collaboration with a medical oncologist. Studies may include positron emission tomography (PET) scan and bone marrow biopsy.

When taking a biopsy of an orbital or conjunctival lymphoproliferative lesion, the ophthalmologist should consult with the pathologist in advance to determine the optimal method for handling the tissue, including the type of fixative to use and the volume of tissue to obtain. Exposure of the biopsy specimen to air for long periods should be avoided. Tissue samples may be wrapped in saline-moistened gauze and transported on ice. It is very important that the tissue be handled gently; crush artifact can prevent the pathologist from rendering a diagnosis. Fresh (unfixed) tissue is required for touch preparations and flow cytometry. Gene rearrangement studies and immunohistochemistry can be performed on fixed tissue. See also Chapter 4, Table 4-1, for a checklist for requesting an ophthalmic pathologic consultation.

Demirci H, Shields CL, Karatza EC, Shields JA. Orbital lymphoproliferative tumors: analysis of clinical features and systemic involvement in 160 cases. *Ophthalmology.* 2008;115(9): 1626–1631.

Swerdlow SH, Campo E, Harris NL, et al. *WHO Classification of Tumours of Haematopoietic and Lymphoid Tissues.* 4th ed. Lyon, France: International Agency for Research on Cancer; 2008.

Lymphoid hyperplasia

Reactive lymphoid hyperplasia is composed of well-differentiated lymphocytes with occasional plasma cells, macrophages, eosinophils, and follicles with germinal centers. The follicles usually contain tingible body macrophages (containing apoptotic debris), and there is mitotic activity; they also often have vessels with endothelial hyperplasia. Atypical lymphoid hyperplasia involves diffuse lymphoid proliferation, generally without reactive germinal centers. It is composed of an admixture of small, mature-appearing lymphocytes and larger lymphoid cells of unknown maturity. RLH and ALH are believed to represent one end of a continuum of lymphoproliferative lesions, with lymphoma at the other end.

Lymphoma

Lymphomas of the orbit may be a presenting manifestation of systemic lymphoma or may arise primarily from the orbit. Extranodal marginal zone B-cell lymphoma of mucosa-associated lymphoid tissue (MALT) is the most common type of lymphoma seen in the orbit. These tumors are generally low-grade B-cell tumors with an excellent prognosis. Other types of lymphoma, such as follicular, large B-cell, and mantle cell lymphoma, occur in the orbit but with a lower incidence. Most of these are non-Hodgkin lymphomas, which constitute one-half of malignant tumors arising in the orbit and the ocular adnexa (Fig 14-8). They have diffuse architecture and contain B-cells with immunopositivity for CD19 and CD20. T-cell lymphomas of the orbit are rare, more aggressive, and immunopositive for CD3, CD4, and CD8. The incidence of secondary orbital involvement in systemic lymphomas is approximately 1%–2%. Interestingly, the incidence of orbital lymphoma is increasing.

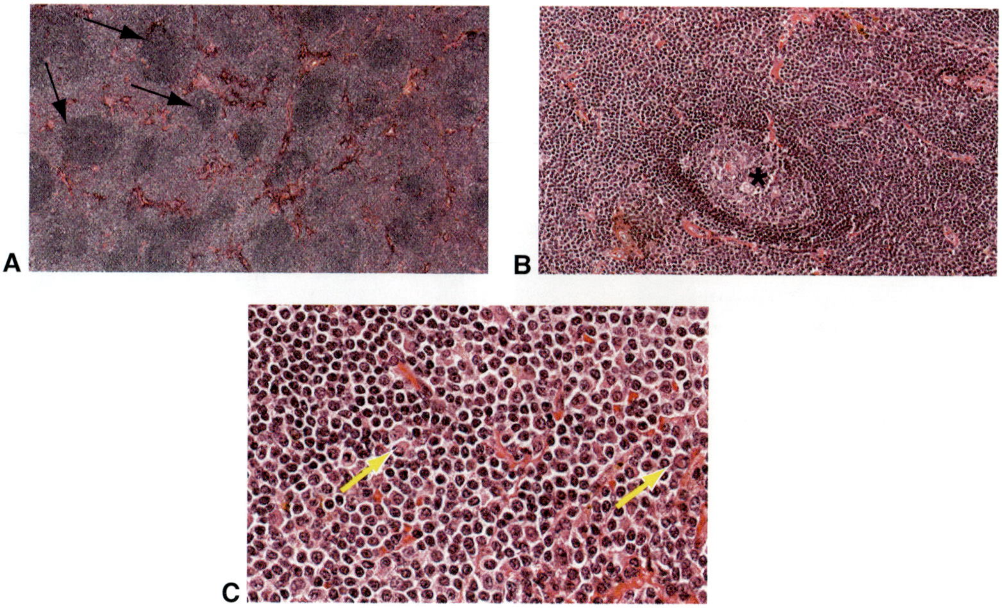

Figure 14-8 Low-grade B-cell lymphoma of the orbit (H&E stain). **A,** Low-magnification photomicrograph shows sheets of dense, small, uniform lymphocytes forming vague follicular arrangements *(arrows)*. **B,** Higher magnification shows a lymphoid follicle with a germinal center *(asterisk)*. **C,** Dutcher bodies with intranuclear inclusions *(arrows)*. *(Courtesy of Heather Potter, MD.)*

Soft-Tissue Tumors

Soft-tissue tumors are diagnosed both by recognition of the histologic patterns (ie, round cell, spindle cell, myxoid, epithelioid, pericytomatous, and pleomorphic) and by immunohistochemistry. The characteristic pathologic features of soft-tissue tumors are described on websites such as PathologyOutlines.com (www.pathologyoutlines.com/eye.html). Typically, a panel of immunohistochemical stains is used for the initial differentiation, and those results direct further studies; however, it may be challenging to classify these tumors.

Vascular Tumors

Orbital lymphatic malformations (previously termed *lymphangiomas*) occur in children and are characterized by fluctuation in proptosis, often enlarging in the setting of illness. They are unencapsulated, diffusely infiltrating tumors that feature lymphatic vascular spaces and lymphoid aggregates in a fibrotic interstitium (Fig 14-9).

Hemangioma in the adult is typically encapsulated and intraconal and consists of cavernous spaces *(cavernous hemangioma)* with variably thick, fibrosed walls (Fig 14-10). Vessels may show thrombosis and calcification. Hemangioma in the child is unencapsulated and more cellular, often with a cutaneous component, and is composed of capillary-sized vessels *(capillary hemangioma)*.

Nassiri N, Rootman J, Rootman DB, Goldberg RA. Orbital lymphaticovenous malformations: current and future treatments. *Surv Ophthalmol.* 2015;60(5):383–405.

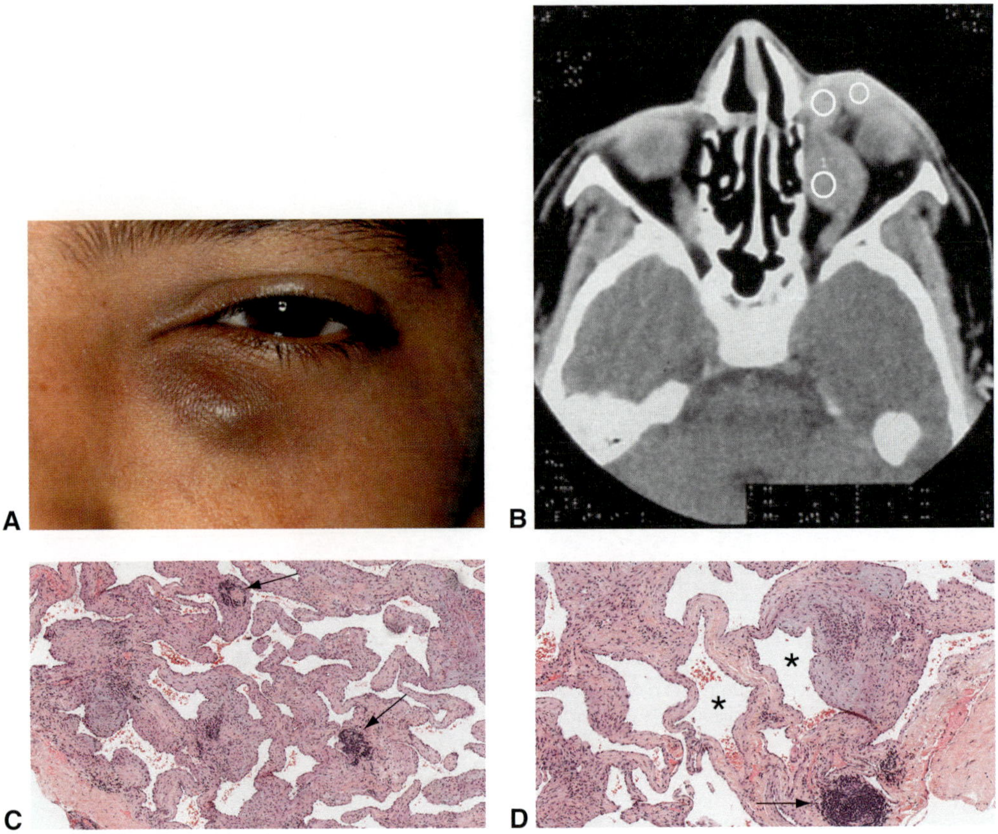

Figure 14-9 Orbital lymphatic malformation. **A,** Clinical appearance. A young boy with an inferior orbital lesion extending anteriorly and nasally below the left lower eyelid. **B,** CT scan (axial view) showing a multilobulated mass *(white circles)* within the left orbit. **C,** Photomicrograph (H&E stain) shows numerous vascular channels with lymphoid follicles *(arrows)*. **D,** Higher magnification (H&E stain) demonstrates endothelial-lined vascular channels *(asterisks)*, a lymphoid follicle *(arrow)*, and scattered lymphocytes and plasma cells within the fibrous walls. *(Parts A and B courtesy of Sander Dubovy, MD; parts C and D courtesy of Heather Potter, MD.)*

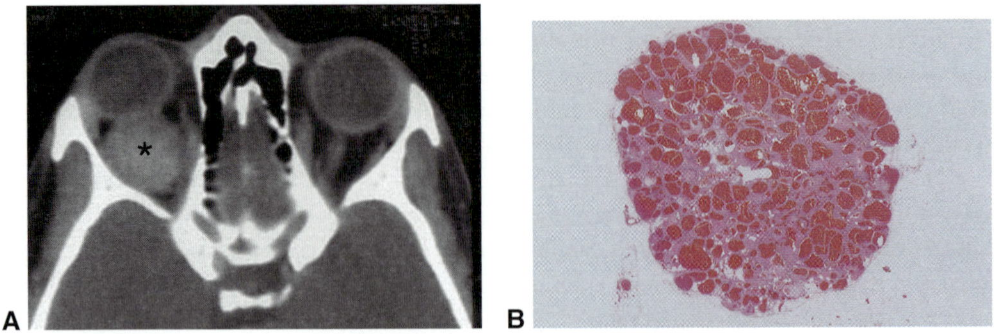

Figure 14-10 Cavernous hemangioma. **A,** CT scan (axial view) showing a well-circumscribed retrobulbar mass *(asterisk)*. **B,** Large blood-filled spaces are separated by thick septa. *(Part A courtesy of Sander Dubovy, MD; part B courtesy of Hans E. Grossniklaus, MD.)*

Tumors With Fibrous Differentiation

Solitary fibrous tumor

Solitary fibrous tumor is the most common mesenchymal tumor of the orbit in adults; presentation occurs in the fifth decade of life on average. Most patients present with an orbital mass causing a combination of symptoms, including proptosis, pain, diplopia, blurred vision, and epiphora. The superonasal orbit is a common site.

Recent research has demonstrated that hemangiopericytomas, fibrous histiocytomas, and giant cell angiofibromas of the orbit share several histologic characteristics and may be better categorized together under the heading of orbital solitary fibrous tumors. Two commonalities among all of these tumors are that they are collagen-rich, contain proliferating CD34-positive fibroblast-like cells, and often demonstrate strong nuclear STAT6 expression.

Classically, the presence of staghorn sinusoidal blood vessels (Fig 14-11) was used to distinguish hemangiopericytoma from other tumors; fibrous histiocytoma demonstrated spindle-shaped, plump histiocyte-like cells with a focal storiform architecture (Fig 14-12); and giant cell angiofibroma was distinguished by the presence of multinucleated floret-type giant cells and angioectatic spaces. However, these findings overlap; for example, 87% of all fibrous tumors show staghorn vessels. Other shared histologic features may include

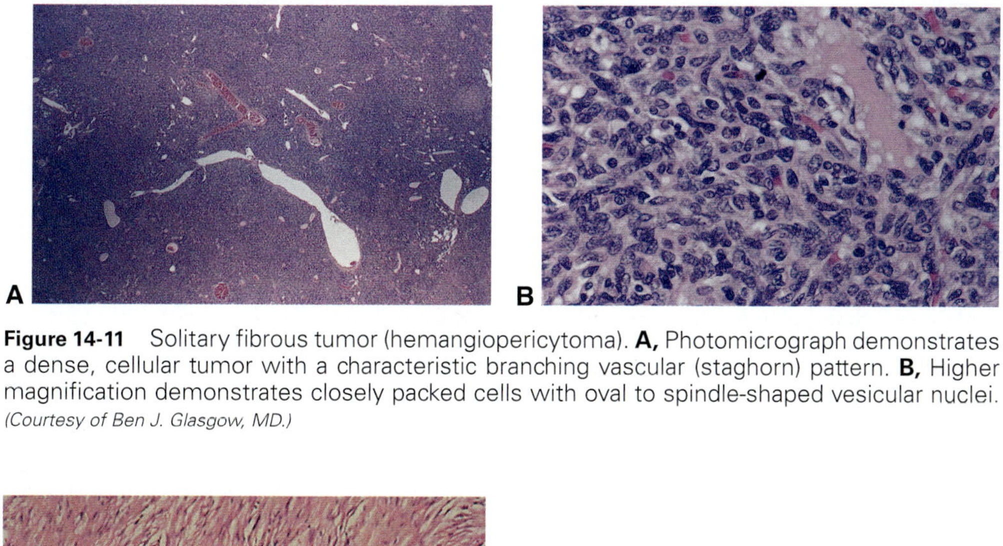

Figure 14-11 Solitary fibrous tumor (hemangiopericytoma). **A,** Photomicrograph demonstrates a dense, cellular tumor with a characteristic branching vascular (staghorn) pattern. **B,** Higher magnification demonstrates closely packed cells with oval to spindle-shaped vesicular nuclei. *(Courtesy of Ben J. Glasgow, MD.)*

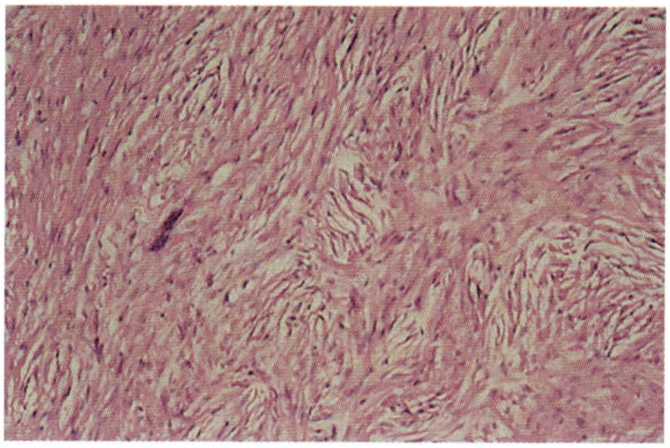

Figure 14-12 Fibrous histiocytoma. Photomicrograph illustrates the storiform (matlike or whorly) pattern.

mild hemorrhage, osteoclast-type cells, stromal myxoid change, mature adipocytes, and mineralization. The presence of overlapping features is the reason that the nomenclature of solitary fibrous tumor is preferred to define all of these tumors.

Most solitary fibrous tumors are benign, but marked cytologic atypia and increased mitotic activity, accentuated by strong staining for Ki-67 and/or p53, support the designation of borderline or low-grade malignant behavior.

Other primary tumors of fibrous connective tissue include nodular fasciitis, fibroma, and fibrosarcoma.

Demicco EG, Harms PW, Patel RM, et al. Extensive survey of STAT6 expression in a large series of mesenchymal tumors. *Am J Clin Pathol.* 2015;143(5):672–682.

Furusato E, Valenzuela IA, Fanburg-Smith JC, et al. Orbital solitary fibrous tumor: encompassing terminology for hemangiopericytoma, giant cell angiofibroma, and fibrous histiocytoma of the orbit: reappraisal of 41 cases. *Hum Pathol.* 2011;42(1):120–128.

Tumors With Muscle Differentiation

Rhabdomyosarcoma

Rhabdomyosarcoma is the most common primary malignant orbital tumor of childhood (average age at onset is 7–8 years). Proptosis is often sudden and rapidly progressive; it requires emergency treatment. Reddish discoloration of the eyelids is *not* accompanied by local heat or systemic fever, as it is in cellulitis. Orbital rhabdomyosarcomas have a better prognosis (overall 5-year survival rate of about 90%) than do their extraorbital counterparts.

Rhabdomyosarcomas arise from primitive mesenchymal cells that differentiate toward skeletal muscle. There are 3 recognized histologic types of orbital rhabdomyosarcoma (Fig 14-13):

1. embryonal (most common)
2. alveolar (worst prognosis)
3. pleomorphic (best prognosis)

Embryonal rhabdomyosarcoma may develop in the conjunctiva and may present as grapelike submucosal clusters (ie, *botryoid variant*). Histologically, spindle cells are arranged in a loose syncytium with occasional cells bearing cross-striations. These cross-striations are found in approximately 60% of embryonal rhabdomyosarcomas. Well-differentiated rhabdomyosarcomas feature numerous cells with striking cross-striations. Immunohistochemical analysis is typically positive for desmin, muscle-specific actin, vimentin, and, less commonly, myogenin. Electron microscopy is helpful for demonstrating the typical sarcomeric banding pattern, especially in cases of embryonal rhabdomyosarcoma, which are not as well-differentiated. Cytogenetic studies are important for identifying genetic translocations such as *FOXO1,* which has prognostic implications.

Hawkins DS, Gupta AA, Rudzinski ER. What is new in the biology and treatment of pediatric rhabdomyosarcoma? *Curr Opin Pediatr.* 2014;26(1):50–56.

Leiomyomas and leiomyosarcomas

Tumors with smooth muscle differentiation are rare. *Leiomyomas* are benign tumors that typically manifest with slowly progressive proptosis in patients in the fourth or fifth decade

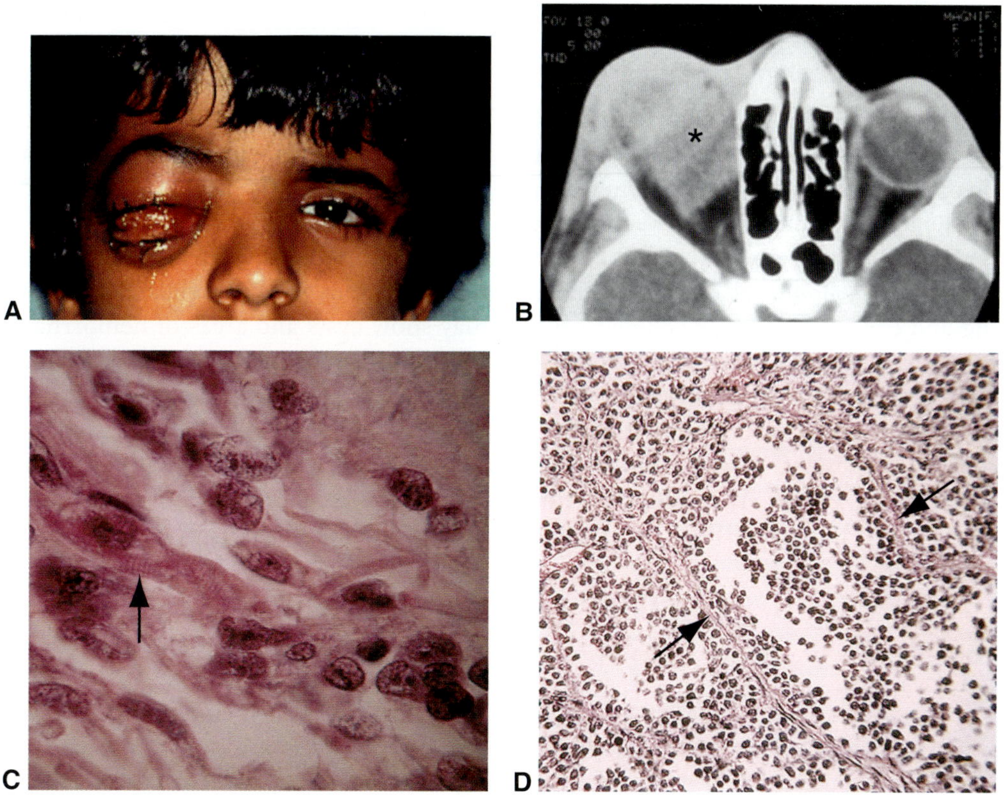

Figure 14-13 Rhabdomyosarcoma. **A,** Child with a large right orbital mass. **B,** CT scan (axial view) showing a large, poorly circumscribed orbital tumor *(asterisk)* and proptosis. **C,** In this embryonal example, cross-striations *(arrow)* representing Z bands of actin–myosin complexes within the cytoplasm of a tumor cell can be identified. **D,** Poorly cohesive rhabdomyoblasts separated by fibrous septa *(arrows)* into "alveoli" are low-magnification histologic features of the alveolar variant of rhabdomyosarcoma. This variant may have a less favorable natural history than the more common embryonal type. *(Parts A and B courtesy of Sander Dubovy, MD.)*

of life. Histologically, these spindle cell tumors show blunt-ended, cigar-shaped nuclei and trichrome-positive filamentous cytoplasm. Immunohistochemistry displays smooth muscle differentiation. *Leiomyosarcomas* are malignant lesions that typically occur in patients in their seventh decade. Histologically, these tumors show more cellularity, necrosis, and nuclear pleomorphism than their benign counterparts. Mitotic figures also appear in leiomyosarcomas but are typically absent in leiomyomas.

Nerve Sheath Tumors

Neurofibroma, which is the most common nerve sheath tumor, is a slow-growing tumor that includes an admixture of endoneural fibroblasts, Schwann cells, and axons. Neurofibromas may be circumscribed but are not encapsulated. They are firm and rubbery. Microscopically, the spindle-shaped cells are arranged in ribbons and cords in a matrix of myxoid tissue and collagen that contains axons. Cytogenetic studies indicate that the most frequent structural rearrangements involve chromosome arm 9p.

Isolated neurofibromas do not necessarily indicate systemic involvement, but the plexiform type of neurofibroma is associated with neurofibromatosis 1 (Fig 14-14). "Plexiform" refers to an intricate network, or "plexus," classically described as a "bag of worms." Studies indicate that a limited number of pathways are potentially involved in tumorigenesis of the plexiform neurofibroma. The *CCN1* gene may be a useful diagnostic or prognostic marker and form the basis for novel therapeutic strategies. The CCNs (cysteine-rich proteins) have been shown to occupy key roles as matricellular proteins, serving as adaptor molecules that connect the cell surface and the extracellular matrix.

A *neurilemoma* (also called *schwannoma*) arises from Schwann cells. Slow growing and encapsulated, this yellowish tumor may show cysts and areas of hemorrhagic necrosis. It may be solitary or associated with neurofibromatosis. Two histologic patterns appear microscopically. Antoni A spindle cells are arranged in interlacing cords, whorls, or palisades that may form Verocay bodies (collections of fibrils resembling sensory corpuscles). The Antoni B pattern is made up of stellate cells that have a mucoid stroma. Vessels are usually prominent and thick-walled, and no axons are present (Fig 14-15). Immunohistochemistry is typically positive for S-100 protein, vimentin, and CD68.

Liu K, DeAngelo P, Mahmet K, Phytides P, Osborne L, Pletcher BA. Cytogenetics of neurofibromas: two case reports and literature review. *Cancer Genet Cytogenet.* 2010;196(1): 93–95.

Pasmant E, Ortonne N, Rittié L, et al. Differential expression of CCN1/CYR61, CCN3/NOV, CCN4/WISP1, and CCN5/WISP2 in neurofibromatosis type 1 tumorigenesis. *J Neuropathol Exp Neurol.* 2010;69(1):60–69.

Adipose Tumors

Lipomas are rare in the orbit. Their pathologic characteristics include encapsulation and a distinctive lobular appearance. Because lipomas are histologically difficult to distinguish from normal or prolapsed fat, their incidence might previously have been overestimated.

Liposarcomas are malignant tumors that are extremely rare in the orbit. Histologic criteria depend on the type of liposarcoma, but the unifying diagnostic feature is the presence of lipoblasts. These tumors tend to recur before they metastasize.

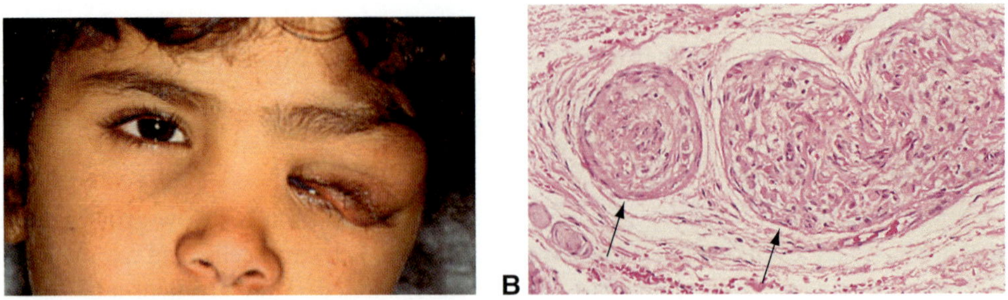

A B

Figure 14-14 Plexiform neurofibroma. **A,** Clinical photograph depicting a typical S-shaped deformity of the upper eyelid. **B,** Note the thickened, tortuous nerves *(arrows)* with proliferation of endoneural fibroblasts and Schwann cells. *(Part A courtesy of Sander Dubovy, MD.)*

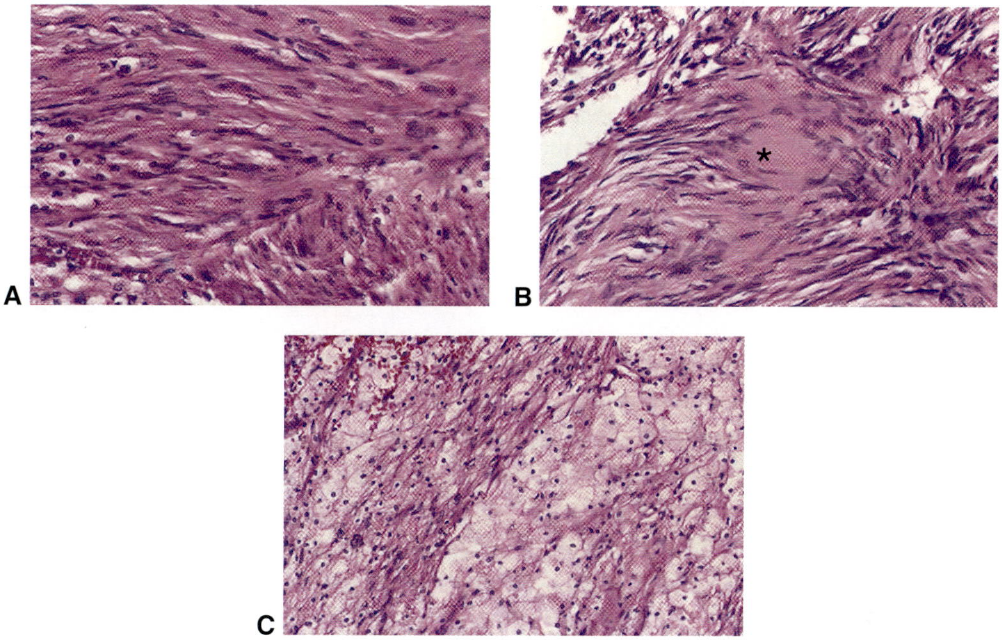

Figure 14-15 Neurilemoma (schwannoma). **A,** The Antoni A pattern. Spindle cells are packed together. **B,** Palisading of nuclei may form a Verocay body *(asterisk).* **C,** The Antoni B pattern consists of a loosely arranged, mucoid stroma and represents degeneration within the tumor.

Bony Lesions of the Orbit

Fibrous dysplasia of bone may be monostotic or polyostotic. When the orbit is affected, the condition is usually monostotic; the patient often presents during the first 3 decades of life. The tumor may cross suture lines to involve multiple orbital bones. Narrowing of the optic canal and lacrimal drainage system can occur. Plain radiographic studies show a ground-glass appearance with lytic foci. Cysts that contain fluid also appear. As a result of arrest in the maturation of bone, trabeculae are composed of woven bone with a fibrous stroma that is highly vascularized rather than lamellar bone. The bony trabeculae often have a C-shaped appearance (Fig 14-16).

Fibro-osseous dysplasia (juvenile ossifying fibroma), a variant of fibrous dysplasia, is characterized histologically by spicules of bone rimmed by osteoblasts (Fig 14-17). At low magnification, ossifying fibroma may be confused with a psammomatous meningioma.

Osseous and cartilaginous tumors are rare; of these, *osteoma* is the most common. It is slow growing and well circumscribed, and it is composed of mature bone. Most commonly, an osteoma arises from the frontal sinus. Other primary tumors in this group include

- osteoblastoma
- giant cell tumor
- chondroma
- Ewing sarcoma
- osteogenic sarcoma
- chondrosarcoma

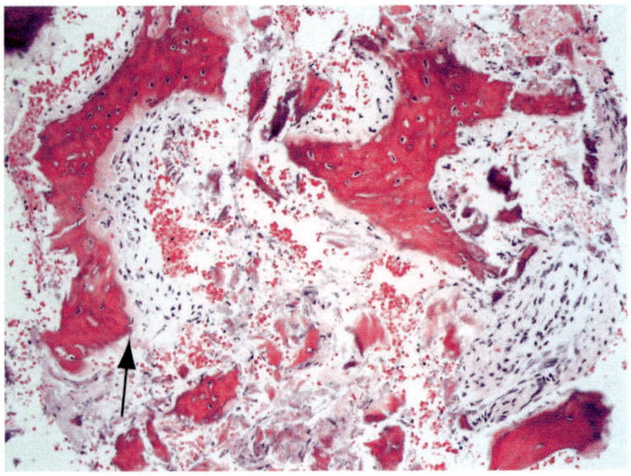

Figure 14-16 Fibrous dysplasia. Bony trabeculae are C-shaped *(arrow)*, composed of immature woven bone, and surrounded by a fibrous stroma. *(Courtesy of Tatyana Milman, MD.)*

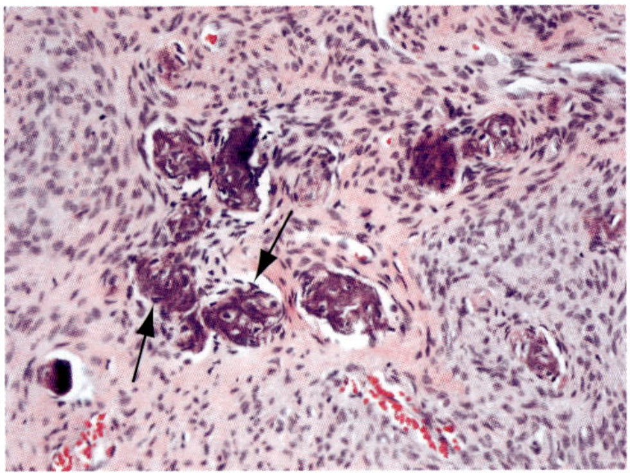

Figure 14-17 Fibro-osseous dysplasia (juvenile ossifying fibroma). Spicules of lamellar bone are set in a cellular fibrous stroma. Note the osteoblasts *(arrows)* lining the bony spicules. *(Courtesy of Tatyana Milman, MD.)*

Secondary Tumors

Secondary malignant orbital tumors are lesions that invade the orbit by direct extension from adjacent structures, such as sinus, bone, or eye. *Metastatic* tumors are malignant lesions that have spread from a distant primary site. The most common primary tumor sites involved in orbital metastasis are the breast in women and the prostate in men. In children, neuroblastoma is the most common primary tumor metastatic to the orbit.

CHAPTER 15

Optic Nerve

Topography

The optic nerve, which is embryologically derived from the optic stalk, is a continuation of the optic tract; thus, the pathology of the optic nerve reflects that of the central nervous system (CNS). The optic nerve extends from the eye to the optic chiasm and is 35–55 mm in its total length; it can be divided into the following 4 topographic areas:

- intraocular 0.7–1.0 mm
- intraorbital 25–30 mm
- intracanalicular 4–10 mm
- intracranial average 10 mm

The cells of the supportive tissue of the CNS, oligodendrocytes, astrocytes, and microglial cells, are glial cells (*glia* = glue). Oligodendrocytes produce and maintain the myelin sheath of the optic nerve; astrocytes are involved with support and nutrition; and microglial cells (CNS histiocytes) have a phagocytic function.

The meningeal coat that covers the optic nerve includes the dura mater (which merges with the sclera), the cellular arachnoid layer, and the vascular pia mater. The pial vessels and connective tissue extend into the optic nerve and subdivide the nerve fibers into fascicles. The subarachnoid space, which contains cerebrospinal fluid, ends at the termination of the meninges (Figs 15-1, 15-2). See BCSC Section 2, *Fundamentals and Principles of Ophthalmology,* and Section 5, *Neuro-Ophthalmology,* for additional discussion of the optic nerve.

Congenital Anomalies

Numerous congenital defects can involve the optic nerve, including optic nerve hypoplasia, optic nerve head (ONH) pits (also called optic disc pits), morning glory disc anomaly, Bergmeister papilla, and optic nerve colobomas. These congenital anomalies are discussed further in BCSC Section 5, *Neuro-Ophthalmology,* and Section 6, *Pediatric Ophthalmology and Strabismus.*

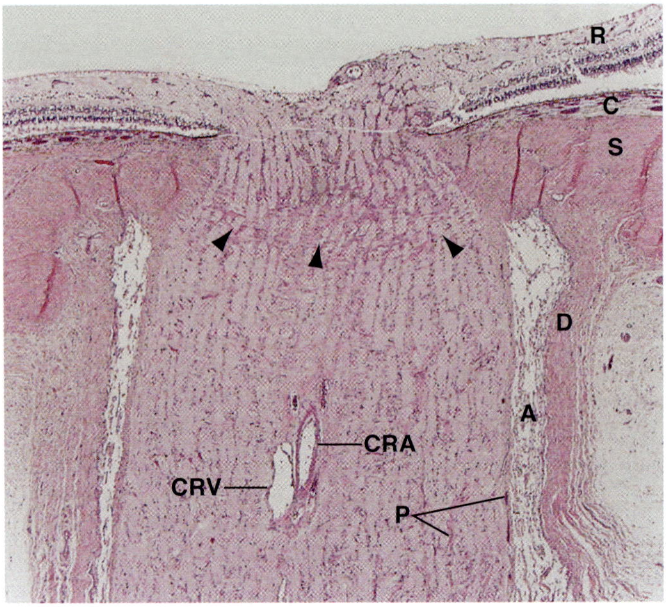

Figure 15-1 Longitudinal section of normal optic nerve. Axons of the retinal ganglion cells (R) become axonal fibers of the optic nerve. Optic nerve axons pass through the fenestrations in the lamina cribrosa *(arrowheads),* which is continuous with the anterior sclera (S). The posterior sclera is continuous with the dura (D). C = choroid, A = arachnoid, P = pial septa, CRA = central retinal artery, CRV = central retinal vein. *(Courtesy of Tatyana Milman, MD.)*

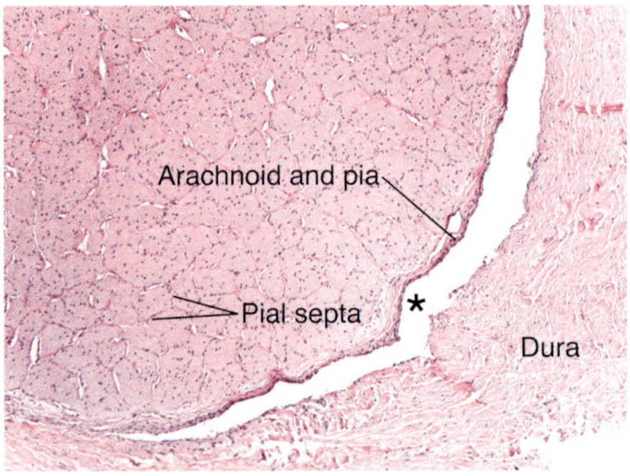

Figure 15-2 Transverse or cross section of the normal optic nerve. The axons of the optic nerve are segregated into fascicles by the delicate fibrovascular pial septa. The nuclei of oligodendrocytes, astrocytes, and microglia are present between the eosinophilic axons. The subdural space *(asterisk)* is relatively narrow in a normal optic nerve. *(Courtesy of Tatyana Milman, MD.)*

Colobomas

Typical colobomas of the ONH result from defective closure of the embryonic fissure. They are often observed inferonasally in the ONH; may be associated with colobomatous defects of the retina/choroid, ciliary body, and iris; and may occur at any point along the course of the embryonic fissure (Fig 15-3A).

Histologically, an optic nerve coloboma consists of a large defect in the optic nerve that involves the retina, retinal pigment epithelium, and choroid. An atrophic, gliotic retina lines the defect. The sclera is ectatic and bowed posteriorly. The wall of the defect may contain adipose tissue and even smooth muscle (see Fig 15-3B).

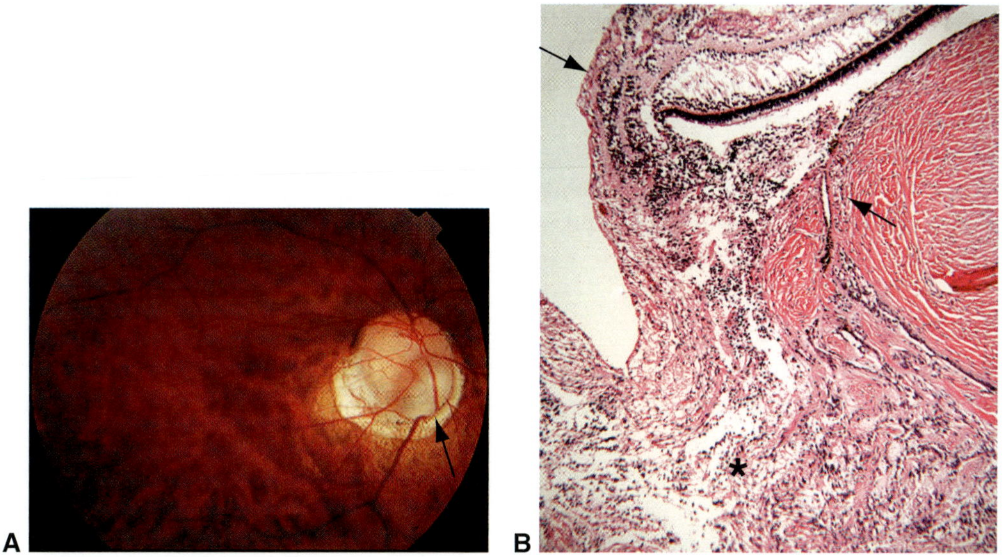

Figure 15-3 Optic nerve coloboma. **A,** Fundus photograph of the right eye shows a colobomatous defect in the inferonasal optic nerve *(arrow).* **B,** Photomicrograph of a gliotic, disorganized retina *(asterisk)* that prolapses into the defect, which is lined by excavated sclera. The normal retina, retinal pigment epithelium, and choroid terminate at the edge of the colobomatous defect *(arrows).* *(Courtesy of Tatyana Milman, MD.)*

Inflammations

Infectious

Bacterial or *fungal* infections of the optic nerve can spread from adjacent anatomical structures, or they may occur as part of a systemic infection, particularly in an immunosuppressed patient. Fungal infections include mucormycosis, cryptococcosis, and coccidioidomycosis. Mucormycosis generally results from contiguous sinus infection. Cryptococcosis results from a direct extension of the infection from the CNS and often produces multiple foci of necrosis with little inflammatory reaction (Fig 15-4). Coccidioidomycosis generally begins

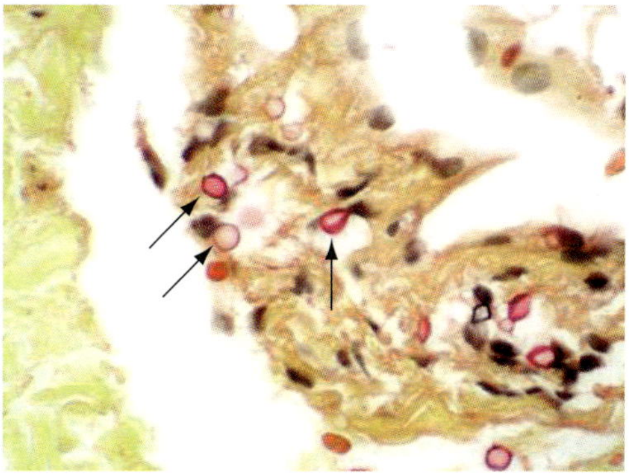

Figure 15-4 Cryptococcosis of the optic nerve in an immunocompromised patient. The dura is infiltrated by cryptococcal organisms *(arrows).* This yeast has a mucopolysaccharide capsule, highlighted with a mucicarmine stain. No inflammatory infiltrate is observed. *(Courtesy of Tatyana Milman, MD.)*

as a primary pulmonary infection, and then spreads to the optic nerve and globe. It produces necrotizing granulomas.

Viral infections of the optic nerve are usually associated with a more diffuse CNS process. *Acute disseminated encephalomyelitis* is an immune-mediated demyelinating disease that often follows bacterial or viral infections. Macrophages remove the damaged myelin. Astrocytic proliferation ultimately produces a glial scar, known as a *plaque.* The findings of acute disseminated encephalomyelitis are almost identical to those of multiple sclerosis (Fig 15-5).

Noninfectious

Noninfectious inflammatory disorders of the optic nerve include giant cell arteritis and sarcoidosis. Giant cell arteritis can produce granulomatous inflammation in the blood vessel wall as well as occlusion of the posterior ciliary vessels, with liquefactive necrosis of the optic nerve. The gold standard for histologic diagnosis of giant cell arteritis is superficial temporal artery biopsy (Fig 15-6). The involvement of the vessel wall in giant cell

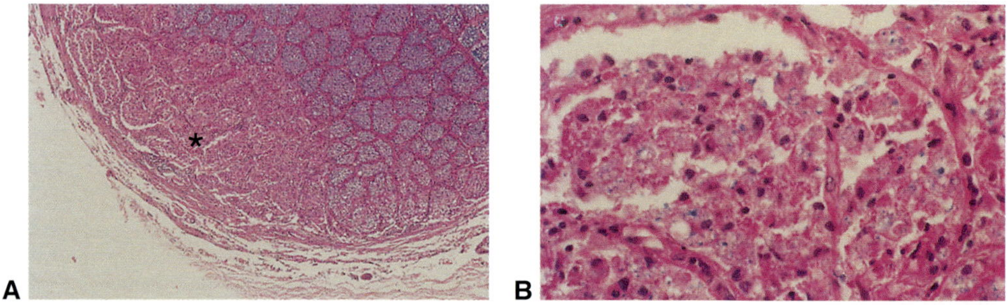

Figure 15-5 Demyelination of the optic nerve. **A,** Luxol fast blue stain, counterstained with H&E. The blue-staining area indicates normal myelin. Note the absence of myelin in the lower left corner of the optic nerve *(asterisk),* corresponding to a focal lesion. **B,** Higher magnification. The blue material (myelin) is engulfed by macrophages.

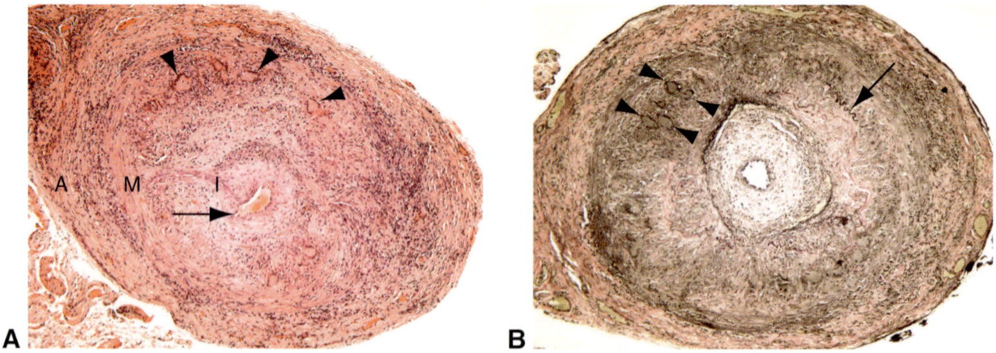

Figure 15-6 Giant cell arteritis, superficial temporal artery. **A,** Vascular lumen *(arrow)* is narrowed by concentric intimal hyperplasia. Prominent transmural inflammatory infiltrate with numerous multinucleated giant cells *(arrowheads)* is observed. **B,** An elastic stain highlights the diffuse loss of the internal elastic lamina. A short segment of remaining internal elastic lamina is marked with an arrow. Giant cells *(arrowheads)* are noted at the level of the internal elastic lamina. I = intima, M = media, A = adventitia. *(Courtesy of Tatyana Milman, MD.)*

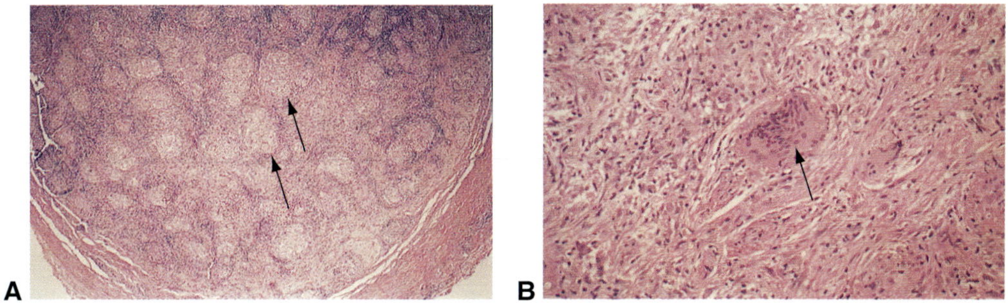

Figure 15-7 Sarcoidosis. **A,** Low-magnification photomicrograph of the optic nerve with discrete noncaseating granulomas *(arrows).* **B,** Higher magnification photomicrograph shows multinucleated giant cells *(arrow)* in the granulomas. *(Courtesy of Hans E. Grossniklaus, MD.)*

arteritis can be patchy (ie, *skip lesions*). Obtaining a biopsy specimen of adequate length (approximately 2 cm) and performing a careful histologic examination of the specimen can increase its diagnostic yield.

Sarcoidosis of the optic nerve is often associated with retinal, vitreal, and uveal lesions (Fig 15-7; see also Chapter 12, Fig 12-8). Unlike the characteristic noncaseating granulomas in the eye, optic nerve lesions may feature necrosis.

Degenerations

Optic Atrophy

Injury to the retinal ganglion cells and the axons of the peripheral optic nerve (that portion of the nerve near the retina) results in axonal swelling. This swelling manifests clinically as ONH edema (Fig 15-8). Axonal swelling and loss of retinal ganglion cells are followed by the retrograde degeneration of axons (ie, *ascending atrophy,* or *Wallerian degeneration*)

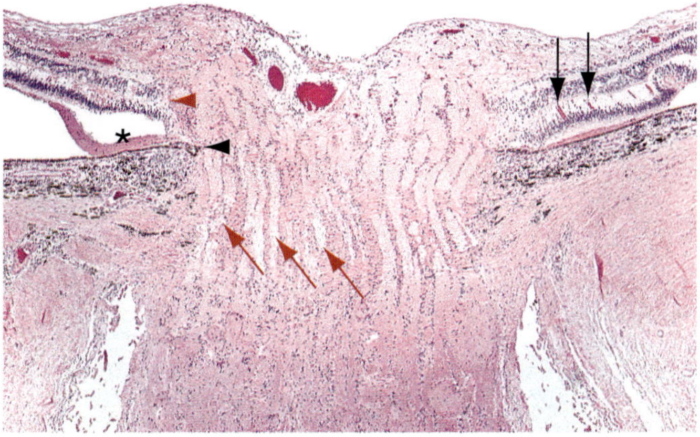

Figure 15-8 Optic nerve head edema. Swollen intralaminar axons demonstrate vacuolar alteration *(red arrows)* and displace the retina laterally *(red arrowhead)* from its normal termination just above the end of Bruch membrane *(black arrowhead).* Juxtapapillary serous intraretinal fluid/hard exudates *(black arrows)* and serous subretinal fluid *(asterisk)* are also observed. *(Courtesy of Tatyana Milman, MD.)*

toward the lateral geniculate body. Pathologic processes within the cranial cavity or orbit result in *descending atrophy* toward the retinal ganglion cells (see BCSC Section 5, *Neuro-Ophthalmology,* for more on optic atrophy).

Axonal degeneration is accompanied by the loss of myelin and oligodendrocytes. The optic nerve also shrinks, despite the proliferation of astrocytes and of fibroconnective tissue in the pial septa (Fig 15-9).

Cavernous optic atrophy of Schnabel is characterized microscopically by large cystic spaces that are posterior to the lamina cribrosa and contain mucopolysaccharides, which stain with alcian blue stain (Fig 15-10). Although the changes associated with cavernous optic atrophy were initially observed in glaucomatous eyes after acute intraocular pressure elevation, the condition has also been increasingly identified in nonglaucomatous elderly patients with generalized arteriosclerotic disease. The mucopolysaccharides were originally thought to be vitreous, forced into the ischemic necrosis–induced cavernous spaces by increased intraocular pressure, but they are more likely produced in situ, within the atrophic spaces of the optic nerve.

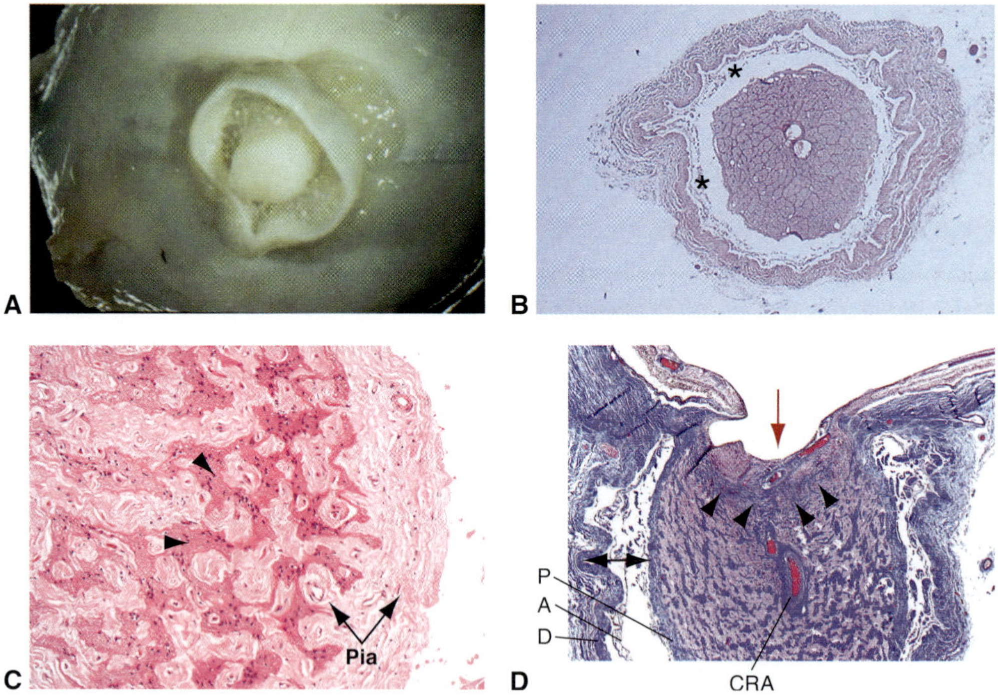

Figure 15-9 Atrophic optic nerve. **A,** Gross appearance. **B,** Low-magnification photomicrograph. Note the widened subdural space *(asterisks).* **C,** High-magnification photomicrograph. Transverse or cross section of atrophic nerve shows loss of axons *(arrowheads),* accompanied by glial proliferation and widening of fibrovascular pial septa *(arrows).* **D,** Glaucomatous optic atrophy. Masson trichrome stains the collagen of the sclera, lamina cribrosa, and meninges dark blue and the axonal fascicles pink. The optic nerve demonstrates advanced cupping *(red arrow),* accompanied by posterior bowing of the lamina cribrosa *(arrowheads).* Axonal atrophy and thickening of pial septa are present. The intermeningeal space is widened due to severe optic nerve atrophy *(double-ended arrow).* CRA = central retinal artery, P = pia, A = arachnoid, D = dura. *(Part A courtesy of Debra J. Shetlar, MD; parts C and D courtesy of Tatyana Milman, MD.)*

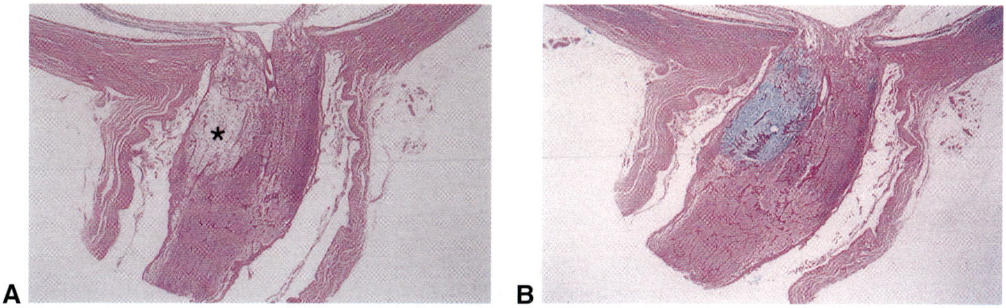

Figure 15-10 Cavernous optic atrophy of Schnabel. **A,** Photomicrograph shows cystic atrophy *(asterisk)* within the optic nerve. **B,** Photomicrograph shows cystic space filled with alcian blue–staining material. *(Courtesy of Hans E. Grossniklaus, MD.)*

Giarelli L, Falconieri G, Cameron JD, Pheley AM. Schnabel cavernous degeneration: a vascular change of the aging eye. *Arch Pathol Lab Med.* 2003;127(10):1314–1319.

Drusen

Drusen of the ONH are calcific, usually bilateral deposits embedded within the parenchyma of small, crowded optic nerve heads with abnormal vasculature. When superficial, ONH drusen appear as refractile, rounded, pale yellow or white deposits. Deeper drusen may be mistaken for papilledema (pseudopapilledema). Most ONH drusen are located anterior to the lamina cribrosa and posterior to Bruch membrane (lamina choroidalis portion of the intraocular optic nerve) (Fig 15-11).

Evidence suggests that abnormal axonal metabolism leads to mitochondrial calcification and drusen formation. Drusen can be associated with angioid streaks, papillitis, optic atrophy, chronic glaucoma, and vascular occlusions, but they are more commonly observed in otherwise normal eyes and are occasionally dominantly inherited. Histologically, ONH drusen appear as basophilic, calcified acellular deposits that contain mucopolysaccharides, amino acids, DNA, RNA, and iron. For more information, see BCSC Section 5, *Neuro-Ophthalmology,* and Section 6, *Pediatric Ophthalmology and Strabismus.*

Lam BL, Morais CG Jr, Pasol J. Drusen of the optic disc. *Curr Neurol Neurosci Rep.* 2008;8(5): 404–408.

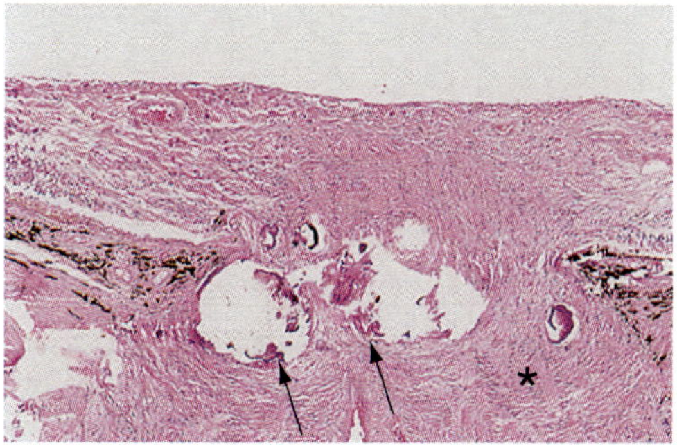

Figure 15-11 Histologically, drusen of the optic nerve head (ONH) appear as discrete basophilic zones of calcification *(arrows)* just anterior to the lamina cribrosa *(asterisk).* The cystic spaces in the ONH are histologic sectioning artifacts associated with the calcific deposits.

Neoplasia

Tumors may affect the ONH (eg, melanocytoma, peripapillary choroidal melanoma, retinal pigment epithelial proliferation, and hemangioma) or the retrobulbar portion of the optic nerve (eg, glioma and meningioma).

Melanocytoma

A melanocytoma is a benign, deeply pigmented melanocytic tumor situated eccentrically on the ONH (Fig 15-12A). It may be elevated, and it typically extends into the adjacent retina as well as posteriorly into the optic nerve. Melanocytomas may grow slowly; however, malignant transformation to melanoma rarely occurs.

Histologically, a melanocytoma is a magnocellular nevus, composed of closely packed, heavily pigmented, plump, polyhedral melanocytes. The dense pigment obscures nuclear detail (Fig 15-12B, C). Thus, bleached preparations (Fig 15-12D) are necessary to demonstrate the bland cytologic features: abundant cytoplasm, small nuclei with finely dispersed chromatin, and inconspicuous nucleoli. Necrosis and melanophagic infiltration within melanocytoma are sometimes observed but are not necessarily indicative of aggressive behavior. See also Chapter 17.

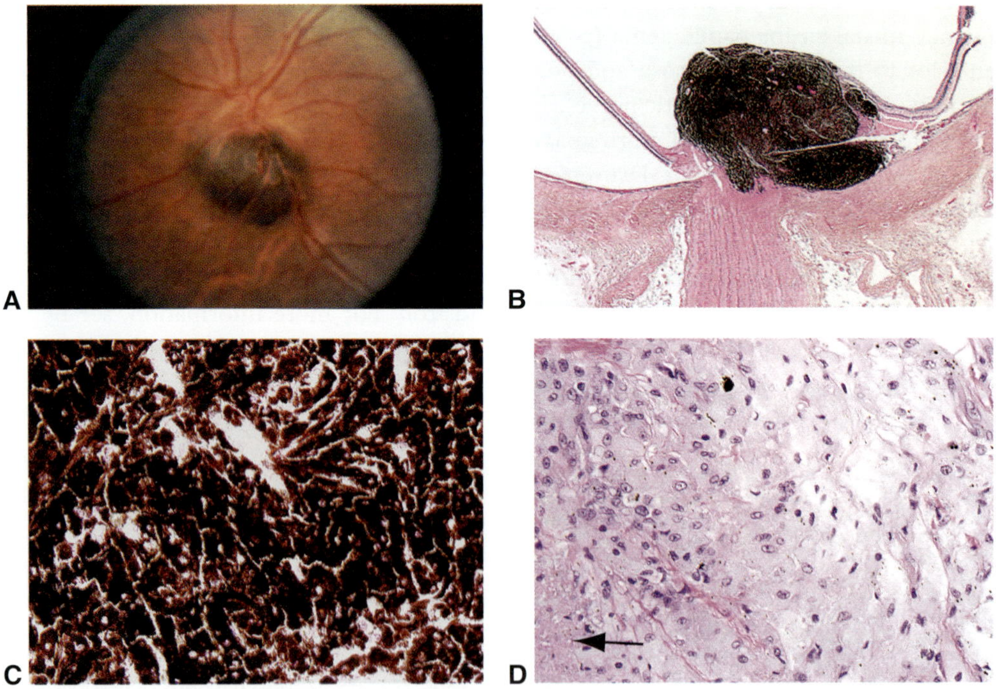

Figure 15-12 Melanocytoma of the optic nerve. **A,** Fundus photograph shows melanocytoma of the ONH. **B,** Low-magnification photomicrograph of melanocytoma shows a dome-shaped, jet-black mass involving the prelaminar optic nerve. The tumor also involves the juxtapapillary choroid and retina. **C,** Higher magnification photomicrograph shows darkly pigmented polyhedral melanocytes with dense intracytoplasmic pigment, obscuring nuclear detail. **D,** Bleached preparation displays the bland nuclear morphology of melanocytoma cells. Note the area of necrosis within the tumor *(arrow)*. *(Part A courtesy of Robert H. Rosa, Jr, MD; parts B–D courtesy of Tatyana Milman, MD.)*

Glioma

A glioma (astrocytoma) may arise in any part of the visual pathway, including the optic nerve head and optic nerve. Optic nerve gliomas are frequently associated with neurofibromatosis 1 (NF1). The tumors most commonly present in the first decade of life and are low-grade *juvenile pilocytic astrocytomas.*

Histologic examination of juvenile pilocytic astrocytomas shows proliferation of spindle-shaped astrocytes with delicate, hairlike (pilocytic) cytoplasmic processes that expand the optic nerve parenchyma. Enlarged, deeply eosinophilic filaments known as *Rosenthal fibers,* which represent degenerating cell processes, may be found in these low-grade tumors (Fig 15-13). In addition, calcification and foci of microcystic degeneration may occur, and the pial septa are thickened. The meninges show a reactive hyperplasia and astrocyte infiltration. Because the dura mater remains intact, the nerve demonstrates fusiform or sausage-shaped enlargement.

High-grade tumors *(Grade IV astrocytomas/glioblastoma multiforme)* rarely involve the optic nerve. When this does occur, the optic nerve is usually involved secondarily from a brain tumor. *Primary malignant gliomas* of the anterior visual pathways occur mainly in adults and are characterized histologically by nuclear pleomorphism, high mitotic activity, necrosis, and hemorrhage. See also BCSC Section 5, *Neuro-Ophthalmology,* and Section 7, *Orbit, Eyelids, and Lacrimal System.*

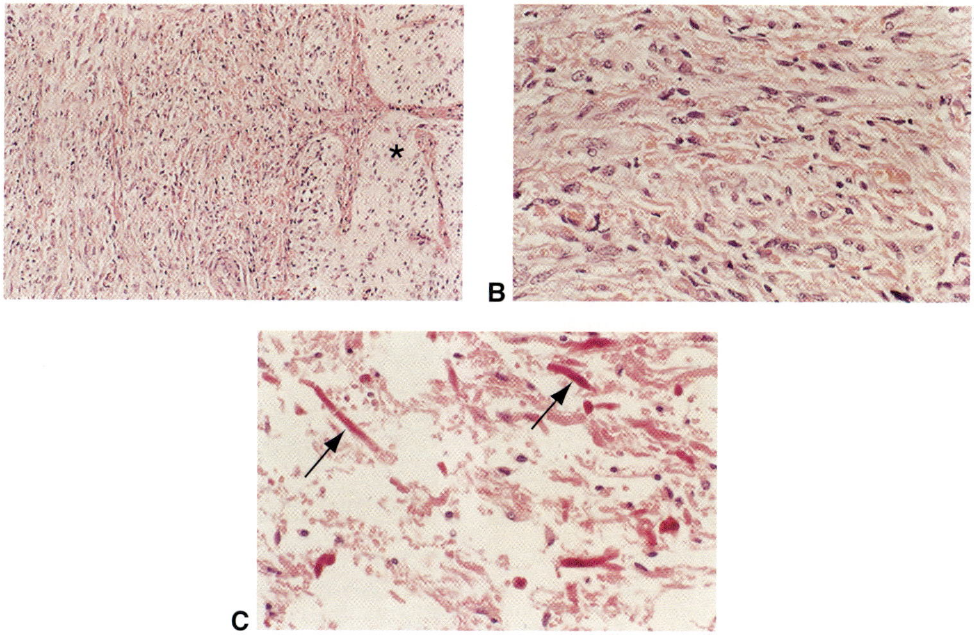

A B C

Figure 15-13 Astrocytoma of the optic nerve. **A,** The right side of this photomicrograph demonstrates a normal optic nerve *(asterisk);* the left side shows a pilocytic astrocytoma. **B,** The neoplastic glial cells are elongated to resemble hairs (hence the term *pilocytic*). **C,** Degenerating eosinophilic filaments, which are known as *Rosenthal fibers (arrows),* may be observed in these tumors.

Meningioma

Primary optic nerve sheath meningiomas arise from the arachnoid sheath of the optic nerve. They are less frequent than *secondary orbital meningiomas,* which extend into the orbit from an intracranial primary site. Although meningioma may, in rare instances, be associated with neurofibromatosis (NF1) in younger patients, optic nerve glioma is a more frequent hallmark of NF1 than meningioma. Primary optic nerve sheath meningiomas may invade the nerve and the eye; rarely, they may also extend through the dura mater to invade the extraocular muscles (Fig 15-14).

Histologically, the tumor (primary or secondary) is usually *meningothelial,* composed of plump cells with indistinct cytoplasmic margins (also called a syncytial growth pattern) arranged in whorls (see Fig 15-14D). *Psammoma bodies,* extracellular rounded calcifications surrounded by a cluster of meningioma cells, tend to be sparse. See BCSC Section 5, *Neuro-Ophthalmology,* and Section 7, *Orbit, Eyelids, and Lacrimal System.*

Miller NR. Primary tumours of the optic nerve and its sheath. *Eye* (Lond). 2004;18(11): 1026–1037.

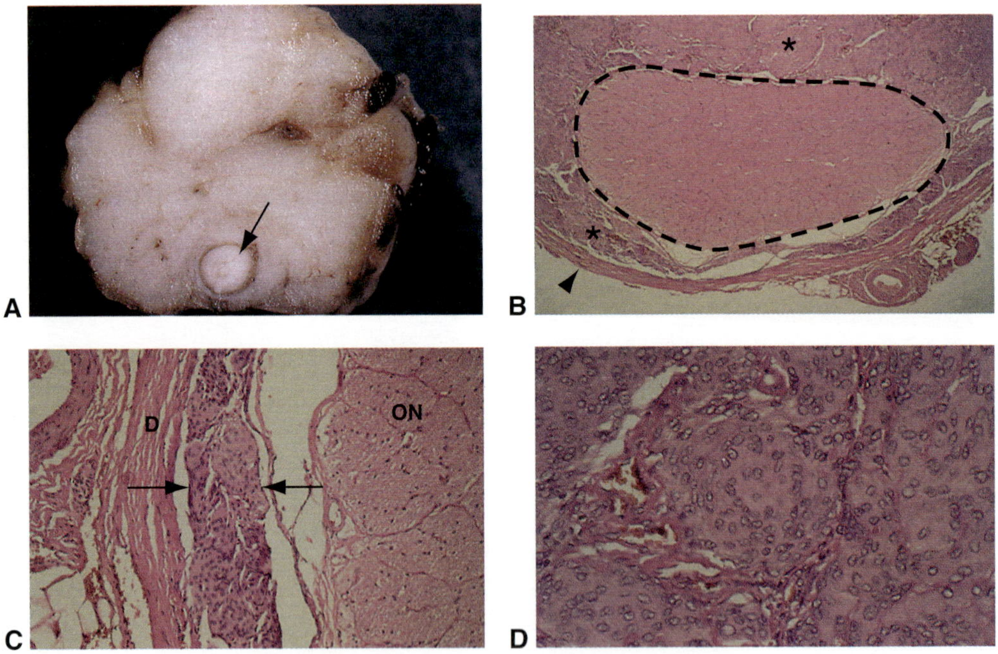

Figure 15-14 Optic nerve meningioma. **A,** The shaggy border of this gross specimen emphasizes the tendency of the perioptic meningioma to invade surrounding orbital tissues. Note the size of the optic nerve *(arrow)* in relation to the tumor. **B,** This meningioma *(asterisks)* has grown circumferentially around the optic nerve *(outlined by dashed line)* and has compressed the nerve (*arrowhead* = dura mater). **C,** Meningioma *(between arrows)* of the optic nerve (ON) originates from the arachnoid. D = dura mater. **D,** Note the whorls of tumor cells, characteristic of meningothelial meningioma, which are the most common histologic variant arising from the optic nerve.

PART II

Intraocular Tumors: Clinical Aspects

CHAPTER **16**

Introduction to Part II

Intraocular tumors make up a broad spectrum of benign and malignant lesions that can lead to loss of vision and/or loss of life. Effective management of these lesions depends on accurate diagnosis. In most cases, experienced ophthalmologists diagnose intraocular neoplasms via clinical examination and ancillary diagnostic tests.

In the past 3 decades, significant advances have been made in managing intraocular tumors and understanding their biology. The Collaborative Ocular Melanoma Study (COMS) gathered important information concerning the most common primary intraocular malignant tumor in adults, choroidal melanoma. The COMS incorporated both randomized clinical trials for patients with medium and large choroidal melanomas and an observational study for patients with small choroidal melanomas. The COMS reported outcomes for enucleation versus brachytherapy for the treatment of medium-sized tumors and for enucleation alone versus pre-enucleation external-beam radiotherapy for large melanomas. In addition to the study's primary objectives, the COMS provided data regarding local tumor failure rates and visual acuity outcomes after iodine-125 brachytherapy, which conserves the globe. The results confirmed that conservative management for well-selected patients does not alter melanoma-related morbidity.

In recent years, there have been several other advances in the management of choroidal melanoma. Researchers have identified key cytogenetic aberrations, specifically monosomy 3 and isochromosome arm 8p, that are associated with metastatic disease. Fine-needle aspiration biopsy (discussed in greater detail in Chapter 4) is available for tumor prognostication and identification of patients at high risk for distant metastasis.

The predisposing gene for retinoblastoma, which is the most common primary intraocular malignant tumor in children, has been isolated, cloned, and sequenced. As with choroidal melanoma, treatment of retinoblastoma has transitioned toward globe-conserving therapy, primarily systemic and focal chemotherapy. The trend away from external-beam radiotherapy and toward chemotherapy has been fueled by growing recognition of the former's potential risk for increasing the incidence of secondary malignancies in children who harbor a germline mutation of the retinoblastoma gene. Advances in the understanding of the molecular genetics of retinoblastoma continue to enhance clinicians' ability to screen and counsel families with this ocular malignancy (see Chapter 19).

The majority of malignancies in the United States and Europe are staged using the classification system developed by the American Joint Committee on Cancer (AJCC). The AJCC system stages cancer in patients based on tumor size, lymph node status, and distant metastasis. Clinical and pathological data may be used to clinically stage a tumor.

It is an important distinction that patients (not a single organ such as the eye) are staged. Other systems are used to group eyes for particular diagnoses, such as retinoblastoma.

Any ophthalmic pathology may result in vision loss, and the appropriate patient education and referral to vision rehabilitation should be provided early, before loss of independence and function occur. The SmartSight patient handout on the American Academy of Ophthalmology website (www.aao.org/smart-sight-low-vision) provides tips on making the most of remaining vision and outlines how patients can identify vision rehabilitation resources in their community.

CHAPTER 17

Melanocytic Tumors

Introduction

Intraocular melanocytic tumors develop from uveal melanocytes in the iris, ciliary body, and choroid. In contrast to melanocytic tumors of the skin and mucosal membranes, which usually initially spread through the lymphatics, uveal melanocytic tumors typically disseminate hematogenously, if there is metastatic spread.

The 2 main groups of melanocytic tumors of the uvea are (1) the benign nevi and (2) the melanomas. Pigmented intraocular tumors that originate in the pigmented epithelium of the iris, ciliary body, and retina constitute another group of melanin-containing tumors of neuroepithelial origin. These rare tumors are discussed separately at the end of this chapter. See also Chapter 12.

Iris Nevus

An iris nevus typically appears as a variably pigmented lesion of the iris stroma that causes minimal distortion of the iris architecture. The true prevalence of iris nevi remains uncertain; many of these lesions are small, produce no symptoms, and are recognized incidentally during routine ophthalmic examination. Iris nevi present in 2 forms:

1. *circumscribed iris nevi,* which are flat to nodular, solitary or multiple, involving a discrete portion of the iris (Fig 17-1A–D)
2. *diffuse iris nevi,* which may involve an entire sector or, in rare instances, the entire iris (Fig 17-1E)

The lesions may cause ectropion iridis (Fig 17-1D, F) and, sometimes, a sectoral cataract. The incidence of iris nevi may be higher in eyes of patients with neurofibromatosis.

Iris nevi are best evaluated by slit-lamp biomicroscopy coupled with gonioscopic evaluation of the anterior chamber angle structures. The clinician should pay specific attention to lesions involving the angle in order to rule out a ciliary body tumor; the most important differential diagnosis is iris or ciliary body melanoma. When melanoma cannot be excluded, close observation with serial slit-lamp photography and, ideally, high-frequency ultrasound biomicroscopy is indicated. Iris nevi do not usually require treatment.

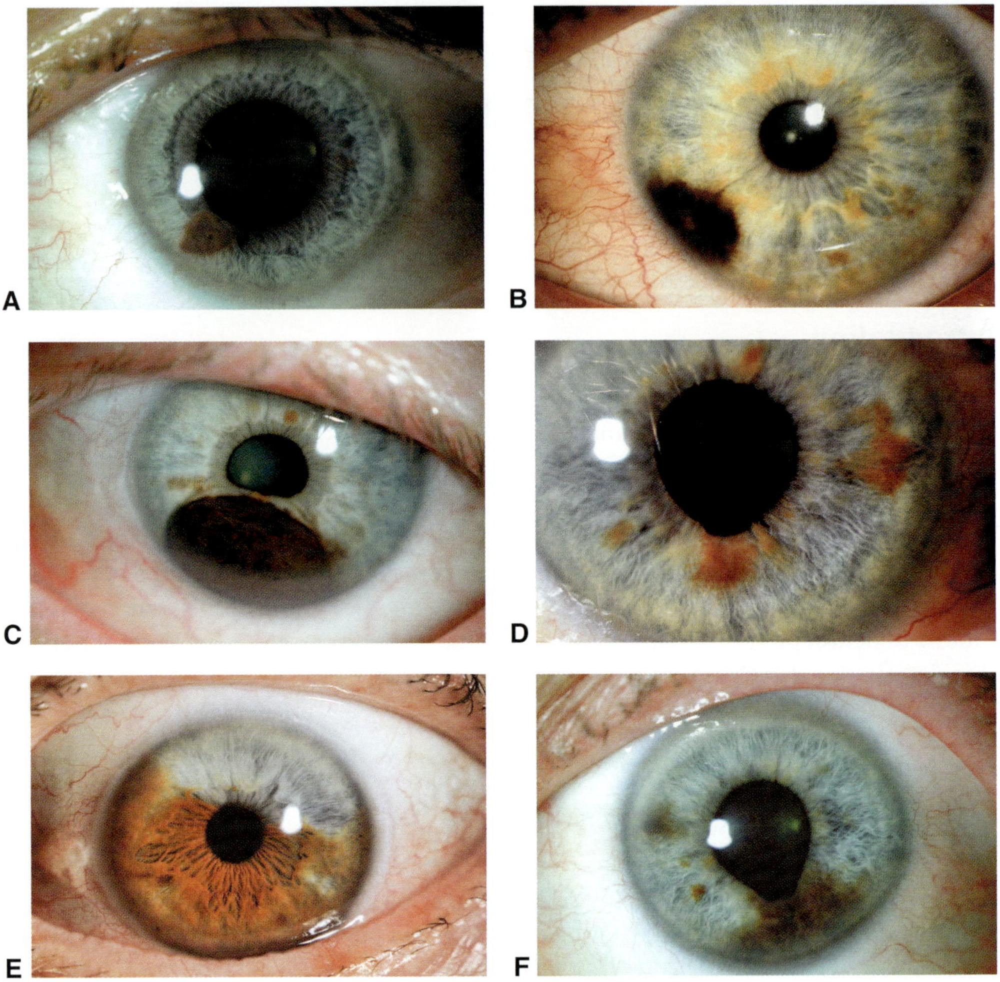

Figure 17-1 Iris nevus, clinical appearance. The lesion is generally only slightly raised from the iris surface and is a homogeneous brown. The chamber angle may be either uninvolved **(A, D)** or involved **(B, C, E, F)**; the lesion may be flat **(A, B, D–F)** or nodular **(C)**, single **(A–C, E)** or multiple **(D, F)**; it may cause ectropion iridis (**D, F**, at 6 o'clock); or it may be diffuse (**E**; note undistorted pupil). *(Courtesy of Tero Kivelä, MD.)*

Nevus of the Ciliary Body and Choroid

Nevi of the ciliary body are mostly small and incidental findings in histologic examination of globes enucleated for other reasons.

Choroidal nevi may occur in up to 8% of the population. Like iris nevi, in most cases, they cause no symptoms and are recognized on routine ophthalmic examination. The typical choroidal nevus appears ophthalmoscopically as a flat or minimally elevated, pigmented (gray to brown) choroidal lesion with soft margins (Fig 17-2A–D). Some nevi are amelanotic and less apparent.

Choroidal nevi are often associated with overlying retinal pigment epithelium (RPE) disturbance and drusen (see Fig 17-2B, C). A minority develop a localized serous retinal

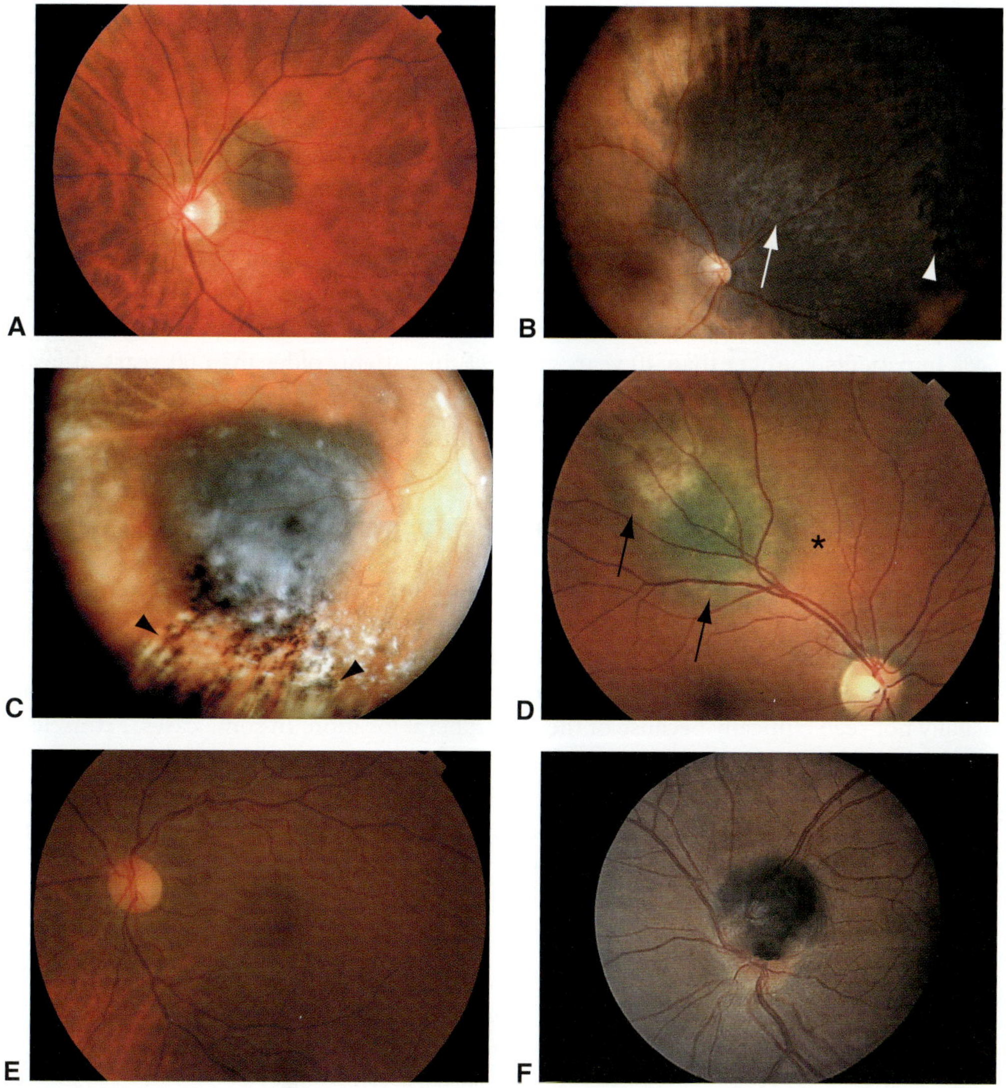

Figure 17-2 Choroidal nevi, clinical appearance. The lesion is generally thinner than 2 mm and variably brown. **A,** Small nevi lack retinal pigment epithelial (RPE) changes. **B,** Large nevi usually exhibit RPE changes (note the drusen *[arrow]* and focal RPE hyperplasia *[arrowhead]*) and **C,** may show tracks *(between arrowheads)* revealing past leakage. **D,** Some nevi display orange pigment *(arrows)* and are associated with subretinal fluid *(asterisk)*. **E,** Congenital ocular melanocytosis produces a diffuse nevus–like appearance. **F,** Melanocytoma, also known as magnocellular nevus, of the optic nerve head. All lesions were followed for several years without evidence of growth. *(Parts A–E courtesy of Tero Kivelä, MD.)*

detachment over and around the nevus, orange pigment, or choroidal neovascular membranes (see Fig 17-2C, D). These nevi may result in reduced vision, metamorphopsia, and visual field defects. Congenital ocular melanocytosis in the choroid is similar in appearance to a diffuse nevus (Fig 17-2E).

Findings from fluorescein angiography are not diagnostic; choroidal nevi may either hypofluoresce or hyperfluoresce, depending on the associated findings. Nevi are distinguished from choroidal melanomas and other pigmented fundus lesions by clinical evaluation and ancillary testing, as described in the section Melanoma of the Ciliary Body and Choroid.

The recommended management of a choroidal nevus is photographic documentation of all lesions, optical coherence tomographic (OCT) measurement of lesions thinner than 1 mm, ultrasonographic measurement of lesions thicker than 1 mm, and regular, lifelong, periodic reassessment for signs of growth. Benign nevi can increase in diameter. According to a long-term follow-up study, nevi enlarged a median of 1 mm overall, but the median yearly rate of enlargement was less than 0.1 mm, and none of the enlarging nevi developed new orange pigment or subretinal fluid. Frequency of enlargement was 54% in patients younger than 40 years and 19% in patients older than 60 years. If faster or more extensive enlargement is documented, especially in patients older than 40 years, malignant change should be ruled out.

Melanocytoma of the Iris, Ciliary Body, and Choroid

Melanocytomas (magnocellular nevi) are rare tumors composed of characteristic large, polyhedron-shaped nevus cells that have small nuclei and abundant cytoplasm filled with large melanin granules (see Chapter 15, Fig 15-12). Iris melanocytoma cells may seed to the anterior chamber angle, causing glaucoma. Melanocytomas of the ciliary body are usually not seen clinically because of their peripheral location. In some cases, extrascleral extension of tumor along an emissary canal appears as a darkly pigmented, fixed subconjunctival mass. Melanocytomas of the choroid and optic nerve head appear as elevated, pigmented tumors, simulating a nevus or a melanoma (Fig 17-2F). There have been reported cases of malignant change in some melanocytomas. When a melanocytoma is suspected, photographic and ultrasonographic studies are appropriate. If growth is documented, melanoma should be excluded.

Mashayekhi A, Siu S, Shields CL, Shields JA. Slow enlargement of choroidal nevi: a long-term follow-up study. *Ophthalmology.* 2011;118(2):382–388.

Shields CL, Furuta M, Berman EL, et al. Choroidal nevus transformation into melanoma: analysis of 2514 consecutive cases. *Arch Ophthalmol.* 2009;127(8):981–987.

Shields CL, Kaliki S, Hutchinson A, et al. Iris nevus growth into melanoma: analysis of 1611 consecutive eyes: the ABCDEF guide. *Ophthalmology.* 2013;120(4):766–772.

Shields JA, Shields CL, Eagle RC Jr. Melanocytoma (hyperpigmented magnocellular nevus) of the uveal tract: the 34th G. Victor Simpson lecture. *Retina.* 2007;27(6):730–739.

Iris Melanoma

Iris melanomas account for 3%–5% of all uveal melanomas. Small melanomas of the iris may be impossible to clinically differentiate from benign iris nevi.

Iris melanomas range in appearance from amelanotic to dark brown lesions, and three-quarters of them involve the inferior iris (Fig 17-3A–C). In rare cases, their growth pattern is diffuse, resulting in unilateral acquired hyperchromic heterochromia and

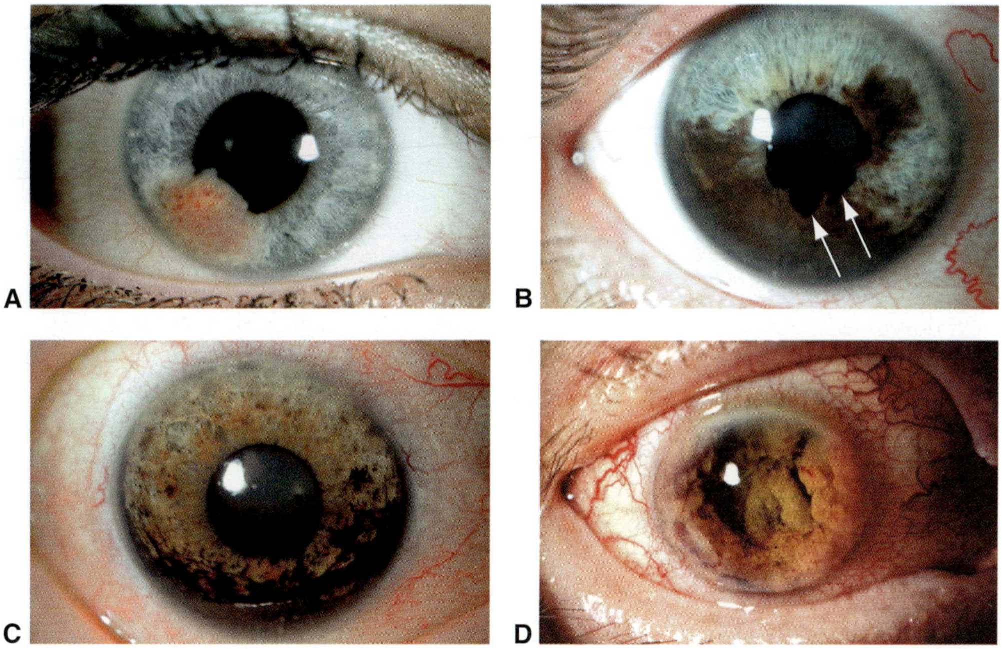

Figure 17-3 Iris melanoma, clinical appearance. **A,** The lesion can be amelanotic and show intrinsic vascularity. **B,** Alternatively, it may be densely pigmented, hiding any blood vessels (note the ectropion uveae *[arrows]* at the lower pupillary margin). **C,** Diffuse iris melanomas disseminate in the anterior chamber and chamber angle. **D,** These melanomas may have a granular, tapioca pudding–like appearance. Anterior chamber angle involvement is associated with secondary glaucoma and risk of metastasis. *(Courtesy of Tero Kivelä, MD.)*

secondary glaucoma. One subtype grows in a pattern that resembles tapioca pudding (Fig 17-3D).

Clinical evaluation of iris melanoma is identical to that for iris nevi. Signs suggesting malignancy include large size, prominent ectropion iridis and vascularity, sectoral cataract, secondary glaucoma, seeding of the peripheral angle structures, extrascleral extension, and documented progressive growth.

The differential diagnosis of iris melanoma may include the following conditions:

- iris freckle (Fig 17-4A)
- iris nevus (see Fig 17-1)
- Lisch nodules (in neurofibromatosis, variably pigmented, multiple, small, flat or nodular nevus-like lesions; Fig 17-4B, C)
- congenital ocular or oculodermal melanocytosis (diffuse iris nevus, episcleral and scleral bluish or slate-gray melanosis, choroidal melanosis, in any combination; may also be sectoral; Fig 17-4D)
- primary iris cyst (pigment epithelial or stromal; Fig 17-4E)
- iridocorneal endothelial (ICE) syndrome (Cogan-Reese iris nevus–type)
- iris pigment epithelial proliferation (after trauma or surgery)
- iris foreign body (secondarily pigmented)

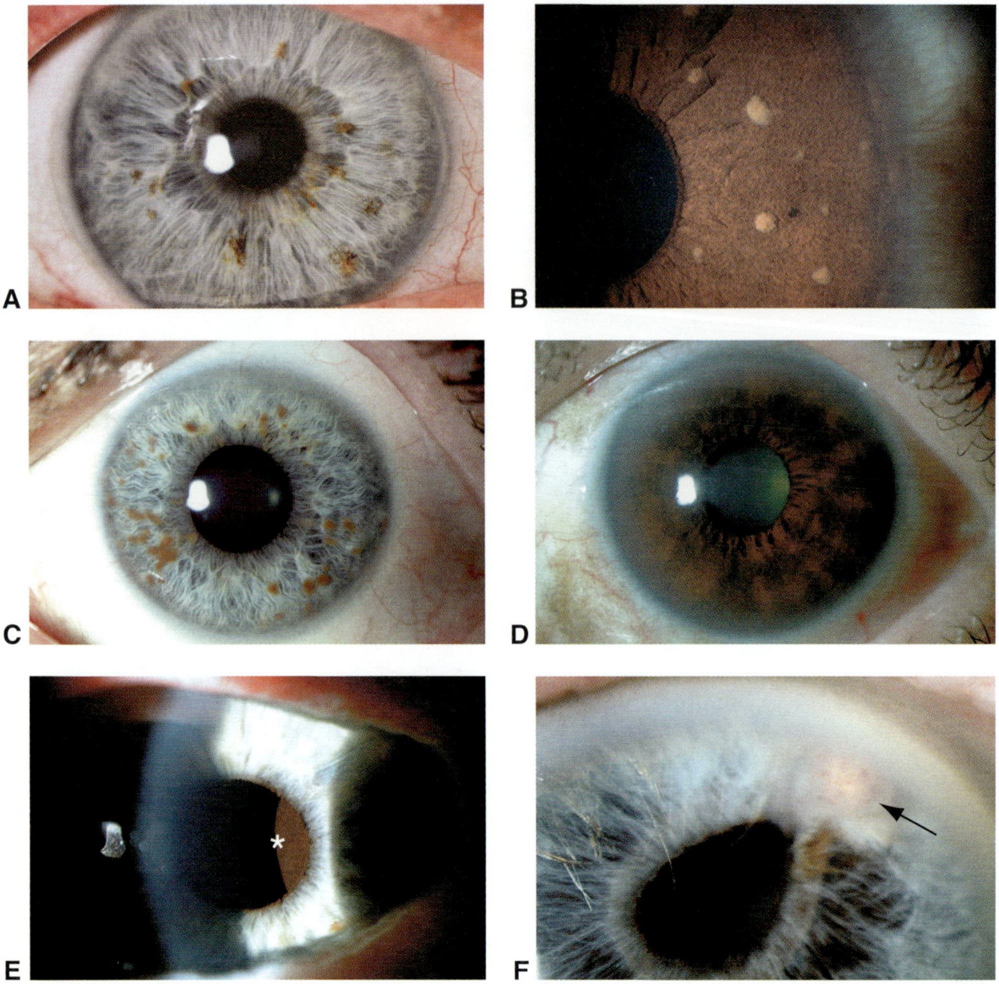

Figure 17-4 Differential diagnosis of iris melanoma. **A,** Iris freckles are small and overlie the stroma. Multiple Lisch nodules in neurofibromatosis on a brown iris **(B)** and a blue iris **(C)**. **D,** Congenital ocular melanocytosis is equivalent to a diffuse nevus, but is associated with pigmented patches in the episclera and sclera. Note the color variation and velvety stromal thickening in the iris. **E,** A pigment epithelial cyst *(asterisk)* can bow the iris forward in the area of the cyst, which is visible after dilation. **F,** Metastasis from pulmonary carcinoma *(arrow)*. *(Parts A, C–F courtesy of Tero Kivelä, MD; part B courtesy of Timothy G. Murray, MD.)*

- iris leiomyoma (amelanotic or lightly pigmented)
- juvenile xanthogranuloma (amelanotic or tan-colored)
- retained lens material simulating iris nodule (amelanotic)
- metastatic carcinoma to the iris (amelanotic; Fig 17-4F)

Advances in high-frequency ultrasonography enable excellent characterization of tumor size and anatomical relationship to normal ocular structures (Fig 17-5A, B). Anterior segment OCT may be helpful, but currently available instrumentation often does not penetrate the full thickness of the lesion (Fig 17-5C). Fluorescein angiography may

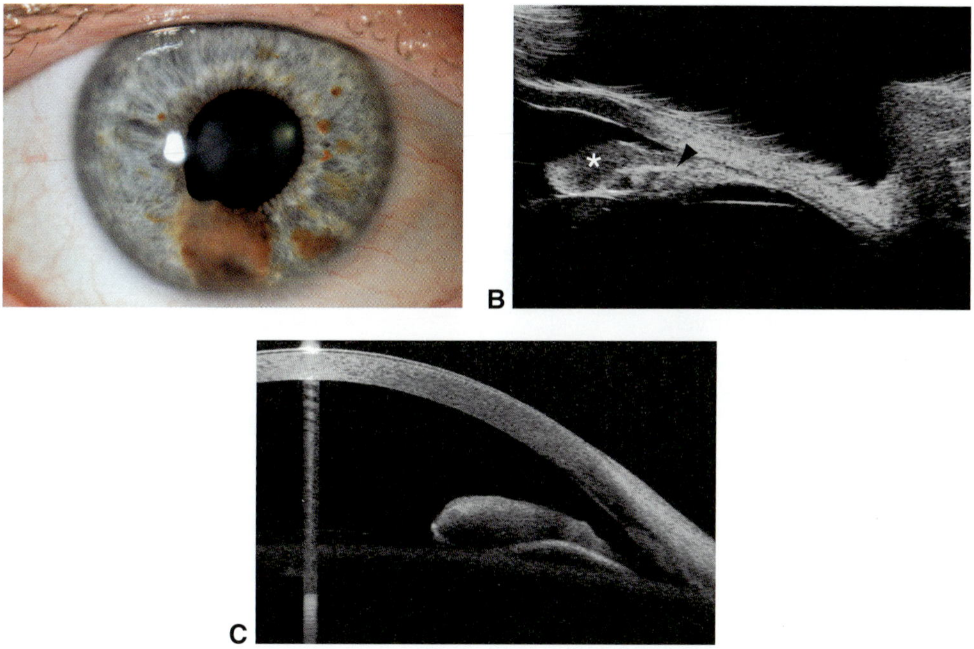

Figure 17-5 Iris tumors. **A,** Clinical appearance. **B,** A corresponding high-frequency ultrasonogram shows a tumor with low internal reflectivity *(asterisk)* in the iris stroma without anterior chamber angle involvement and with ciliary processes behind the iris. The iris pigment epithelium is highly reflective *(arrowhead)*. **C,** A corresponding anterior segment optical coherence tomography (OCT) scan shows a tumor with initial high signal intensity; the signal becomes attenuated, leading to signal loss from the deeper tumor and from the part of the iris pigment epithelium posterior to the tumor; ciliary processes are not imaged. *(Courtesy of Tero Kivelä, MD.)*

document intrinsic vascularity; however, this finding is of limited value in differential diagnosis. Biopsy may be considered when the diagnosis is not clear. If there is documented growth, or if secondary glaucoma occurs, diagnostic and therapeutic excision is indicated. Alternatively, brachytherapy using custom-designed plaques or proton-beam radiotherapy may be used.

The prognosis for most patients with iris melanoma is excellent; the mortality rate is low (1%–4%), possibly because the tumor is usually smaller and its biological behavior may be distinct from that of choroidal and ciliary body melanomas. The main risk factor for metastatic death is anterior chamber angle invasion, which may present as poorly controlled glaucoma, mimicking pigmentary glaucoma.

Hau SC, Papastefanou V, Shah S, Sagoo MS, Restori M, Cohen V. Evaluation of iris and iridociliary body lesions with anterior segment optical coherence tomography versus ultrasound B-scan. *Br J Ophthalmol.* 2015;99(1):81–86.

Henderson E, Margo CE. Iris melanoma. *Arch Pathol Lab Med.* 2008;132(2):268–272.

Jakobiec FA, Silbert G. Are most iris 'melanomas' really nevi? A clinicopathologic study of 189 lesions. *Arch Ophthalmol.* 1981;99(12):2117–2132.

Khan S, Finger PT, Yu GP, et al. Clinical and pathologic characteristics of biopsy-proven iris melanoma: a multicenter international study. *Arch Ophthalmol.* 2012;130(1):57–64.

Melanoma of the Ciliary Body and Choroid

Ciliary body and choroidal melanomas (posterior melanomas) are the most common primary intraocular malignancies in adults. Approximately 6700–7100 uveal melanomas are diagnosed annually, of which 65% affect non-Hispanic whites; 87,000–106,000 survivors are under follow-up care. The incidence varies by age, ethnicity, and latitude, ranging from 0.2 cases per million in people of Asian descent to 8.6 per million in whites living in regions at higher latitudes. The incidence in the United States increases from 4.6 to 7.5 per million and the incidence in Europe increases from 2.6 to 8.4 per million from south to north, respectively.

Less than 1% of ciliary body and choroidal melanomas are diagnosed in children younger than 18 years. Approximately 80% of these melanomas are found in adults between 45 and 80 years of age. In the United States and Europe, the mean age at diagnosis is 60–65 years, whereas in Asia it is 45–50 years.

Risk factors in addition to race and ethnicity, age, and latitude have not been conclusively identified, but they may include the following:

- light-colored complexion (white skin, blue eyes, blond hair) and an inability to tan (associated with white race)
- ocular melanocytic abnormalities including nevi (lifetime risk = 1:500) and congenital ocular and oculodermal melanocytosis (lifetime risk = 1:400)
- dysplastic nevus syndrome (threefold risk)
- *BAP1* germline mutation or other genetic predisposition

Ultraviolet radiation is not a risk factor for posterior melanoma; it might even be protective because it increases production of vitamin D, which is thought to lower the risk of cancers in tissues not exposed to direct sunlight.

Clinical Characteristics

Because of their location behind the iris, *ciliary body melanomas* often remain asymptomatic until they become rather large (Fig 17-6A). Symptoms and signs eventually include episcleral sentinel vessels (Fig 17-6B); reduced vision from induced astigmatism or cataract when the tumor touches the lens (see Fig 17-6A); photopsia and visual field alterations from the associated, usually late retinal detachment; and, rarely, secondary glaucoma.

Ciliary body melanomas are not usually visible unless the pupil is widely dilated. Some erode through the iris root into the anterior chamber and become visible during gonioscopic (Fig 17-6C) or external examination (Fig 17-6D). Eventually, the tumor extends through the sclera along aqueous channels, producing an epibulbar nodule (Fig 17-6E). Some ciliary body melanomas assume a diffuse growth pattern and extend up to 360° around the eye; in this case, they are known as *ring melanomas* (Fig 17-6F).

The typical *choroidal melanoma* is a variably pigmented, elevated, initially flat or dome-shaped subretinal mass (Fig 17-7A–C). Initial symptoms and signs may deceptively resemble those of vitreous detachment, but eventually metamorphopsia, reduced vision, and a visual field defect from direct tumor growth or secondary retinal

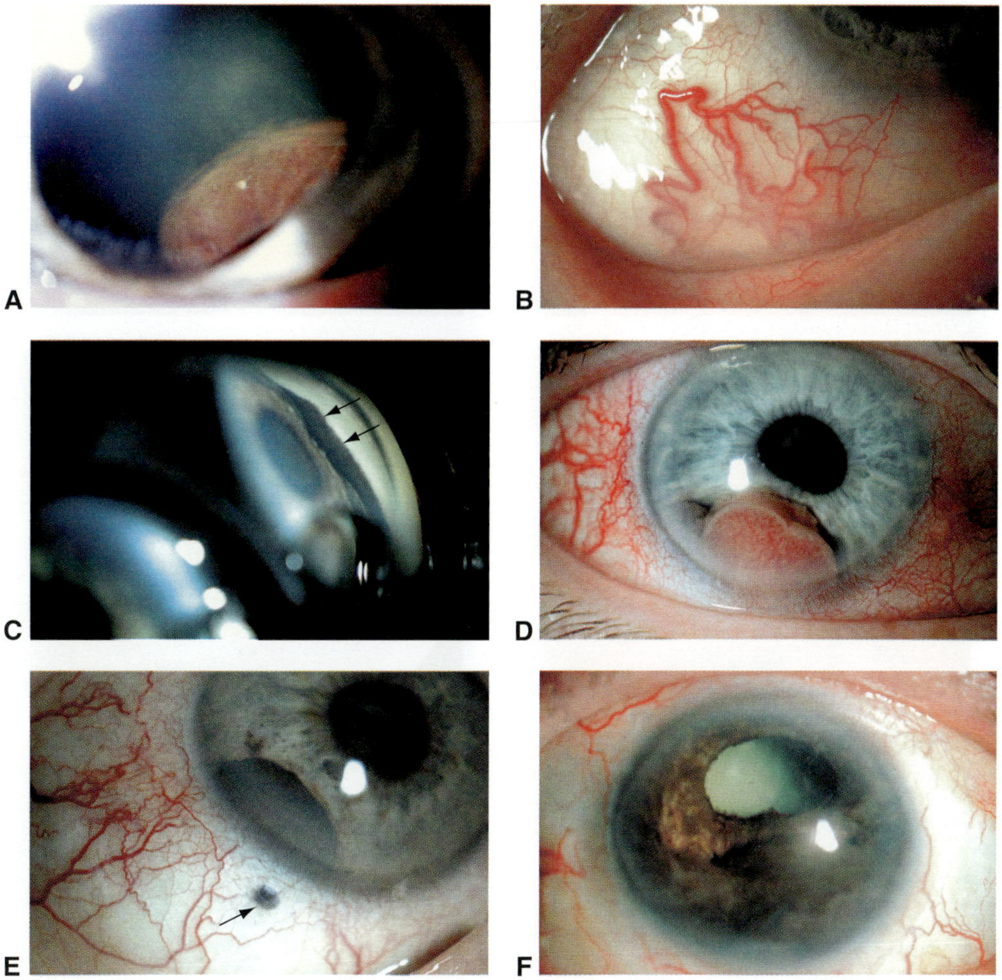

Figure 17-6 Ciliary body melanoma, clinical appearance. **A,** Such tumors may not be evident unless the pupil is widely dilated. They may indent the lens. **B,** Sentinel vessels. Anterior extension of a ciliary body melanoma may be visible only by gonioscopy *(arrows)* **(C),** or the tumor may invade the anterior chamber **(D)** and extrasclerally *(arrow)* through emissary channels **(E),** whereas a ring melanoma **(F)** grows circumferentially within the ciliary body and may extend into the anterior chamber. *(Courtesy of Tero Kivelä, MD.)*

detachment develop. The degree of pigmentation ranges from amelanotic to dark brown (Fig 17-7C, D). At the RPE level, clumps of orange pigment may appear over the surface of smaller tumors (see Fig 17-7A) and serous detachment of the neurosensory retina is common (see Fig 17-7C, D). With time, 50% of tumors erupt through Bruch membrane and assume a mushroom shape; some also erode through the retina, causing subretinal or vitreous hemorrhage (Fig 17-7E, F). If an extensive retinal detachment develops, anterior displacement of the lens–iris diaphragm and secondary angle-closure glaucoma occasionally occur. In advanced cases, neovascularization of the iris may occur.

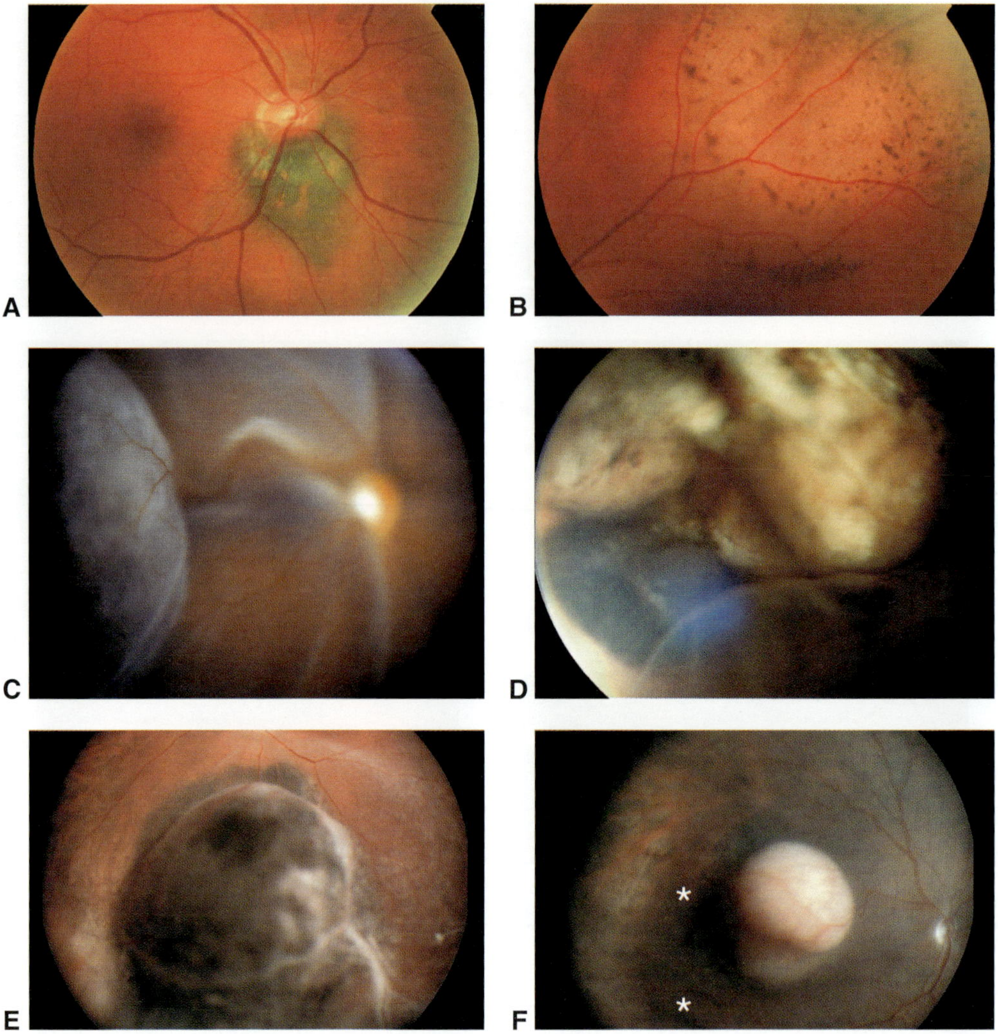

Figure 17-7 Choroidal melanoma, clinical appearance. **A,** Small choroidal melanoma with orange pigmentation, abutting the optic nerve head. **B,** Amelanotic melanoma with dark-appearing orange pigmentation. **C,** Medium-sized choroidal melanoma with exudative retinal detachment. **D,** Large, variably pigmented choroidal melanoma with exudative retinal detachment. **E,** Mushroom-shaped choroidal melanoma extending through Bruch membrane. **F,** Amelanotic melanoma with invasion into the retina, surrounded by dark subretinal blood *(asterisks)*. *(Courtesy of Tero Kivelä, MD.)*

Diagnostic Evaluation

Clinical evaluation of suspected posterior uveal melanomas includes obtaining a history (including family history of cancer), performing an ophthalmoscopic evaluation, and ancillary testing. When used appropriately, the tests described in this chapter enable accurate diagnosis of melanocytic tumors in almost all cases. Atypical lesions may need to be characterized via other testing modalities, including fine-needle aspiration or vitrectomy biopsy; alternatively, when appropriate, lesions may be closely observed for characteristic changes in clinical behavior in order to establish a correct diagnosis.

The most important diagnostic technique for evaluating patients with intraocular tumors is *indirect ophthalmoscopic viewing;* it provides stereopsis and a wide field of view and facilitates visualization of the peripheral fundus, particularly when performed with scleral depression. Indirect ophthalmoscopy and wide-field fundus photography enable clinical assessment of tumor basal dimension and apical height. However, eyes with opaque media require ultrasonography, computed tomography (CT), or magnetic resonance imaging (MRI).

Slit-lamp biomicroscopy, used in combination with *gonioscopy,* offers the best clinical method for establishing the presence and extent of anterior involvement of the tumor (see Fig 17-6C). High-frequency ultrasound biomicroscopy also enables excellent visualization of anterior ocular structures. To evaluate lesions of the posterior fundus under high magnification, Goldmann 3-mirror and newer wide-field contact lenses can be used with the slit lamp, enabling a detailed assessment of neurosensory retinal detachment, orange pigment, rupture of Bruch membrane, retinal tumor invasion, and vitreous involvement.

Fundus photography is valuable for documenting the appearance of choroidal melanoma and for identifying changes in its shape and basal dimensions in follow-up examinations. Wide-angle (60°–200°) fundus photographs (see Fig 17-6C–F) can reveal the full extent of many tumors and document their relationship to intraocular landmarks. The relative positions of retinal blood vessels may be helpful markers of changes in the size of a lesion. Wide-angle fundus photographs allow clinicians to use intrinsic scales to measure the basal diameter of a choroidal melanoma.

Fundus autofluorescence (FAF) imaging helps highlight orange pigment, which is brightly autofluorescent (Fig 17-8A, B). FAF is especially helpful in confirming the presence of orange pigment over amelanotic melanomas. In addition, any recent leakage of subretinal fluid produces increased autofluorescence (see Fig 17-8B), whereas long-standing or past leakage may result in decreased autofluorescence from secondary RPE atrophy.

OCT is generally more accurate than ultrasonography when used for measuring and following changes in the thickness of choroidal lesions thinner than 1 mm, especially in the enhanced depth imaging (EDI) mode. OCT is also helpful in differential diagnosis because it can reveal degenerative RPE and photoreceptor changes in long-standing lesions, as well as orange pigment and subretinal fluid in suspicious pigmented lesions.

Fluorescein angiography findings are not pathognomonic for choroidal melanoma. *Indocyanine green angiography* is not more accurate for diagnosis, but it does often show alterations in choroidal blood flow in the region of the tumor. Wide-field angiography can also be used to assess vascular compromise after radiotherapy of choroidal melanomas.

Ultrasonography is the most important ancillary tool for evaluating ciliary body and choroidal melanomas. The growth and regression of an intraocular tumor can be documented with serial examination. Standardized A-scan ultrasonography usually reveals a solid tumor pattern with high-amplitude initial echoes and low-amplitude internal reflections (low internal reflectivity; Fig 17-8C). Spontaneous vascular pulsations can be demonstrated in most cases. B-scan examination provides information about the size (thickness

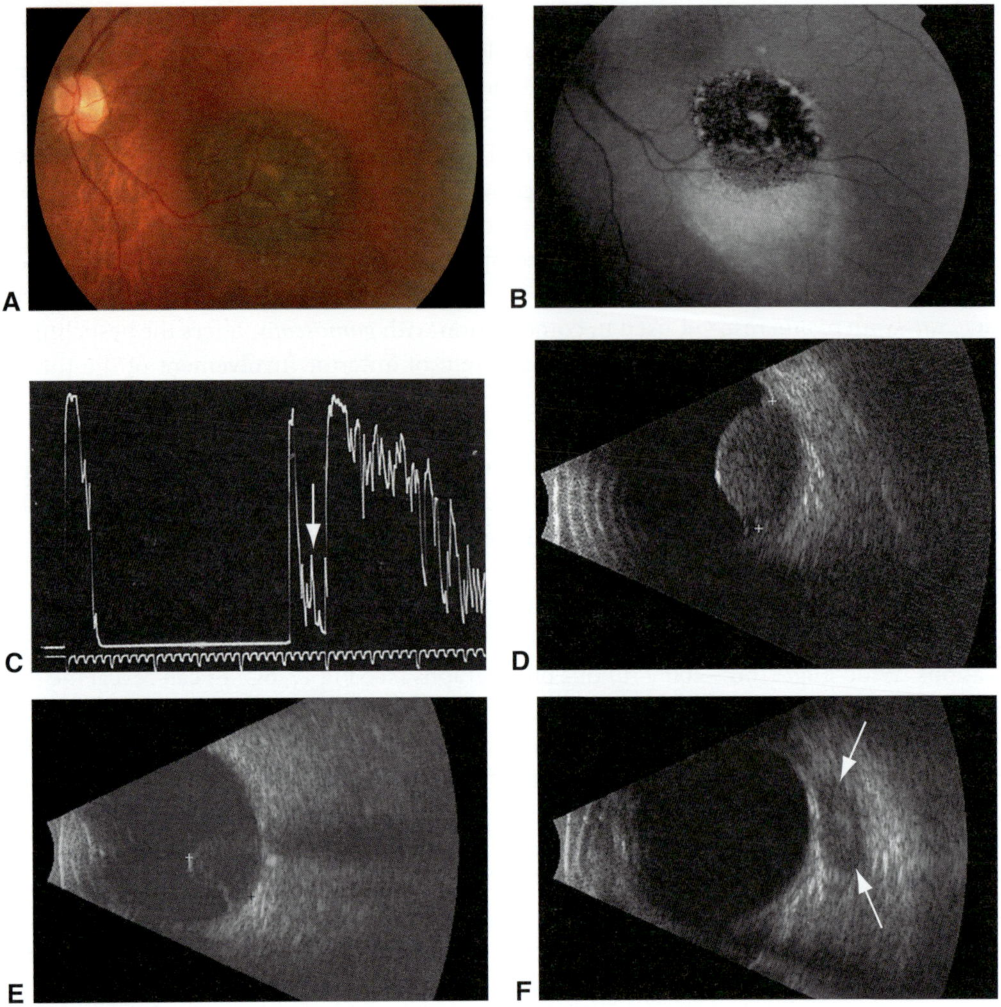

Figure 17-8 Imaging of choroidal tumors. Choroidal melanoma with orange pigment **(A)** that exhibits increased autofluorescence with fundus autofluorescence imaging **(B).** Note also increased autofluorescence associated with recent leakage (subretinal fluid) inferior to the tumor. The tumor's center shows decreased autofluorescence due to RPE loss. The A-scan ultrasonogram shows characteristic low internal reflectivity *(arrow)* of a choroidal melanoma **(C).** B-scan ultrasonography is used primarily to show the tumor location and its topography. Typical features include low internal reflectivity, leading to apparent choroidal excavation relative to the surrounding more reflective healthy choroid **(D),** and a mushroom or collar-button shape of larger tumors **(E).** Posterior extrascleral extension of tumor *(between arrows)* is apparent as a low-reflective orbital lesion in contact with the sclera **(F).** *(Parts A–B, D–F courtesy of Tero Kivelä, MD.)*

and basal diameter), general shape, and position of intraocular tumors (Fig 17-8D, E). B-scan ultrasonography is the best technique for detection of posterior extrascleral extension associated with intraocular malignancies (Fig 17-8F). Occasionally, tumor shape and associated retinal detachment can be evaluated more easily with ultrasonography than with ophthalmoscopy. B-scan ultrasonography typically shows a dome-shaped (see Fig 17-8D) or collar button–shaped (see Fig 17-8E) choroidal mass that has a highly reflective anterior border, acoustic hollowness, and choroidal excavation. The peripheral location of ciliary body melanomas makes standard ultrasonography more difficult to perform. High-frequency ultrasound biomicroscopy, which does not share these limitations, enables excellent imaging of the anterior segment and ciliary body (see Fig 17-5). Although ultrasonography is generally considered highly reliable in the differential diagnosis of posterior uveal melanoma, it may be difficult or impossible to differentiate a necrotic melanoma from a subretinal hemorrhage or a melanoma from an atypical metastatic tumor.

Although *CT* and *MRI* are not widely used to assess uncomplicated intraocular melanocytic tumors, they are useful in identifying tumors in eyes with opaque media and in determining extrascleral extension and involvement of other organs. MRI may help differentiate intraocular hemorrhage and atypical vascular lesions from melanocytic tumors.

If high-frequency ultrasonography is not available, *transillumination* may be helpful in assessing the degree of pigmentation and in determining basal diameters of suspected ciliary body or anterior choroidal melanomas. The shadow of a tumor is visible with a transilluminating light source, preferably a high-intensity fiber-optic device, placed either on the surface of the topically anesthetized eye in a quadrant opposite the lesion or directly on the cornea, using a dark corneal cap (Fig 17-9). Fiber-optic transillumination is also routinely used during surgery for radioactive applicator insertion to locate the uveal melanoma and delineate its borders.

Differential Diagnosis

This section describes the most common lesions to be considered in the differential diagnosis of posterior uveal melanoma.

Diagnostic accuracy for *choroidal nevus,* discussed earlier in this chapter, is associated with clinical experience and availability of ancillary testing facilities. For the evaluation and management of posterior pigmented lesions with characteristics predictive of growth, patients may be referred to ocular oncology centers. No single clinical factor is pathognomonic for benign versus malignant choroidal melanocytic lesions. Specifically, 6%–10% of benign choroidal nevi show orange pigment and 9%–15% are associated with subretinal fluid. Only 11%–58% of these nevi, increasing in frequency with the age of the

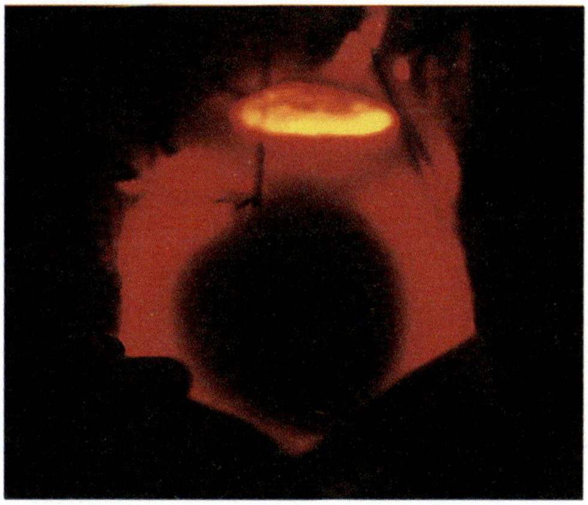

Figure 17-9 Transillumination of the eye reveals a shadow at the site of a choroidal melanoma. This technique may be used to mark the tumor base to ensure accurate placement of a radioactive plaque.

patient, have overlying drusen. More than 20% of choroidal melanocytic tumors thicker than 3 mm are melanomas, and far less than 1% of those thinner than 1 mm are melanomas. Tumors that are 1–3 mm in thickness are difficult to classify with certainty. The risk of malignancy increases substantially for lesions larger than 6 mm in basal diameter.

Clinical risk factors for the growth of small choroidal melanocytic lesions have been well characterized; they include 5 clinical features that have given rise to the mnemonic "*to f*ind *s*mall *o*cular *m*elanomas":

- *t*hickness of the tumor greater than 2 mm
- *f*luid under the retina
- *s*ymptoms (eg, metamorphopsia, photopsia, visual field loss)
- *o*range pigmentation overlying the tumor
- *m*argin of the tumor touching the optic nerve head

The following risk factors are also important:

- larger size at presentation
- absence of drusen or degenerative RPE changes
- homogeneous low internal reflectivity on ultrasonography
- hot spots on fluorescein angiography

To document growth, the clinician may periodically photograph and measure the tumor with OCT (using the EDI mode) or ultrasonography. Slow growth does not necessarily suggest or confirm malignancy. Of 284 benign choroidal nevi, 31% showed enlargement (median increase in diameter = 1 mm) over long observation periods (7 years or more). The frequency of enlargement may be higher in patients younger than 40 years (54%) compared with those older than 60 years (19%). Enlarging nevi may not develop any new orange pigment or subretinal fluid suggestive of malignant change. Thus, if rapid or progressive growth occurs, or new risk factors appear, definitive treatment should be considered. When risk factors for growth are identified, transscleral or transvitreal fine-needle aspiration or vitrectomy biopsy is an alternative to follow-up. Monosomy 3 or a gene expression profile other than class 1A is generally interpreted as a melanoma with significant metastatic potential.

Melanocytoma (magnocellular nevus) of the ciliary body or optic nerve head typically appears as a dark brown to black lesion. It is usually located eccentrically over the optic nerve head, and it may be elevated. It often has fibrillar or feathery margins as a result of extension into the nerve fiber layer (see Fig 17-2F; see also Chapter 15, Fig 15-12). Because a melanocytoma rarely transforms into melanoma, it is important to differentiate the two. Melanocytomas can produce an afferent pupillary defect and visual field abnormalities ranging from an enlarged blind spot to extensive nerve fiber layer defects.

Congenital hypertrophy of the RPE (CHRPE) refers to a sharply defined, flat, very darkly pigmented lesion that ranges from 1 mm to greater than 10 mm in diameter. Patients are asymptomatic, and the lesion can be noted during ophthalmic examination at any age. In younger patients, CHRPE often appears homogeneously black; in older individuals, foci of depigmentation (lacunae) often develop (Fig 17-10B, C), and the lesion

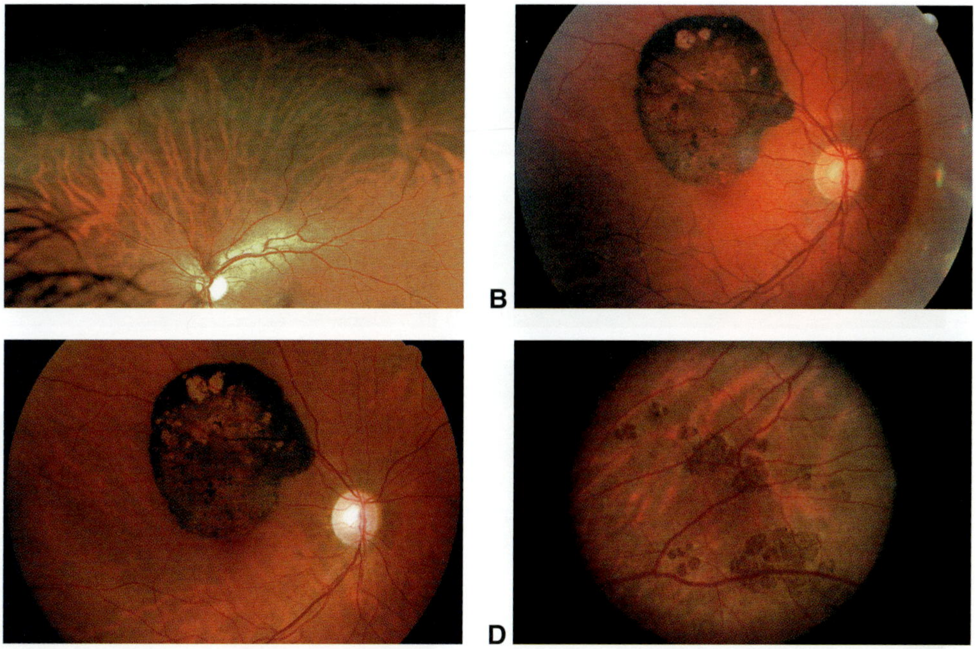

Figure 17-10 Congenital hypertrophy of the retinal pigment epithelium (CHRPE), various clinical appearances. **A,** Large, homogeneous black CHRPE lesion posterior to the ora serrata. **B,** CHRPE with atrophic lacunae. **C,** Note the slight enlargement of the lesion from part B, observed 8 years later, with larger and more numerous lacunae. **D,** Grouped pigmentation of the RPE represents a variant of CHRPE. *(Parts A–C courtesy of Tero Kivelä, MD.)*

may slowly enlarge (Fig 17-10C; see also Fig 17-10B). The histologic findings are identical to that of *grouped pigmentation of the retina,* also known as *bear tracks* (Fig 17-10D). The presence of multiple, atypical CHRPE-like patches in patients with *Gardner syndrome,* a subtype of *familial adenomatous polyposis,* appears to be a marker for the development of colon carcinoma. Fundus findings enable the ophthalmologist to help the gastroenterologist determine which family members should participate in colon carcinoma screening (see Chapter 11).

Patients with *age-related macular degeneration (AMD)* may present with macular or extramacular subretinal neovascularization, hemorrhage, and fibrosis, accompanied by varying degrees and patterns of pigmentation (Fig 17-11A). Hemorrhage, a finding commonly associated with exudative AMD, usually does not occur with melanomas unless they have broken through Bruch membrane. Clinical evaluation of the fellow eye is helpful in documenting AMD. OCT shows predominantly subretinal and intraretinal abnormalities. Ultrasonography reveals high or heterogeneous reflectivity rather than low internal reflectivity, as well as a lack of intrinsic vascularity. When in doubt, the clinician may use fluorescein angiography to help reveal early hypofluorescence secondary to blockage from the hemorrhage, which is often followed by late hyperfluorescence in the distribution of the choroidal neovascular membrane (Fig 17-11B). Serial observation shows involutional alterations of the evolving disciform lesion.

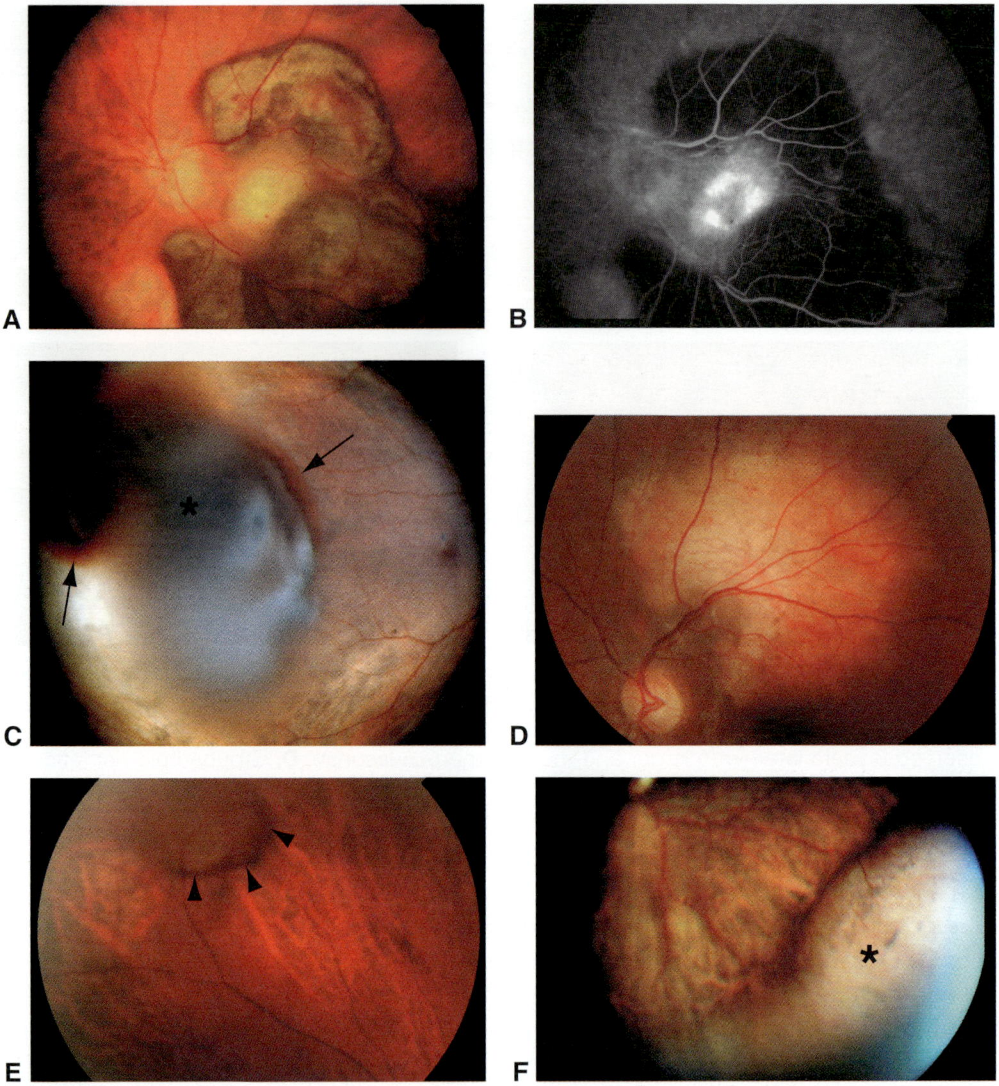

Figure 17-11 Differential diagnosis of posterior uveal melanoma. **A,** Subretinal hemorrhage secondary to exudative macular degeneration. **B,** Fluorescein angiography reveals hyperfluorescence and late fluorescein leakage in the central macula associated with the choroidal neovascular membrane and hypofluorescence associated with blockage of fluorescein transmission due to subretinal blood. **C,** Peripheral exudative hemorrhagic chorioretinopathy (PEHCR); note the red subretinal *(arrows)* and dark sub-RPE blood *(asterisk).* **D,** Choroidal osteoma with yellow-orange color and well-defined pseudopod-like margins. **E,** Varix of the vortex vein *(arrowheads).* These lesions are more likely to be developmental rather than degenerative. **F,** Metastasis *(asterisk)* to the choroid from pancreatic cancer. *(Courtesy of Tero Kivelä, MD.)*

Choroidal detachments can be hemorrhagic or serous. They are often associated with hypotony and may develop in the early postoperative period after ophthalmic surgery. Hemorrhagic detachments are often dome shaped, involve multiple quadrants, and may be associated with breakthrough vitreous bleeding. Ultrasonographic findings may closely resemble those of melanoma but reveal absence of intrinsic vascularity and involution of the hemorrhage over time. Observational management is indicated in most cases. MRI with gadolinium enhancement may be beneficial in suspicious cases.

Peripheral exudative hemorrhagic chorioretinopathy (PEHCR) is a spontaneously developing, often asymptomatic peripheral lesion in elderly individuals that resembles a choroidal detachment. It is often associated with suprachoroidal or subretinal bleeding and lipid exudation; associated retinal detachment is uncommon (Fig 17-11C). PEHCR is thought to be analogous to AMD, and the fellow eye often shows a similar or a nonexudative chorioretinal degeneration. PEHCR almost always involutes spontaneously.

Choroidal osteomas are benign, presumably acquired bony tumors that typically arise from the juxtapapillary choroid in young adults (more commonly in women) and are bilateral in 20%–25% of cases. The characteristic lesion appears yellow to orange and has well-defined margins (Fig 17-11D). Ultrasonography reveals a high-amplitude echo corresponding to the bony plate and loss of the normal orbital echoes behind the lesion (acoustic shadowing). CT can reveal calcification but is not needed for diagnosis. Choroidal osteomas typically enlarge slowly over many years and can decalcify with time. If they involve the macula, vision is generally impaired. Subretinal neovascularization is a common complication. The etiology of these lesions is unknown, but chronic low-grade choroidal inflammation has been suspected (see Chapter 12).

Choroidal hemangiomas (see Chapter 18) resemble the surrounding fundus in color and may appear to be lightly pigmented. Over time, a serous retinal detachment may develop. These lesions, which are often associated with overlying cystic retinal degeneration, are hyperechogenic on ultrasonography and show a characteristic vascular pattern on fluorescein and indocyanine green angiography.

Varix of the vortex vein (Fig 17-11E) is found predominantly in the nasal quadrants and can reach 4–5 mm in diameter. When filled with blood, it appears dark in color. The clinician can easily diagnose this condition by observing its coincidence with the vortex vein ampulla and by gently compressing the eye during indirect ophthalmoscopy, which causes the varix to deflate.

Intraocular metastases (Fig 17-11F; see also Chapter 20) are generally amelanotic and thus pale or yellowish, unless they originate from cutaneous melanoma. Most show moderately high or heterogeneous reflectivity on ultrasonography.

Table 17-1 lists additional conditions to be considered in cases with *amelanotic* choroidal masses.

Classification

Melanomas of the ciliary body and choroid have been categorized by size in several different ways. Although a size classification based on tumor volume would be logical, no simple and reliable method for assessing tumor volume is available. The *Collaborative Ocular Melanoma Study (COMS)* classified posterior uveal melanomas as small, medium, or large on the basis of thickness and basal diameter.

The recently revised, evidence-based, and validated Tumor, Node, Metastasis (TNM) staging system developed by the American Joint Committee on Cancer (AJCC) is recommended. The seventh and forthcoming eighth editions both categorize posterior

Table 17-1 Differential Diagnosis of Amelanotic Choroidal Mass

Amelanotic melanoma
Chorioretinal granuloma
Choroidal detachment
Choroidal hemangioma
Choroidal metastasis
Choroidal osteoma
Leiomyoma
Neurilemoma
Posterior scleritis
Sclerochoroidal calcification

Modified from Shields JA, Shields CL. Differential diagnosis of posterior uveal melanoma. In: Shields JA, Shields CL. *Intraocular Tumors: A Text and Atlas*. Philadelphia: Saunders; 1992:137–153.

melanomas as small (T1), medium (T2), large (T3), or very large (T4) according to tumor thickness and basal diameter, extension to the ciliary body, and extrascleral growth. These categories are used to assign melanomas into 7 stages (I, IIA, IIB, IIIA–C, and IV) that differ in prognosis (Table 17-2).

Metastatic Evaluation

The incidence of metastatic uveal melanoma is as high as 50% at 25 years after treatment for ciliary body or choroidal melanoma. The COMS reported an incidence of metastatic disease of 25% at 5 years after initial treatment and 34% at 10 years. However, metastatic disease at the time of initial presentation can be detected in less than 2% of patients. It is likely that many patients have undetectable micrometastases at the time of their primary treatment.

The liver is the primary organ involved in metastatic uveal melanoma; in 90% of patients, liver involvement is the first manifestation of metastatic disease. Other relatively frequent sites, generally after liver metastasis, include the lungs, bones, and skin. In cases that were autopsied, liver involvement was found in 100% and lung involvement in 50% of patients with metastases. All patients require metastatic evaluation prior to definitive treatment of intraocular melanoma (Table 17-3). The purpose of this evaluation is twofold:

1. To determine whether the patient has any other medical conditions that contraindicate surgical treatment or need to be treated. The COMS and smaller studies have found a second primary cancer in approximately 10% of patients. If there is any question regarding whether the lesion in the eye is a metastatic tumor, the clinician should conduct a thorough medical evaluation to determine the site of primary malignancy.
2. To rule out the possibility of detectable metastatic melanoma from the eye, especially for AJCC T3 melanomas (metastasis found in 3%) and T4 melanomas (metastasis found in 20%). If metastatic disease is clinically present during the pretreatment evaluation, enucleation is inappropriate unless the eye is painful.

In order to detect metastatic disease at an early phase, metastatic evaluation is often performed on all patients with uveal melanoma on a yearly basis. Some centers initially provide surveillance every 3 to 6 months if the risk of metastasis is considered to be high (eg, AJCC stage III; presence of epithelioid cells, monosomy 3, or class 2 gene expression

Table 17-2 AJCC Staging of Ciliary Body and Choroidal (Posterior) Melanoma

Stage	Percentage of Patients	5-Year Survival	10-Year Survival
Stage I	21%–32%	96%–97%	88%–94%
Stage IIA	31%–34%	89%–98%	80%–84%
Stage IIB	22%–23%	79%–81%	67%–70%
Stage IIIA	9%–17%	66%–67%	45%–60%
Stage IIIB	3%–8%	45%–50%	27%–50%
Stage IIIC	1%	25%–26%	0%–10%
Stage IV (metastasis)	<2%	<5%	<1%

Modified from Kujala E, Damato B, Coupland SE, et al. Staging of ciliary body and choroidal melanomas based on anatomic extent. *J Clin Oncol.* 2013;31(22):2825–2831, and AJCC Ophthalmic Oncology Task Force. International Validation of the American Joint Committee on Cancer's 7th Edition Classification of Uveal Melanoma. *JAMA Ophthalmol.* 2015;133(4)376–383.

Table 17-3 Clinical Evaluation of Metastatic Uveal Melanoma

Liver imaging—ultrasonography in routine evaluation
Liver function tests
Chest x-ray

If any of the above are abnormal:
- Triphasic liver CT
- PET-CT of the abdomen/chest
- MRI of the abdomen

CT = computed tomography; MRI = magnetic resonance imaging; PET-CT = positron emission tomography–computed tomography.

profile). Metastatic evaluation should include a comprehensive physical examination; however, liver imaging is the most important component of the evaluation. Ultrasonography of the abdomen is usually sufficient, but if metastatic disease is suspected, triphasic CT, MRI, or positron emission tomography–computed tomography (PET-CT) is usually recommended in order to evaluate the extent of the disease.

Liver function tests are usually performed; however, they have recently become less reliable in the evaluation of liver metastases because of increasingly common fatty liver disease and the widespread use of cholesterol-lowering statins, which may alter liver enzyme levels. Chest x-ray is also usually performed at the time of diagnosis, although its yield is low. Possible novel blood markers for early detection of metastatic uveal melanoma are being explored.

A liver or other organ-site biopsy may confirm metastatic disease. Biopsy is appropriate before the institution of any treatment for metastatic disease.

The interval between the diagnosis of primary uveal melanoma and its metastasis depends on many clinical, histologic, cytogenetic, and molecular genetic factors. It varies from a few months to more than 25 years. When metastatic disease is diagnosed early enough, the options for treatment include surgical resection; chemotherapy, including intra-arterial hepatic chemotherapy and chemoembolization; immunotherapy or biological therapy; and hepatic selective internal radiation therapy (SIRT, also known as intrahepatic radioembolization).

AJCC Ophthalmic Oncology Task Force. International Validation of the American Joint Committee on Cancer's 7th Edition Classification of Uveal Melanoma. *JAMA Ophthalmol.* 2015;133(4)376–383.

Francis JH, Patel SP, Gombos DS, Carvajal RD. Surveillance options for patients with uveal melanoma following definitive management. *Am Soc Clin Oncol Educ Book.* 2013:382–387.

Kujala E, Damato B, Coupland SE, et al. Staging of ciliary body and choroidal melanomas based on anatomic extent. *J Clin Oncol.* 2013;31(22):2825–2831.

Kujala E, Mäkitie T, Kivelä T. Very long-term prognosis of patients with malignant uveal melanoma. *Invest Ophthalmol Vis Sci.* 2003;44(11):4651–4659.

Mashayekhi A, Siu S, Shields CL, Shields JA. Slow enlargement of choroidal nevi: a long-term follow-up study. *Ophthalmology.* 2011;118(2):382–388.

Treatment

For many years, management of posterior uveal melanomas was controversial for 2 reasons: (1) data on the natural history of untreated patients with posterior uveal melanoma were limited, and (2) there were insufficient data on patients who were matched for known and unknown risk factors and managed by different therapeutic techniques to assess the comparative effectiveness of those treatments. Currently, both surgical and radiotherapeutic techniques are used to treat posterior uveal melanoma. The COMS reported outcomes of randomized, prospectively administered treatment of patients with medium and large choroidal melanomas. The choice of treatment depends on 4 factors:

1. size, location, and extent of the tumor
2. vision status of the affected eye and of the fellow eye
3. age and general health of the patient
4. patient and physician preference

Observation

Most benign choroidal tumors (eg, nevus, osteoma, and hemangioma) can be managed with observation. Significant controversy persists regarding the diagnosis and management of small choroidal melanomas. Lesions with any of the 5 main risk factors for growth (thickness >2 mm, subretinal fluid, symptoms, orange pigment, or tumor margin touching the optic nerve head), and all lesions with documented growth, should be considered for treatment. Short-term observation to verify growth of a suspected small uveal melanoma has traditionally been considered appropriate, especially when the tumor is located in the macular area. As mentioned earlier, a fine-needle aspiration or vitrectomy biopsy can be considered as an alternative. Observation of active and larger melanomas may be appropriate in very elderly patients and those with systemic illness who are poor candidates for any kind of therapeutic intervention.

Enucleation

Historically, enucleation has been the gold standard in the treatment for malignant intraocular tumors. A past hypothesis that surgical manipulation of eyes containing a melanoma would lead to tumor dissemination and increased mortality is no longer accepted. Enucleation remains appropriate for some small to medium (T1 and T2), many large (T3), and most very large (T4) choroidal melanomas, especially when useful vision has been lost or when the patient declines other treatments. The COMS found no evidence that pre-enucleation external-beam radiotherapy performed on patients with large choroidal melanomas improves 5-year mortality rates. However, local orbital recurrence was more frequent after enucleation alone.

Hawkins BS; Collaborative Ocular Melanoma Study Group. The Collaborative Ocular Melanoma Study (COMS) randomized trial of pre-enucleation radiation of large choroidal melanoma: IV. Ten-year mortality findings and prognostic factors. COMS report no. 24. *Am J Ophthalmol.* 2004;138(6):936–951.

Brachytherapy with a radioactive plaque

The application of a radioactive plaque to the sclera overlying an intraocular tumor is probably the most common way to treat uveal melanoma. With this technique, which has been widely available since the 1950s, a very high dose of radiation can be delivered to the tumor (typically 80–100 gray [Gy] to the tumor apex and up to 1000 Gy to the tumor base), while a relatively low dose is delivered to the surrounding normal structures of the eye. Although various isotopes can be used (eg, cobalt-60, strontium-90, iridium-192, and palladium-103), the most common are iodine-125 (γ-rays) and ruthenium-106 (β-rays). In the United States, iodine-125 is the most frequently used isotope in the treatment of uveal melanomas of any size; whereas in Europe, ruthenium-106 is preferred for smaller melanomas. Advances in intraoperative localization, especially the use of ultrasonography, have increased local tumor control rates, which typically reach 90%. In most patients, the tumor decreases in size (Fig 17-12A); in others, the result could be total flattening of the tumor or little change in size, although clinical and ultrasound changes may be evident. Regrowth is diagnosed in approximately 10% of treated tumors, usually at 1 tumor margin, but sometimes diffusely.

Radiation-related adverse effects, especially optic neuropathy and maculopathy, limit vision in as many as 50% of patients, depending on tumor size and location. These adverse

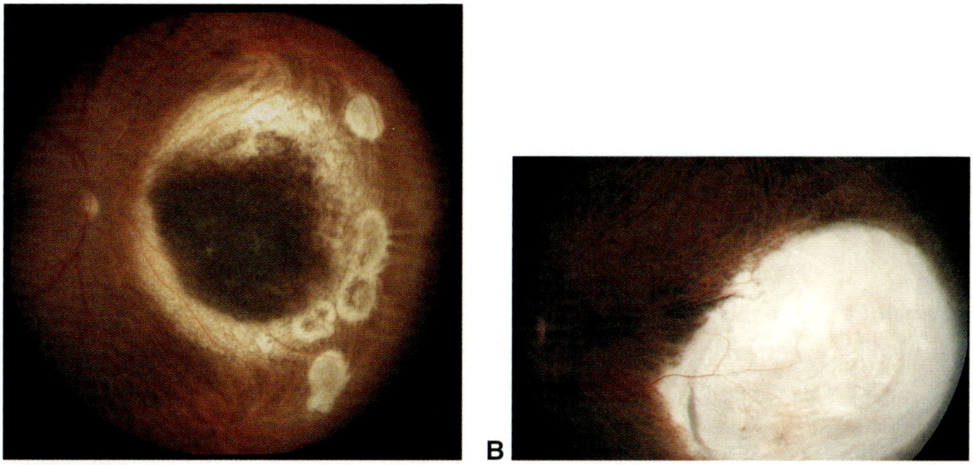

Figure 17-12 Choroidal melanoma, treated. **A,** Mildly elevated remnant of a melanoma surrounded by atrophic chorioretinal scarring after plaque brachytherapy, nasal to the optic nerve head. **B,** RPE and choroid are absent (and the outer retina likely atrophic) but the inner retina is present, as evidenced by its blood vessels, after transscleral resection of choroidal melanoma located temporal to the macula. *(Part A courtesy of Jacob Pe'er, MD; part B courtesy of Tero Kivelä, MD.)*

effects may or may not respond to intravitreal anti–vascular endothelial growth factor (anti-VEGF) treatment. When the tumor is anteriorly located, radiation cataract is common and can be managed with routine cataract extraction. After initial radiotherapy, large tumors may cause a chronic exudative retinal detachment or become "toxic," often leading to neovascular glaucoma, which may respond to intravitreal anti-VEGF, intraocular pressure–lowering medication, cyclophotocoagulation, or resection of the residual tumor. Radiation complications appear to be dose-dependent and typically develop after a delay of 1 to several years.

American Brachytherapy Society–Ophthalmic Oncology Task Force. The American Brachytherapy Society consensus guidelines for plaque brachytherapy of uveal melanoma and retinoblastoma. *Brachytherapy.* 2014;13(1):1–14.

Bergman L, Nilsson B, Lundell G, Lundell M, Seregard S. Ruthenium brachytherapy for uveal melanoma, 1979–2003: survival and functional outcomes in the Swedish population. *Ophthalmology.* 2005;112(5):834–840.

Collaborative Ocular Melanoma Study Group. The COMS randomized trial of iodine 125 brachytherapy for choroidal melanoma: V. Twelve-year mortality rates and prognostic factors: COMS report no. 28. *Arch Ophthalmol.* 2006;124(12):1684–1693.

Charged-particle radiation

High–linear energy transfer radiation with charged particles (protons or helium ions) is effective in managing ciliary body and choroidal melanomas. In this technique, tantalum clips are surgically attached to the sclera to mark the basal margins of the tumor prior to the first radiation fraction. The charged-particle beams deliver a more homogeneous dose of radiation energy to a tumor than a radioactive plaque would, and the lateral spread of radiation energy is less extensive; the energy loss of ionizing radiation during its travel through matter is known as the *Bragg peak effect.* Local tumor control rates of up to 98% have been reported. The tumor response is similar to that observed after brachytherapy. Radiation complications, usually anterior, lead to neovascular glaucoma in 10% and some vision loss in up to 50% of treated eyes, depending on tumor size and location. Chronic dry eye may develop.

External-beam radiotherapy

Conventional external-beam radiotherapy is ineffective for uveal melanoma. In recent years, some centers have used fractionated stereotactic radiotherapy and gamma knife radiosurgery as the primary treatment. The results and adverse effects are comparable to those of other irradiation methods.

Alternative treatments

Transpupillary thermotherapy and photodynamic therapy In the past, laser photocoagulation played a limited role in the treatment of melanocytic tumors. Today, transpupillary thermotherapy (TTT), in which a long-duration, large–spot size, relatively low-energy infrared diode laser raises the temperature of the choroid, is used to manage selected small choroidal melanomas and, more frequently, to augment plaque brachytherapy or to control a local recurrence at the tumor margin. Reports suggest that TTT alone is associated with a higher rate of local tumor recurrence compared with brachytherapy. Some of these recurrences are extraocular.

Surgical excision Surgical transscleral resection or endoresection during vitrectomy has been successfully performed in eyes with malignant and benign intraocular tumors (Fig 17-12B). Concerns regarding surgical excision include the inability to evaluate tumor margins for residual disease, the high incidence of pathologically recognized scleral and retinal involvement in medium and large choroidal melanomas, and the possibility of spreading the tumor intraocularly and extraocularly. The surgical techniques are generally quite demanding, requiring an experienced surgeon with specialized training. Today, local excision of uveal melanoma is coupled with adjuvant radiotherapy, such as brachytherapy or proton-beam therapy, to reduce local recurrence rates to levels comparable to those after radiotherapy.

Damato BE. Local resection of uveal melanoma. *Dev Ophthalmol.* 2012;49:66–80.

Chemotherapy Currently, chemotherapy is not effective in the treatment of primary uveal melanoma. However, various regimens are available to treat patients with metastatic disease.

Immunotherapy In immunotherapy, systemic cytokines, immunomodulatory agents, or vaccine therapy is used to try to activate a tumor-directed T-cell immune response. This treatment is theoretically appropriate for uveal melanoma, because primary tumors arise in an immune-privileged organ and may express antigens to which the host is not sensitized. Currently, however, immunotherapy for primary uveal melanoma is not available. Immunotherapy for metastatic disease is under investigation.

Exenteration Traditionally advocated for patients with extrascleral extension of a posterior uveal melanoma, exenteration is rarely employed today. The current trend is toward more conservative treatment for these patients, with either enucleation plus a limited tenonectomy, or modified plaque brachytherapy or proton-beam therapy, unless orbital invasion is very advanced.

Prognosis and Prognostic Factors

There are 6 main clinical risk factors for melanoma-related mortality:

- larger tumor size (part of TNM staging)
- ciliary body extension (part of TNM staging)
- extraocular extension (part of TNM staging)
- older age
- faster tumor growth
- tumor regrowth after globe-conserving therapy, especially radiotherapy

The histologic and molecular features associated with a higher rate of metastases include the following:

- epithelioid cells
- high mitotic or cell proliferation index
- specific extravascular matrix patterns (loops and networks of loops) and high microvascular density
- mean diameter of the 10 largest nucleoli
- large numbers of tumor-infiltrating lymphocytes and macrophages

The prognostic factors most strongly associated with risk of metastasis are genetic:

- monosomy 3, especially with gains in chromosome 8
- gene expression profiling class 1B and, especially, class 2
- *BAP1* mutation and absence of *SF3B1* and *EIF1AX* mutations within tumor tissue

Table 17-2 lists 10-year survival estimates based on the current evidence-based staging system of the seventh edition of the AJCC *Cancer Staging Manual.* Stage IV implies that metastasis is present at the time of diagnosis of the primary tumor.

See Chapter 12 for a more detailed discussion.

Damato B, Eleuteri A, Taktak AF, Coupland SE. Estimating prognosis for survival after treatment of choroidal melanoma. *Prog Retin Eye Res.* 2011;30(5):285–295.

Edge S, Byrd DR, Compton CC, Fritz AG, Greene FL, Trotti A, eds. Malignant melanoma of the uvea. In: AJCC *Cancer Staging Manual.* 7th ed. New York: Springer; 2010:part X, pp 547–559.

Harbour JW. Molecular prognostic testing and individualized patient care in uveal melanoma. *Am J Ophthalmol.* 2009;148(6):823–829.

Shields CL, Furuta M, Thangappan A, et al. Metastasis of uveal melanoma millimeter-by-millimeter in 8033 consecutive eyes. *Arch Ophthalmol.* 2009;127(8):989–998.

Collaborative Ocular Melanoma Study

Data from the prospective, randomized, international COMS trials provide an additional framework for patient discussions concerning long-term survival and rates of globe conservation with enucleation and iodine-125 brachytherapy.

The COMS Large Choroidal Melanoma Trial

- evaluated 1003 patients with choroidal melanomas greater than 16 mm in basal diameter and/or greater than 10 mm in apical height (greater than 8 mm if peripapillary)
- compared enucleation alone with enucleation preceded by external-beam radiotherapy
- reported no significant difference in 5-year and 10-year all-cause mortality rates (approximately 60% and 40%, respectively)
- concluded that adjunctive radiotherapy did not improve overall survival but reduced risk of orbital recurrence
- established the appropriateness of primary enucleation alone in managing large choroidal melanomas not amenable to globe-conserving therapy

The COMS Medium Choroidal Melanoma Trial

- evaluated 1317 patients with choroidal melanomas 6–16 mm in basal diameter and/or 2.5–10 mm in apical height (up to 8 mm if peripapillary)
- compared enucleation with iodine-125 brachytherapy
- reported no significant difference in 5-year and 10-year all-cause mortality rates (approximately 20% and 35%, respectively)
- reported no significant difference in 5-year and 10-year frequencies of histologically confirmed metastases (approximately 10% and 18%, respectively)

- reported the following ancillary findings: (1) only 2 of 660 enucleated eyes were misdiagnosed as having a choroidal melanoma, (2) at 5 years the local tumor recurrence rate was 10% and the secondary enucleation rate was 13%, and (3) at 3 years there was a decline in visual acuity to 20/200 in approximately 40% of patients, and the visual angle quadrupled (ie, there were 6 lines of visual loss) in approximately 50% of patients

The COMS Small Choroidal Melanoma Study was an observational study of 204 patients with tumors measuring 4.0–8.0 mm in basal diameter and/or 1.0–2.4 mm in apical height, but many of the tumors were nongrowing.

Pigmented Epithelial Tumors of the Uvea and Retina

Adenoma and Adenocarcinoma

Benign adenomas of the nonpigmented and pigmented ciliary epithelium may appear clinically indistinguishable from amelanotic and pigmented melanomas arising in the ciliary body. Benign adenomas of the RPE are rare. These lesions are oval, deeply melanotic tumors that arise abruptly from the RPE. Adenomas rarely enlarge and seldom undergo malignant change. Adenocarcinomas of the RPE are also very rare; only a few cases have been reported. They typically have feeder retinal vessels and may be associated with yellowish lipid exudates. Although these lesions display malignant features on histologic examination, their metastatic potential is minimal. Adenomas and adenocarcinomas show high internal reflectivity by ultrasonography.

Fuchs adenoma (also called *pseudoadenomatous hyperplasia*) is usually an incidental finding at autopsy and rarely becomes apparent clinically. It appears as a glistening, white or tan, irregular tumor arising from the ciliary crest. It consists of benign proliferation of the nonpigmented ciliary epithelium with accumulation of basement membrane–like material.

Acquired Hyperplasia

Hyperplasia of the pigmented ciliary epithelium or the RPE usually develops in response to trauma, inflammation, or other ocular insults (Fig 17-13A). Because of their location, ciliary body lesions often do not become evident clinically. Occasionally, however, they may reach a large size and simulate a ciliary body melanoma. Posteriorly located lesions may be more commonly recognized and can lead to diagnostic uncertainty. In the early management of these atypical lesions, observation is often appropriate to document stability of the lesion. In rare cases, adenomatous hyperplasia may mimic a choroidal melanoma.

Simple Hamartoma

Simple hamartoma of the RPE is a small (up to 1 mm), sharply demarcated transretinal lesion that is located close to the center of the macula, arising from the RPE (Fig 17-13B). These lesions do not change over time.

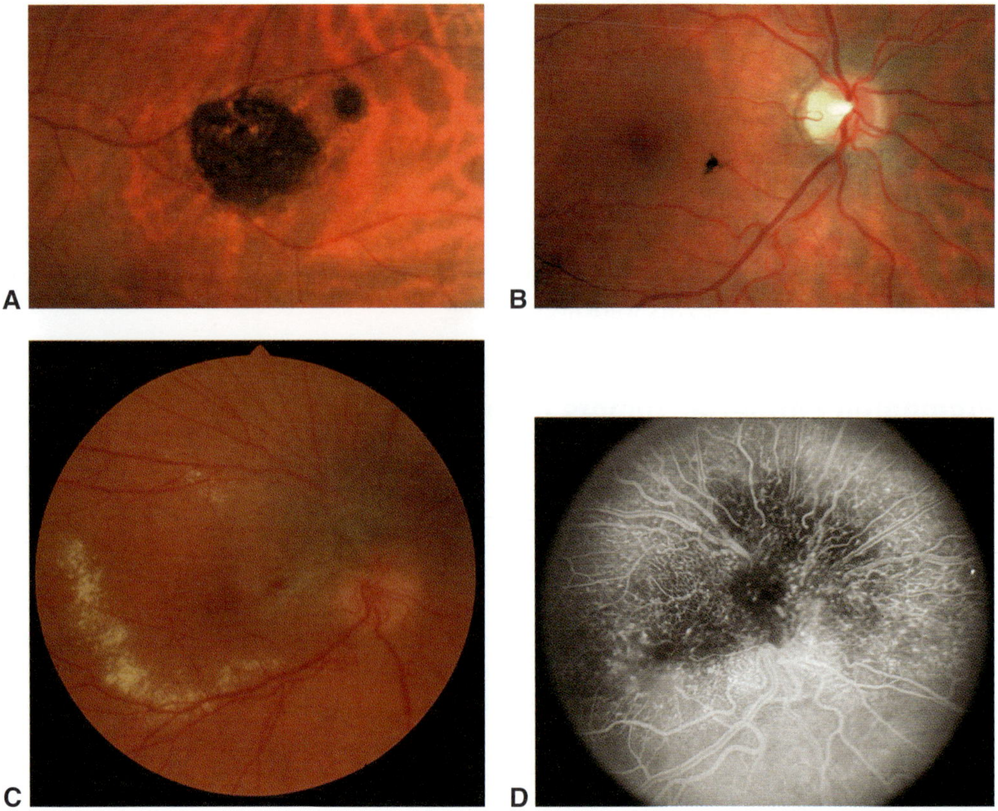

Figure 17-13 Lesions of the RPE. **A,** Reactive hyperplasia. **B,** Simple hamartoma. **C,** Clinical appearance and **D,** fluorescein angiogram of a peripapillary combined hamartoma of the retina and RPE. Note obscuration of the retinal vessels in superior aspect of the lesion, moderate deep pigmentation, and secondary hard exudates. The fluorescein angiogram shows the vascular component of the hamartoma, composed of small capillary-like telangiectatic vessels. Note the relative hypofluorescence superior to the optic nerve head due to the RPE component of this lesion. *(Parts A and B courtesy of Tero Kivelä, MD; parts C and D courtesy of Robert H. Rosa, Jr, MD.)*

Combined Hamartoma

Combined hamartoma of the RPE and retina is a rare disorder that occurs most frequently near the optic nerve head margin, though it may also be observed in the peripheral fundus. Typically, the hamartoma appears as a pigmented, slightly elevated lesion with vitreoretinal traction and tortuous retinal vessels (Fig 17-13C, see also Fig 11-49). Glial cells within this lesion may contract, producing traction lines seen clinically in the retina. Exudative complications associated with the vascular component of the lesion may be seen. These lesions have been mistaken for melanomas because of their pigmentation, slight elevation, and propensity to change in young individuals.

Kálmán Z, Tóth J. Two cases of congenital simple hamartoma of the retinal pigment epithelium. *Retin Cases Brief Rep.* 2009;3(3):283–285.

Shields CL, Thangappan A, Hartzell K, Valente P, Pirondini C, Shields JA. Combined hamartoma of the retina and retinal pigment epithelium in 77 consecutive patients' visual outcome based on macular versus extramacular tumor location. *Ophthalmology.* 2008;115(12):2246–2252.

CHAPTER **18**

Angiomatous Tumors

Hemangiomas

Choroidal Hemangiomas

Hemangiomas of the choroid occur in circumscribed and diffuse forms.

A *circumscribed choroidal hemangioma* typically occurs in patients with no systemic disorders. This dome-shaped, often inconspicuous vascular hamartoma is generally located in the postequatorial fundus, often in the macular area (Fig 18-1A, B). It may initially be difficult to distinguish from the surrounding fundus, but eventually degenerative changes occur in the overlying retinal pigment epithelium (RPE). These tumors also cause cystoid degeneration of the overlying outer retinal layers. In some cases, the tumors produce a secondary exudative retinal detachment that often extends into the foveal region, resulting in blurred vision and metamorphopsia.

Circumscribed choroidal hemangioma may be difficult to diagnose, because it can resemble other choroidal lesions, including

- amelanotic choroidal melanoma
- choroidal osteoma
- carcinoma metastatic to the choroid
- granuloma of the choroid

Ancillary diagnostic studies are helpful in evaluating both types of choroidal hemangiomas. A-scan ultrasonography shows a high-amplitude initial echo and high-amplitude broad internal echoes (high internal reflectivity; Fig 18-1C). B-scan ultrasonography reveals localized or diffuse choroidal thickening with prominent internal reflections without choroidal excavation or acoustic shadowing. Optical coherence tomography shows minimal internal signal (Fig 18-1D). Fluorescein angiography and indocyanine green angiography reveal large choroidal vessels in the prearterial or arterial phases, with late staining of the tumor and late leakage or pooling in the cystoid spaces of the overlying retina (Fig 18-1E–H).

Diffuse choroidal hemangioma is generally seen in patients with Sturge-Weber syndrome (ie, encephalofacial angiomatosis). It may also be associated with congenital ocular melanocytosis (ie, phakomatosis pigmentovascularis). This tumor produces diffuse reddish-orange coloration of the fundus, resulting in an ophthalmoscopic pattern referred to as *tomato ketchup fundus* (Fig 18-2). Secondary glaucoma and exudative retinal detachment often develop in eyes with this lesion. See also Chapter 12 in this

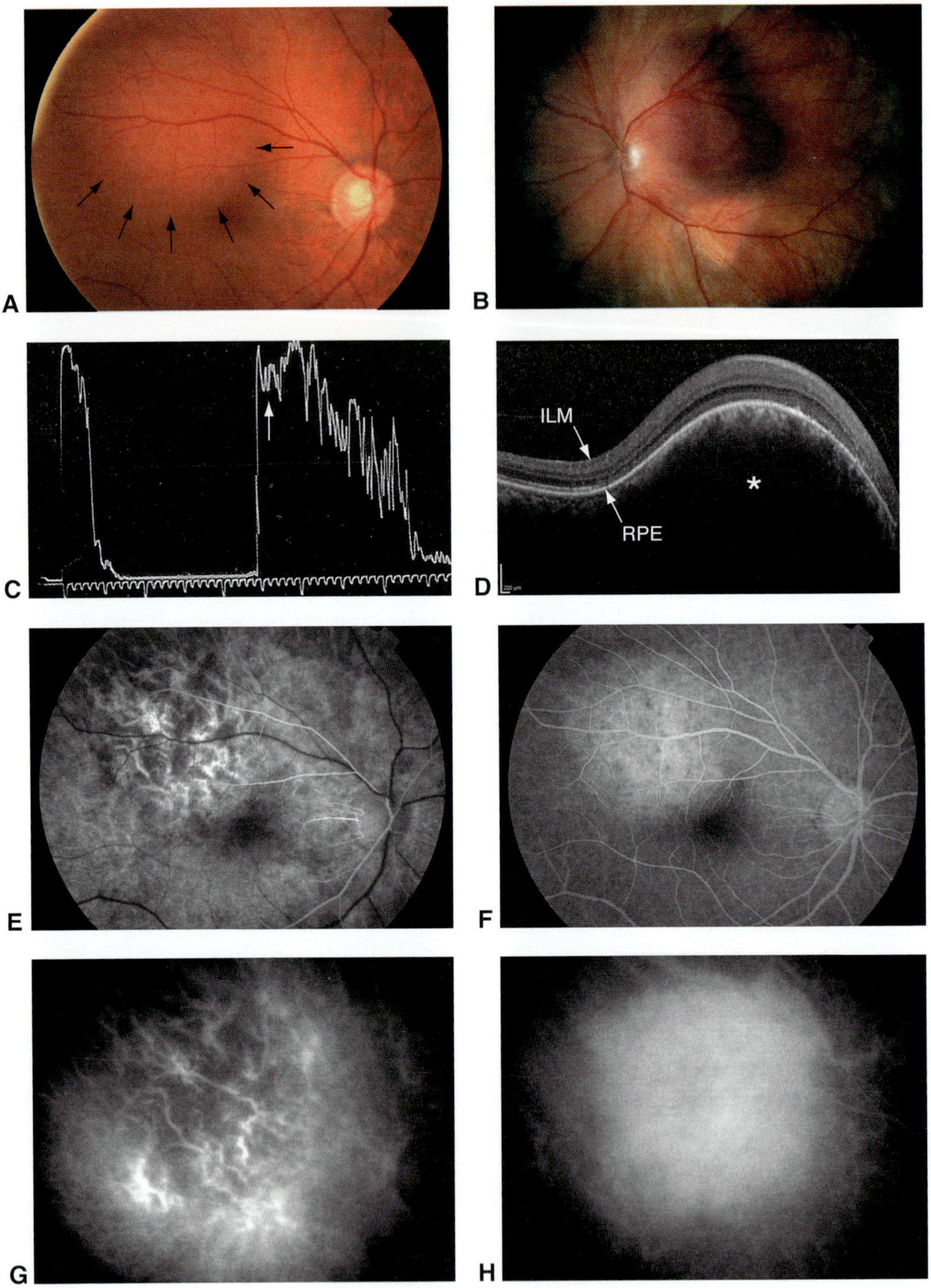

Figure 18-1 Circumscribed choroidal hemangioma. **A,** Dome-shaped tumor (inferior edge outlined by *arrows*) resembles the surrounding fundus in color. **B,** Wide-angle fundus photograph in which the eye is illuminated transclerally from one side shows the reddish color of the hemangioma. **C,** A-scan ultrasonography shows characteristic high internal reflectivity *(arrow)*. **D,** Optical coherence tomography shows a very-low-signal intensity lesion *(asterisk)*. ILM = internal limiting membrane; RPE = retinal pigment epithelium. **E,** Early fluorescein angiogram from the arterial phase shows intratumoral vessels. **F,** In the late phase of the angiogram, the tumor is hyperfluorescent. **G, H,** Indocyanine green angiography produces comparable findings. Compare **E–H** with **A** (same lesion). *(Parts A, B, and E–H courtesy of Tero Kivelä, MD; part D courtesy of Robert H. Rosa, Jr, MD.)*

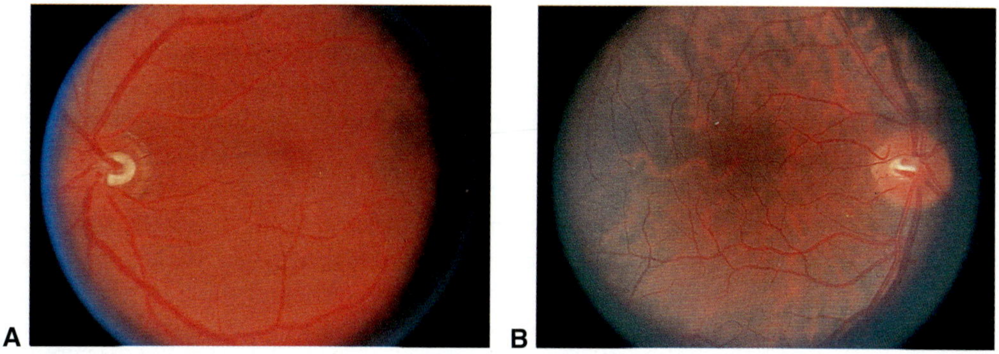

Figure 18-2 Diffuse choroidal hemangioma, clinical appearance. The saturated red color of the affected fundus **(A)** contrasts markedly with the color of the unaffected fundus **(B)** of the same patient.

volume, BCSC Section 12, *Retina and Vitreous,* and Section 6, *Pediatric Ophthalmology and Strabismus.*

Asymptomatic choroidal hemangiomas require no treatment. The most common indication for treatment is exudative detachment of the retina. Symptomatic circumscribed choroidal hemangiomas were traditionally managed with laser photocoagulation that created chorioretinal adhesions. However, photocoagulation was often unsuccessful and created scars. Recurrent detachments were common. The primary treatment of choice for symptomatic circumscribed choroidal hemangioma is photodynamic therapy (PDT).

PDT for circumscribed choroidal hemangioma is administered using the same standard parameters as PDT for exudative age-related macular degeneration. Most hemangiomas respond to PDT with resolution of the subretinal fluid and regression of the lesion, often with associated improvement in vision. However, cystoid macular edema may persist, and any degenerative changes in the overlying RPE may limit visual recovery.

Low-dose radiation (most commonly 20 gray [Gy]) via brachytherapy or radiotherapy (charged-particle, stereotactic, or external beam) has been successfully used to treat choroidal hemangiomas, including those unresponsive to PDT. All of these methods can be used to treat patients with circumscribed choroidal hemangioma; for diffuse choroidal hemangiomas, only external beam radiotherapy is used. Complications from the radiation and from the exudative retinal detachment may limit vision.

To date, there is little published evidence to support the use of vascular endothelial growth factor (VEGF) inhibitors to treat choroidal hemangiomas.

Boixadera A, García-Arumí J, Martínez-Castillo V, et al. Prospective clinical trial evaluating the efficacy of photodynamic therapy for symptomatic circumscribed choroidal hemangioma. *Ophthalmology.* 2009;116(1):100–105.

Retinal Angiomas

Hemangioblastoma

Retinal hemangioblastoma (previously known as *angiomatosis retinae* and *retinal capillary hemangioma*) is a rare sporadic or autosomal dominant condition with a reported incidence of 1 in 40,000. Although retinal lesions may be present at birth, diagnosis is typically made in the second to third decades of life. Retinal hemangioblastomas may be solitary or multiple; they appear as red to orange tumors arising within the retina with large-caliber, tortuous afferent and efferent retinal blood vessels (Fig 18-3A, B). Associated yellow-white retinal and subretinal lipid exudates that often involve the fovea may appear. Exudative detachments often occur in eyes with hemangioblastomas. Atypical variations include tumors arising from the optic nerve head (Fig 18-3C) and in the retinal periphery, where vitreous traction may elevate the tumor from the surface of the retina. Fluorescein angiography, which is not needed for diagnosis, demonstrates a rapid arteriovenous transit (Fig 18-3D), with immediate filling of the feeding arteriole, subsequent filling of the numerous fine blood vessels that constitute much of the tumor, and drainage by the dilated venule. Massive leakage of dye into the tumor and vitreous can occur.

When a hemangioblastoma of the retina occurs as the only finding, the condition is generally known as *von Hippel disease.* This condition is familial in about 20% of cases and bilateral in about 50%. The lesions may be multiple.

If retinal hemangioblastomas are associated with a cerebellar or spinal hemangioblastoma, then the condition is called *von Hippel–Lindau syndrome.* The gene for von Hippel–Lindau syndrome has been isolated to chromosome 3. A number of other tumors

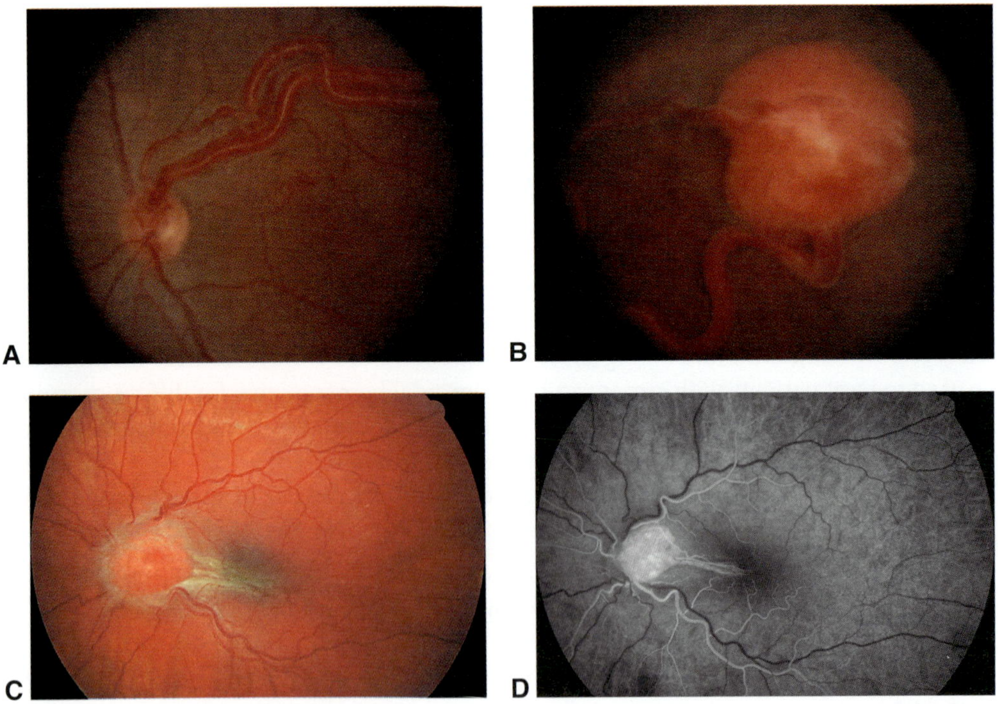

Figure 18-3 Retinal hemangioblastoma, clinical appearance. Dilated, tortuous retinal feeder artery and draining vein emanating from the optic nerve head **(A)** lead to the red- to orange-colored retinal tumor **(B).** An optic nerve head hemangioblastoma causes traction in the macular area **(C).** In the early arterial phase of fluorescein angiography, the lesion is brightly hyperfluorescent **(D).** *(Parts A and B courtesy of Robert H. Rosa, Jr, MD; parts C and D courtesy of Tero Kivelä, MD.)*

and cysts may develop in patients with this syndrome; the most serious of these lesions are renal cell carcinoma and pheochromocytoma.

When von Hippel–Lindau syndrome is suspected, appropriate genetic consultation and screening are critical for long-term follow-up of ocular manifestations and systemic complications. Patients with this syndrome can now undergo genetic screening that determines whether they are at risk for developing systemic manifestations of the disease. By identifying the retinal lesions, the ophthalmologist is often the first medical specialist to identify affected family members. Screening for systemic vascular anomalies (eg, cerebellar hemangioblastomas) and malignancies may reduce mortality, and aggressive screening for and early treatment of retinal hemangioblastomas may reduce complications and improve long-term visual outcomes.

The treatment of retinal hemangioblastomas includes photocoagulation for smaller lesions; cryotherapy for larger and more peripheral lesions; and either plaque brachytherapy or proton beam radiotherapy or scleral buckling with cryotherapy for larger lesions with more extensive retinal detachment. Both standard and modified PDT protocols have been successfully used to treat selected retinal hemangioblastomas. The use of VEGF inhibitors in the treatment of retinal hemangioblastomas is still experimental. Reports suggest that the principal efficacy of VEGF inhibitors is in reducing macular edema, but the impact on the size of the hemangioblastomas has been variable. Although most optic nerve head hemangioblastomas are notoriously resistant to treatment, some have responded to the same conservative therapies used on peripheral lesions, or have been resected using vitrectomy.

The visual prognosis remains guarded for patients with optic nerve head and large retinal lesions.

Cavernous hemangioma

Cavernous hemangioma of the retina is an uncommon lesion that resembles a cluster of grapes (Fig 18-4). These lesions may also occur on the optic nerve head. Retinal cavernous hemangiomas may be associated with similar skin and central nervous system

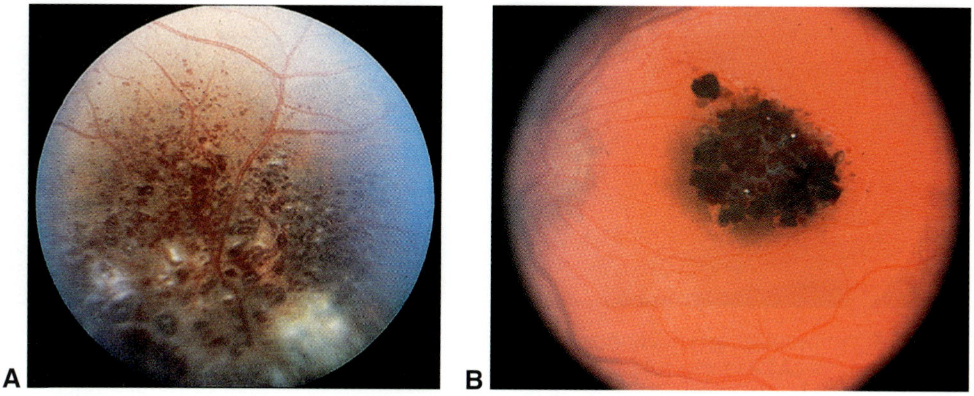

Figure 18-4 Retinal cavernous hemangioma, clinical appearance. **A,** Multiple tiny vascular saccules and associated white fibrovascular tissue. **B,** A smaller lesion consisting of a grapelike cluster of clumped vascular saccules. *(Part B courtesy of Timothy G. Murray, MD.)*

lesions. Patients that have intracranial lesions may experience associated seizures. Unlike retinal hemangioblastomas, cavernous hemangiomas are not typically associated with exudation, and therefore treatment is rarely required. However, small hemorrhages as well as gliotic and fibrotic areas may appear on the surface of the lesion. Fluorescein angiography may reveal plasma–erythrocyte separation within the vascular spaces of the cavernous hemangioma; this separation is virtually diagnostic of these lesions. In contrast to retinal hemangioblastomas, retinal cavernous hemangiomas fill very slowly. The fluorescein remains in the vascular spaces for an extended period without apparent leakage (see BCSC Section 12, *Retina and Vitreous,* Fig 7-12).

Arteriovenous Malformations

Congenital retinal arteriovenous malformation (also known as racemose hemangioma) is an anomalous artery-to-vein anastomosis that can range from a small, localized vascular communication in the iris, near the optic nerve head or in the retinal periphery to a prominent tangle of large, tortuous blood vessels throughout most of the fundus (Fig 18-5A, B).

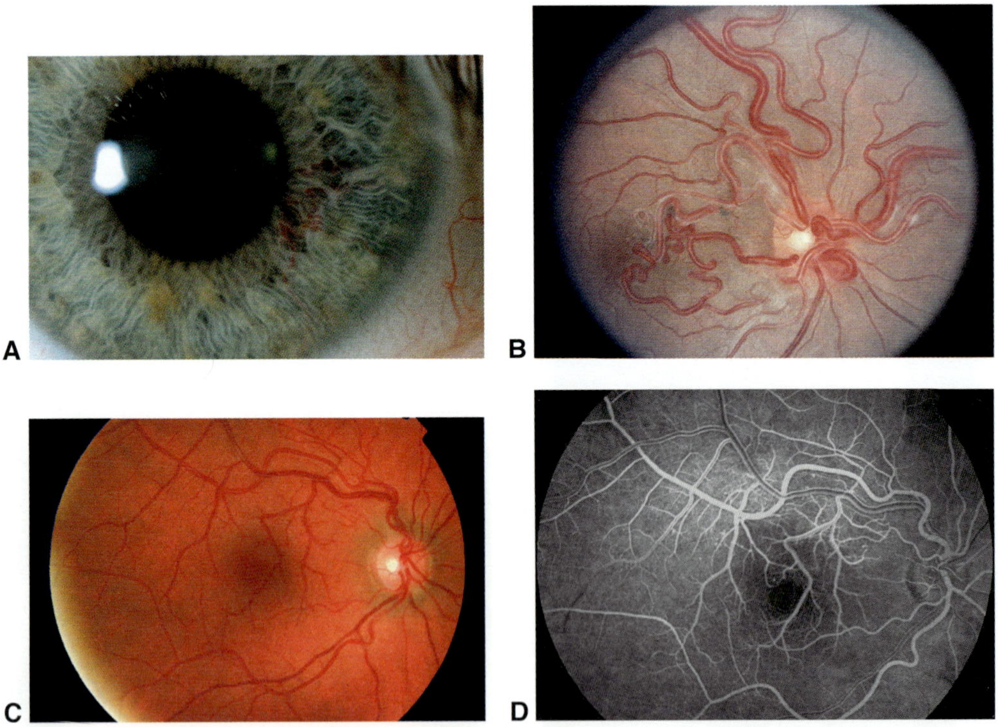

Figure 18-5 Intraocular arteriovenous malformations, clinical appearance. Racemose hemangioma in the iris **(A)** and the retina **(B)** in 2 different patients. **C,** Although it can occasionally have an arteriovenous communication, a retinal macrovessel is distinct from racemose hemangioma. **D,** Fluorescein angiography highlights the macrovessel, which crosses the macular area and the horizontal midline. Absence of leakage is characteristic of retinal arteriovenous malformations. *(Parts A, C, and D courtesy of Tero Kivelä, MD; part B courtesy of Robert H. Rosa, Jr, MD.)*

Racemose refers to the clustered or bunched nature of the vessels. When associated with an arteriovenous malformation of the midbrain region, this condition is generally referred to as *Wyburn-Mason syndrome* (also known as Bonnet-Dechaume-Blanc syndrome; see BCSC Section 5, *Neuro-Ophthalmology,* and Section 6, *Pediatric Ophthalmology and Strabismus*). Associated similar arteriovenous malformations may appear in the orbit and mandible.

A racemose hemangioma of the retina is different from a congenital retinal macrovessel, which is a large aberrant retinal vessel that crosses the midline and often also the macular area (Fig 18-5C, D). Retinal macrovessels occasionally show arteriovenous communications.

CHAPTER 19

Retinoblastoma

Retinoblastoma is the most common primary intraocular malignant tumor of childhood and is the second most common (after uveal melanoma) primary intraocular malignant tumor in all age groups. The frequency of retinoblastoma ranges from 1 in 14,000 to 1 in 20,000 live births. It is estimated that 250–300 new cases occur in the United States each year. Both sexes and all races are equally affected, and the tumor occurs bilaterally in 30%–40% of cases. Approximately 90% of cases are diagnosed in patients younger than 3 years. The mean age at diagnosis depends on family history and the laterality of the disease:

- patients with a known family history of retinoblastoma: 8 months
- patients with bilateral disease: 12 months
- patients with unilateral disease: 24 months

Globally, incidence data for retinoblastoma show an approximately 50-fold variation. Registries with the highest incidence of retinoblastoma include countries in Africa.

Abramson DH, Beaverson K, Sangani P, et al. Screening for retinoblastoma: presenting signs as prognosticators of patient and ocular survival. *Pediatrics.* 2003;112(6 Pt. 1):1248–1255.

Orjuela M. Epidemiology. In: C Rodriguez-Galindo, MW Wilson, eds. *Retinoblastoma,* Pediatric Oncology. New York: Springer; 2010:11–23.

Wong JR, Tucker MA, Kleinerman RA, Devesa SS. Retinoblastoma incidence patterns in the US Surveillance, Epidemiology, and End Results program. *JAMA Ophthalmol.* 2014;132(4): 478–483.

Genetic Counseling

In nearly all cases, retinoblastoma is caused by a mutation in the *RB1* tumor suppressor gene located on the long arm of chromosome 13 at locus 14 (13q14). In order for a tumor to form, both copies of the *RB1* gene must be mutated. If a patient has bilateral retinoblastoma, there is an approximately 98% chance that it represents a germline mutation. About 10% of retinoblastoma patients have a family history of retinoblastoma. The children of a patient who has the hereditary form of retinoblastoma have a 45% chance of being affected (50% chance of inheriting and 90% chance of penetrance). In these cases, the child inherits an abnormal gene from the affected parent, which, when coupled with somatic mutations in the remaining normal *RB1* allele, leads to the development of multiple tumors in 1 or both eyes.

Sporadic cases constitute approximately 90% of all retinoblastomas. Of these, 60% of patients have unilateral disease with no germline mutations. The remaining patients have new germline mutations and multiple tumors will develop. Approximately 15% of the sporadic unilateral patients are carriers of a germline *RB1* mutation. Unless there are multiple tumors in the affected eye, these patients cannot be distinguished from those without a germline mutation. Much like their counterparts with bilateral retinoblastoma, children with unilateral retinoblastoma and a germline mutation are more likely to present at an earlier age. Commercial laboratories are able to test retinoblastoma patients' blood for germline mutations. Methods of genetic testing used in retinoblastoma screening include gene sequencing via quantitative polymerase chain reaction (PCR), karyotyping, fluorescence in situ hybridization (FISH), multiplex ligation-dependent probe amplification (MLPA), and ribonucleic acid (RNA) analysis. With these screening methods, there is a 96% chance of finding a new tumor mutation, if one exists. The success rate can be further increased if blood and freshly harvested tumor are available for analysis.

Between 1% and 3% of retinoblastomas in children younger than 6 months are associated with a mutation in *N-MYC* (not *RB1*).

Counseling with a genetic specialist is recommended for all families afflicted with or a risk for developing retinoblastoma. Genetic counseling for retinoblastoma can be very complex (Fig 19-1). As mentioned earlier, a bilateral retinoblastoma survivor has a 45% chance of having an affected child, whereas a unilateral survivor has a 7%–15% chance of having an affected child. Unaffected parents of a child with bilateral involvement have less than a 5% risk of having another child with retinoblastoma. If 2 or more siblings are affected, the chance that another child will be affected increases to 45%. See also Chapter 11 and BCSC Section 6, *Pediatric Ophthalmology and Strabismus.*

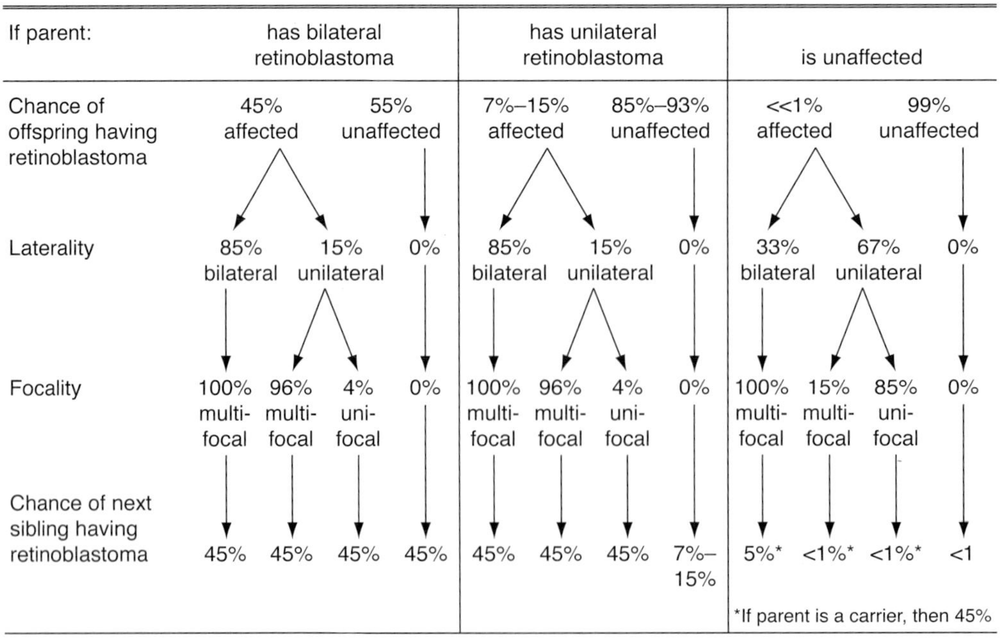

Figure 19-1 Genetic counseling for retinoblastoma. *(Chart created by David H. Abramson, MD.)*

Abramson DH, Mendelsohn ME, Servodidio CA, Tretter T, Gombos DS. Familial retinoblastoma: where and when? *Acta Ophthalmol Scand.* 1998;76(3):334–338.

Murphree AL. Molecular genetics of retinoblastoma. *Ophthalmol Clin North Am.* 1995;8: 155–166.

Thériault BL, Dimaras H, Gallie BL, Corson TW. The genomic landscape of retinoblastoma: a review. *Clin Exp Ophthalmol.* 2014;42(1):33–52.

Diagnostic Evaluation

Retinoblastoma is a clinical diagnosis. Fine-needle aspiration biopsy (FNAB) should be undertaken only with extreme caution and only by an experienced ocular oncologist, because of the risk of systemic dissemination of tumor.

Clinical Examination

The presenting signs and symptoms of retinoblastoma are determined by the extent and location of the tumor at the time of diagnosis. In the United States, the most common presenting signs of retinoblastoma are leukocoria (white pupillary reflex), strabismus, and ocular inflammation (Fig 19-2, Table 19-1). Other presenting features, such as iris

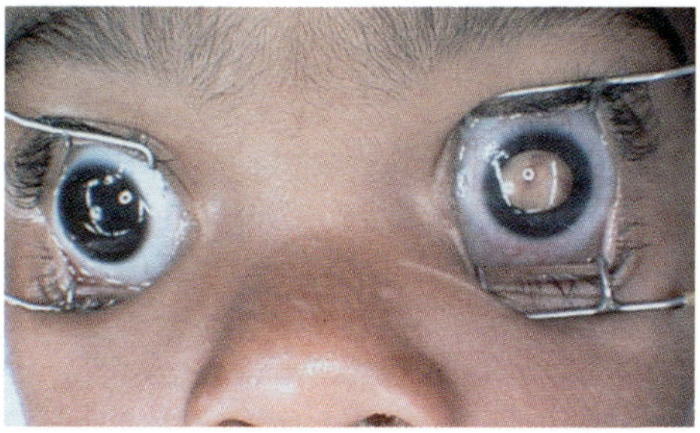
A

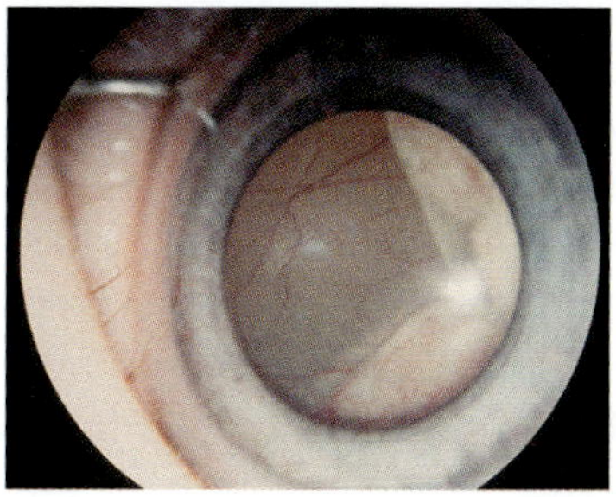
B

Figure 19-2 Retinoblastoma. **A,** Clinical appearance shows leukocoria and strabismus associated with advanced intraocular tumor. **B,** High magnification. Note the large retrolental tumor and secondary total exudative retinal detachment. *(Courtesy of Timothy G. Murray, MD.)*

Table 19-1 Presenting Signs and Symptoms of Retinoblastoma

Among Patients <5 Years	Among Patients ≥5 Years
Leukocoria (most common)	Leukocoria (35%)
Strabismus (≈20%)	Decreased vision (35%)
Ocular inflammation (≈5%)	Strabismus (15%)
Pseudohypopyon	Floaters (5%)
Hyphema	Pain (5%)
Iris heterochromia	
Spontaneous globe perforation	
Proptosis	
Cataract	
Glaucoma	
Nystagmus	
Tearing	
Anisocoria	

heterochromia, spontaneous hyphema, and orbital cellulitis or inflammation, are uncommon. In rare instances, a small lesion may be found on routine examination. Reported vision problems are infrequent because most patients are preschool-aged children.

The diagnosis of retinoblastoma can generally be made on the basis of an office examination that includes documented visual acuity. An examination under anesthesia (EUA) is needed for all patients suspected of having retinoblastoma in order to completely assess the extent of ocular disease prior to treatment (Fig 19-3). The intraocular pressure and corneal diameter of both eyes should be measured intraoperatively. The location of all tumors in each eye should be clearly documented.

Retinoblastoma begins as a translucent, gray to white intraretinal tumor, fed and drained by dilated, tortuous retinal vessels (Figs 19-4, 19-5). As the tumor grows, foci of calcification develop, giving the tumor its characteristic chalky white appearance. Exophytic tumors grow beneath the retina and may have an associated serous retinal detachment. As these tumors grow, the retinal detachment may become extensive, obscuring visualization of the tumor (Fig 19-6). Endophytic tumors grow on the retinal surface into the vitreous cavity. Blood vessels may be difficult to discern in endophytic tumors. Endophytic tumors are more likely to give rise to *vitreous seeds* (Fig 19-7), which are cells shed from retinoblastoma that remain viable in the vitreous and subretinal space and may eventually result in tumor implants throughout the eye. Vitreous seeds may also enter the anterior chamber, where they can aggregate on the iris to form nodules or settle inferiorly to form a pseudohypopyon (Fig 19-8). Secondary glaucoma and rubeosis iridis occur in approximately 50% of such cases.

Diffuse infiltrating retinoblastoma is a rare variant of retinoblastoma that is detected later in childhood (>5 years); it is typically unilateral. Diffuse infiltrating retinoblastoma presents a diagnostic dilemma, as the retina may be difficult to see through the dense vitreous cells. This variant is often mistaken for an intermediate uveitis of unknown etiology.

Ultrasonography can aid the diagnosis of retinoblastoma by demonstrating characteristic calcifications within the tumor. Although these calcifications can also be seen on

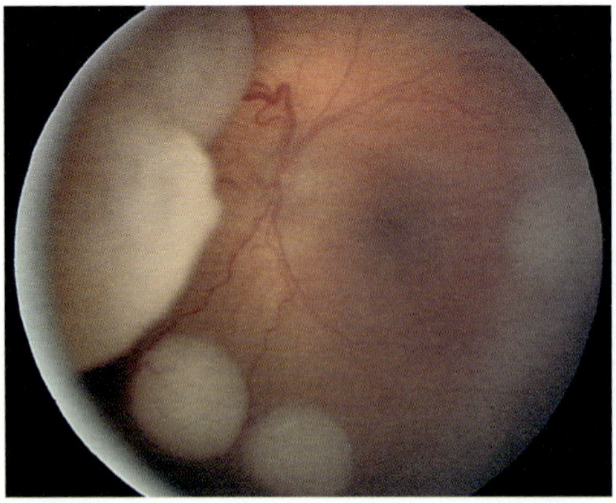

Figure 19-3 Retinoblastoma. Multiple tumor foci in an eye of a patient with a germline *RB1* mutation. *(Courtesy of Matthew W. Wilson, MD.)*

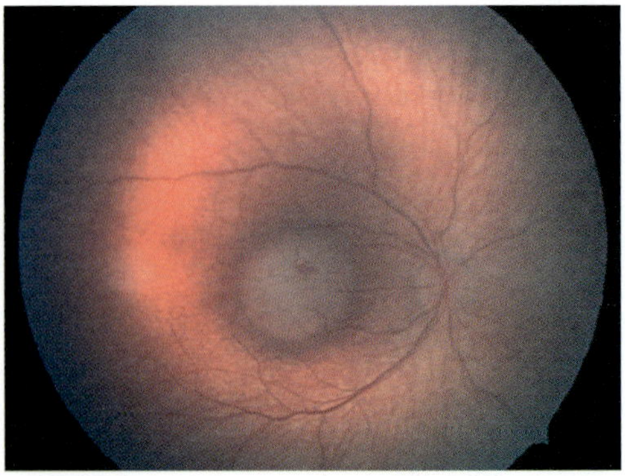

Figure 19-4 Retinoblastoma, clinical appearance. Small, discrete white tumor supplied by dilated retinal blood vessels. *(Courtesy of Timothy G. Murray, MD.)*

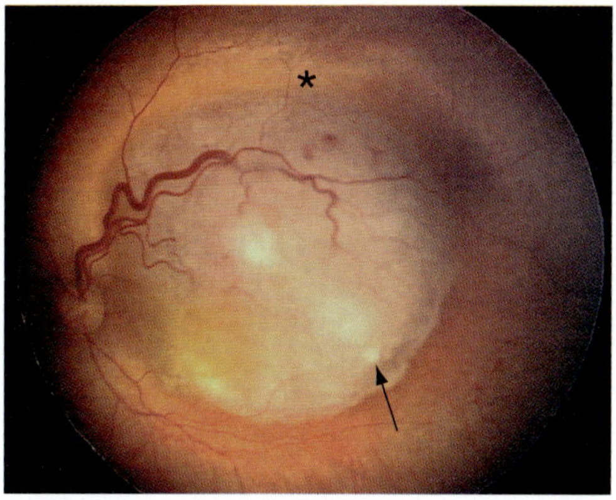

Figure 19-5 Retinoblastoma. Note the dilated retinal blood vessels, foci of calcification *(arrow)*, and cuff of subretinal fluid *(asterisk)*. *(Courtesy of Matthew W. Wilson, MD.)*

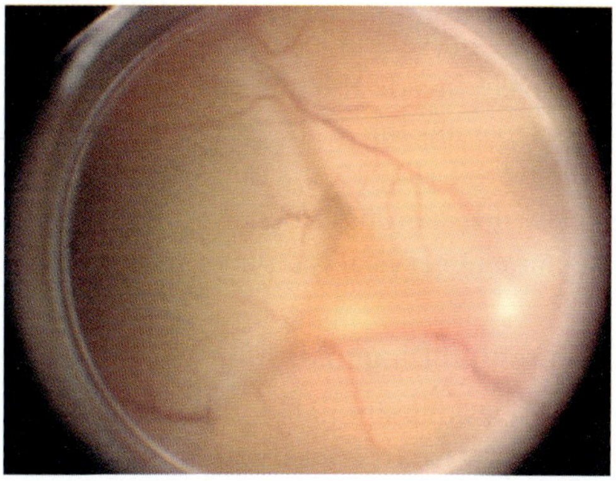

Figure 19-6 Retinoblastoma. Complete exudative detachment obscures tumor visualization. Note normal-appearing retinal vessels, as opposed to those found in Coats disease. *(Courtesy of Matthew W. Wilson, MD.)*

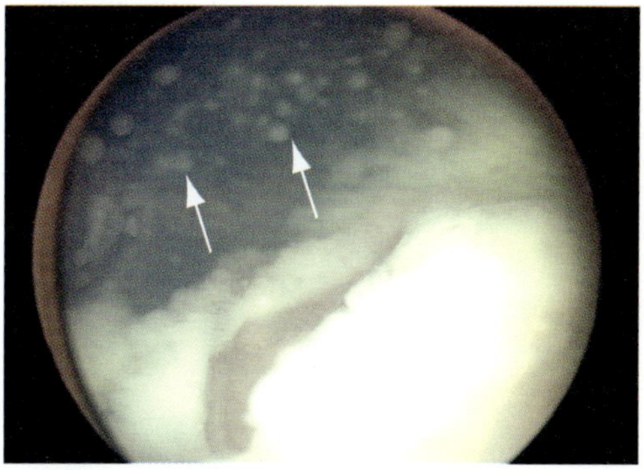

Figure 19-7 Retinoblastoma. Large endophytic tumor with extensive vitreous seeding *(arrows)*. *(Courtesy of Matthew W. Wilson, MD.)*

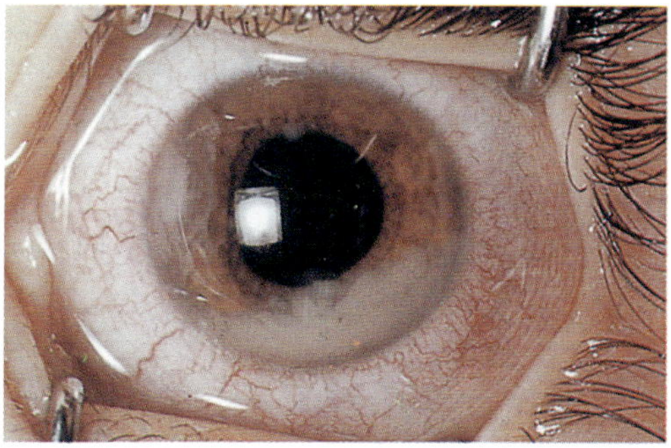

Figure 19-8 Retinoblastoma, clinical appearance. Pseudohypopyon resulting from migration of tumor cells into the anterior chamber.

computed tomography (CT) scan, magnetic resonance imaging (MRI) has become the preferred diagnostic modality for evaluating the optic nerve, orbits, and brain. MRI not only offers better soft-tissue resolution but also avoids exposing the patient to potentially harmful radiation. Recent studies have suggested that systemic metastatic evaluation, typically via bone marrow and lumbar puncture, is not indicated in children without neurologic abnormalities or evidence of extraocular extension. If optic nerve extension is suspected, lumbar puncture may be performed. Parents and siblings should be examined for evidence of untreated retinoblastoma or retinocytoma, which would represent evidence of a hereditary predisposition to the disease. Children with retinoblastoma should have a complete history and physical examination done by a pediatric oncologist.

In the United States, patients rarely present with metastases or intracranial extension at the time of diagnosis. The most frequently identified sites of metastatic involvement in children with retinoblastoma include abdominal viscera, brain, distal bones, lymph nodes, skull bones, and spinal cord. Retinoblastoma cells may escape the eye by invading the optic nerve and extending into the subarachnoid space. In addition, tumor cells may massively invade the choroid before traversing emissary canals or eroding through the sclera to enter the orbit. Extraocular extension may result in proptosis as the tumor grows in the orbit (Fig 19-9). In the anterior chamber, tumor cells may invade the trabecular meshwork, gaining access to the conjunctival lymphatics. Subsequently, palpable preauricular and cervical lymph nodes may develop.

Differential Diagnosis

Several lesions simulate retinoblastoma (Table 19-2). Most of these conditions can be differentiated from retinoblastoma on the basis of a comprehensive history, clinical examination, and results from appropriate ancillary diagnostic testing.

Persistent fetal vasculature

Persistent fetal vasculature (PFV), also known as *persistent hyperplastic primary vitreous (PHPV),* is typically recognized within days or weeks of birth. The condition is unilateral in two-thirds of cases and is associated with microphthalmos, a shallow or flat anterior chamber, a hypoplastic iris with prominent vessels, and a retrolenticular fibrovascular mass that draws the ciliary body processes inward. On indirect ophthalmoscopy, a vascular stalk may be seen arising from the optic nerve head and attaching to the posterior lens capsule. Ultrasonography confirms the diagnosis by showing persistent hyaloid remnants

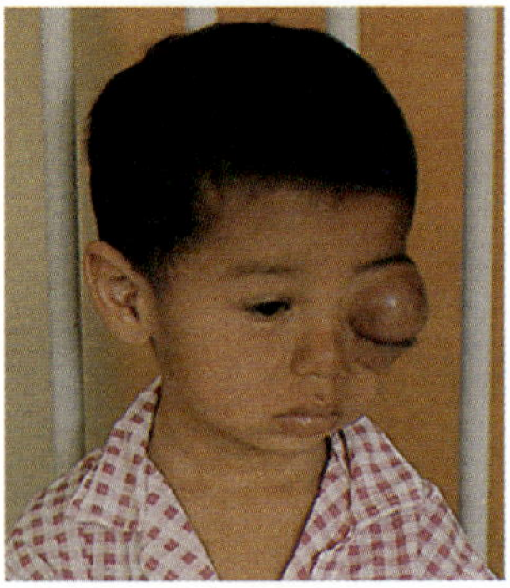

Figure 19-9 Retinoblastoma, clinical appearance. Proptosis caused by retinoblastoma with orbital invasion.

Table 19-2 Differential Diagnosis of Retinoblastoma

Astrocytic hamartoma
Coats disease
Coloboma of choroid or optic nerve head
Congenital retinal fold
Organizing vitreous hemorrhage
Persistent fetal vasculature
Posterior cataract
Retinal dysplasia
Retinopathy of prematurity
Toxocariasis (larval granuloma)
Uveitis

arising from the optic nerve head, usually in association with a closed funnel retinal detachment. No retinal tumors are seen, and the axial length of the eye is shortened. Calcification may be present. See also Chapter 10 and BCSC Section 6, *Pediatric Ophthalmology and Strabismus.*

Coats disease

Coats disease is clinically evident within the first decade of life and is more common in boys. The lesion is typically characterized by unilateral retinal telangiectasia associated with intraretinal yellow exudation without a distinct mass (Fig 19-10). The progressive leakage of fluid may result in extensive retinal detachment and neovascular glaucoma. Ultrasonography documents the absence of retinal tumors and shows the collection of cholesterol in the subretinal fluid. Fluorescein angiography shows classic telangiectatic vessels and areas of retinal ischemia (see BCSC Section 12, *Retina and Vitreous*).

Ocular toxocariasis

Ocular toxocariasis typically occurs in older children who have a history of soil ingestion or exposure to puppies or kittens. Toxocariasis presents with posterior and peripheral granulomas, with associated uveitis. Exudative retinal detachment, organized vitreoretinal traction, and cataracts may be present. Ultrasonography shows vitritis, retinal detachment, granulomas, retinal traction, and the absence of calcium. See BCSC Section 9, *Intraocular Inflammation and Uveitis,* for additional discussion.

Astrocytoma

Retinal astrocytoma, or astrocytic hamartoma, generally appears as a small, smooth, white, glistening tumor located in the nerve fiber layer of the retina (Fig 19-11). It may be single or multiple, unilateral or bilateral. In some cases, it may grow and calcify, typically having a mulberry appearance. Astrocytomas occasionally arise from the optic nerve head; such tumors are often referred to as *giant drusen.* Retinal astrocytomas commonly occur in patients with tuberous sclerosis and may also be found in patients with neurofibromatosis; most are not associated with a phakomatosis.

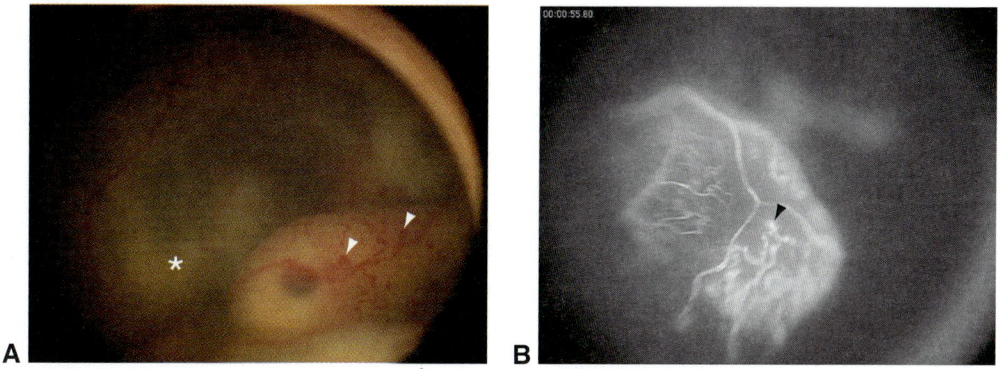

Figure 19-10 Coats disease. **A,** Clinical appearance of characteristic lightbulb aneurysms *(arrowheads).* Note the associated exudative retinal detachment with subretinal exudate *(asterisk).* **B,** Fluorescein angiogram showing classic telangiectatic vessels *(arrowhead). (Courtesy of Matthew W. Wilson, MD.)*

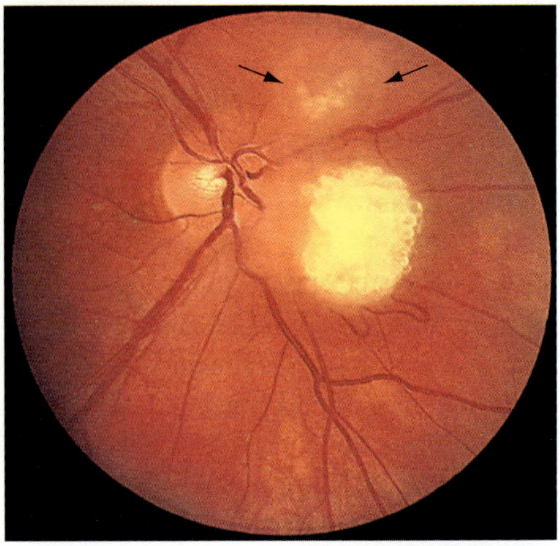

Figure 19-11 Retinal astrocytic hamartomas, clinical appearance. Note the more subtle opalescent lesion *(between arrows)* superonasal to the optic nerve head and the larger "mulberry" lesion that is inferonasal to the nerve head.

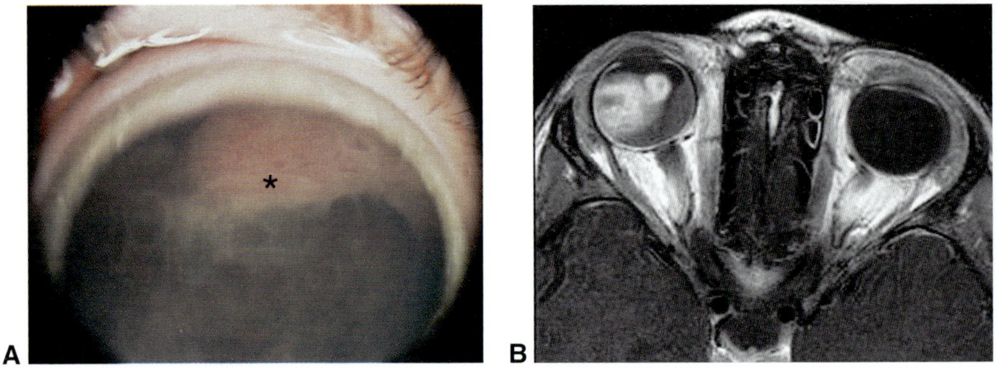

Figure 19-12 Medulloepithelioma. **A,** Pigmented lesion arising in the ciliary body, with an amelanotic apex *(asterisk)*. **B,** T1-weighted magnetic resonance image (MRI) with gadolinium, showing diffuse enhancement and multiple cystic spaces. *(Courtesy of Matthew W. Wilson, MD.)*

Medulloepithelioma

Medulloepithelioma is a tumor derived from the inner layer of the optic cup (medullary epithelium); it can be either benign or malignant (see Chapter 11, Fig 11-48). This type of tumor typically becomes clinically evident in children aged 4–12 years, but it may also occur in adults. It usually appears as a variably pigmented mass arising from the ciliary body (Fig 19-12A), but it has also been documented in the retina and optic nerve. Smaller lesions may present with unexplained neovascular glaucoma accompanied by iris heterochromia. The tumor may erode through the iris root or grow along the lens zonular fibers, entering the anterior chamber. Diagnostic imaging may reveal large cysts on the surface of the tumor or within the lesion (Fig 19-12B). See Chapter 11 for a discussion of the histologic features of medulloepithelioma.

Management of medulloepithelioma usually consists of enucleation or observation. Small lesions have been successfully treated with plaque brachytherapy, but most eyes treated in this fashion succumb to enucleation. For most of these tumors, surgical resection is specifically avoided because of late complications and documented metastases associated with this treatment. Fortunately, metastasis is rare with appropriate management, even if the tumor appears frankly malignant on histologic examination.

Classification

The Reese-Ellsworth Classification for Intraocular Tumors is the historic method of grouping intraocular retinoblastomas. The system takes into account the number, size, and location of tumors and the presence or absence of vitreous seeding. This classification sorts eye tumors into groups from very favorable (group I) to very unfavorable (group V) by probability of eye preservation when treated with external-beam radiation alone. The Reese-Ellsworth classification does not stage extraocular disease, nor does it provide prognostic information about patient survival or vision.

The use of external-beam radiotherapy for the treatment of retinoblastoma has been supplanted by the use of primary local and/or systemic chemotherapy. As a result, the International Classification System for Intraocular Retinoblastoma is now the most commonly used system worldwide. In this system, eyes are grouped on the basis of the size of the tumor and the presence of subretinal fluid, as well as the extent of vitreous and subretinal seeding. Eyes are assigned a letter from A to E (most to least salvageable with chemotherapy). Eyes with anterior chamber involvement, neovascular glaucoma, vitreous hemorrhage, and/or necrosis are considered unsalvageable (Table 19-3).

The American Joint Committee on Cancer (AJCC) also has a staging system for retinoblastoma that relates to both intraocular and extraocular disease, but it is not used clinically by most ocular oncologists.

Murphree AL. Intraocular retinoblastoma: the case for a new group classification. *Ophthalmol Clin North Am.* 2005;18(1):41–53.

Reese AB. *Tumors of the Eye.* 3rd ed. Hagerstown, MD: Harper & Row; 1976:90–132.

Shields CL, Mashayekhi A, Demirci H, Meadows AT, Shields JA. Practical approach to management of retinoblastoma. *Arch Ophthalmol.* 2004;122(5):729–735.

Table 19-3 International Classification for Intraocular Retinoblastoma (ABC System)

Group A	Small tumors (<3 mm) confined to the retina; >3 mm from the fovea; >1.5 mm from the optic nerve head
Group B	Tumors (>3 mm) confined to the retina in any location, with clear subretinal fluid up to 5 mm from the tumor margin
Group C	Localized vitreous and/or subretinal seeding
Group D	Diffuse vitreous and/or subretinal seeding
Group E	No visual potential or presence of 1 or more of the following: • tumor in the anterior segment • tumor in or on the ciliary body • neovascular glaucoma • vitreous hemorrhage obscuring the tumor or significant hyphema • phthisical or prephthisical eye • orbital cellulitis–like presentation

Associated Conditions

Retinocytoma

Retinocytoma is clinically indistinguishable from retinoblastoma. Chapter 11 describes the histologic characteristics that distinguish retinocytoma from retinoblastoma (see Fig 11-47). The developmental biology of retinocytoma is controversial; some authorities believe that retinocytoma is retinoblastoma that has undergone differentiation, analogous to ganglioneuroma, the differentiated form of neuroblastoma. Other authorities contend that retinocytoma is a benign counterpart of retinoblastoma.

Although histologically benign, retinocytoma carries the same genetic implications as retinoblastoma. A child harboring a retinoblastoma in 1 eye and a retinocytoma in the other should be considered capable of transmitting an *RB1* mutation to offspring.

Singh AD, Santos MM, Shields CL, Shields JA, Eagle RC, Jr. Observations on 17 patients with retinocytoma. *Arch Ophthalmol.* 2000;118(2):199–205.

Primitive Neuroectodermal Tumor

The term *primitive neuroectodermal tumor (PNET),* or *trilateral retinoblastoma,* is reserved for cases of bilateral retinoblastoma associated with ectopic intracranial disease. The ectopic focus is usually located in the pineal gland or the parasellar region and has historically been known as a *pinealoblastoma.* This tumor affects up to 5% of children with a germline *RB1* mutation. In rare cases, a child may present with ectopic intracranial retinoblastoma prior to ocular involvement. More commonly, this independent malignancy presents months to years after treatment of the intraocular retinoblastoma.

Several observations support the concept of primary intracranial pinealoblastoma. CT findings helped establish that intracranial tumors in some patients with terminal retinoblastoma are anatomically separate from the primary tumors in the orbit. These intracranial tumors are not associated with metastatic disease elsewhere in the body, and unlike metastatic retinoblastoma, they often demonstrate features of differentiation such as *Flexner-Wintersteiner rosettes* (see Chapter 11, Fig 11-43). Embryologic, immunologic, and phylogenic evidence of photoreceptor differentiation in the pineal gland offers further support for the concept of trilateral retinoblastoma.

All patients with retinoblastoma should undergo baseline neuroimaging studies to exclude intracranial involvement. Experts disagree on the role of serial imaging in screening for PNETs. Reports suggest a decline in their incidence; whether this is due to the prophylactic effect of systemic chemotherapy or a decrease in the use of radiation therapy is unclear.

Friedman DN, Sklar CA, Oeffinger KC, et al. Long-term medical outcomes in survivors of extra-ocular retinoblastoma: the Memorial Sloan-Kettering Cancer Center (MSKCC) experience. *Pediatr Blood Cancer.* 2013;60(4):694–699.

Jubran RF, Erdreich-Epstein A, Butturini A, Murphree AL, Villablanca JG. Approaches to treatment for extraocular retinoblastoma: Children's Hospital Los Angeles experience. *J Pediatr Hematol Oncol.* 2004;26(1):31–34.

Moll AC, Imhof SM, Schouten-Van Meeteren AY, Kuik DJ, Hofman P, Boers M. Second primary tumors in hereditary retinoblastoma: a register-based study, 1945–1997: is there an age effect on radiation-related risk? *Ophthalmology.* 2001;108(6):1109–1114.

Treatment

When treating retinoblastoma, the ophthalmologist must understand that it is a malignancy. In industrialized countries, survival rates exceed 95% when the disease is contained within the eye. However, with extraocular spread, survival rates decrease to below 50%. Therefore, when determining the treatment strategy, the clinician's first goal must be preservation of life, then preservation of the eye, and finally preservation of vision. Modern management of intraocular retinoblastoma incorporates a combination of different treatment modalities, including enucleation, local and systemic chemotherapy, laser therapy, cryotherapy, external-beam radiation therapy, and plaque brachytherapy. Metastatic disease is managed using intensive chemotherapy, radiation, and bone marrow transplantation. Treating children with retinoblastoma requires a team composed of an ocular oncologist, pediatric ophthalmologist, pediatric oncologist, and radiation oncologist.

Enucleation

Enucleation remains the definitive treatment for retinoblastoma, providing, in most cases, a complete surgical resection of the disease. Typically, enucleation is considered an appropriate intervention when

- the tumor involves more than 50% of the globe
- orbital or optic nerve involvement is suspected
- anterior segment involvement is present
- neovascular glaucoma is present
- the affected eye has limited vision potential

The goal of enucleation techniques is to minimize the potential for inadvertent globe penetration while obtaining the greatest possible length of resected optic nerve, typically longer than 10 mm. Most surgeons use porous integrated implants, such as hydroxyapatite or porous polyethylene.

Attempts at globe-conserving therapy should be undertaken only by ophthalmologists well versed in the management of this rare childhood tumor and in conjunction with similarly experienced pediatric oncologists. Failed attempts at eye salvage may place a child at risk of metastatic disease.

Chemotherapy

Over the past 30 years, systemic intravenous chemotherapy has replaced primary external-beam radiation as the preferred globe-salvaging method. Most treatment regimens include various combinations of carboplatin, vincristine, and etoposide and are most successful in curing eyes belonging to group A, B, or C. After initial regression, tumors are consolidated with laser therapy, cryotherapy, or brachytherapy (Fig 19-13) (see the following sections for discussion of these treatments). Due in part to concerns associated with systemic toxicity (such as second tumors and ototoxicity), local methods such as intra-arterial and intravitreal chemotherapy have gained acceptance in some centers. Intra-arterial chemotherapy involves selective cannulation of the ophthalmic artery and direct injection of chemotherapy to the ocular vasculature (Fig 19-14). Various drugs have been used for this

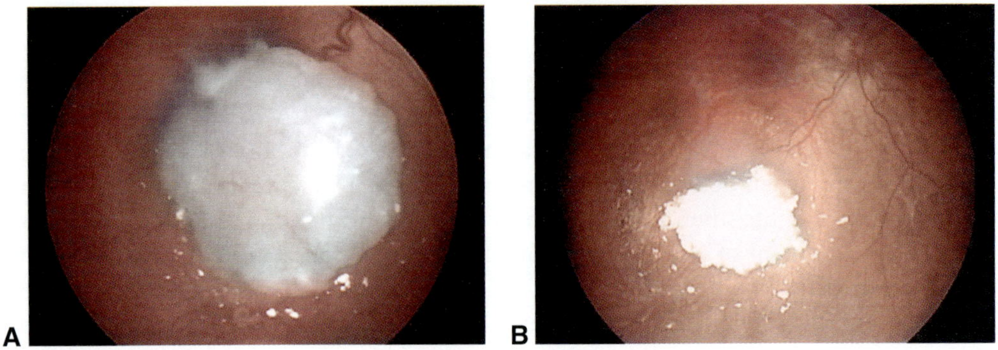

Figure 19-13 Retinoblastoma. **A,** Appearance before chemotherapy. **B,** Reduced tumor volume after 2 cycles of chemotherapy alone.

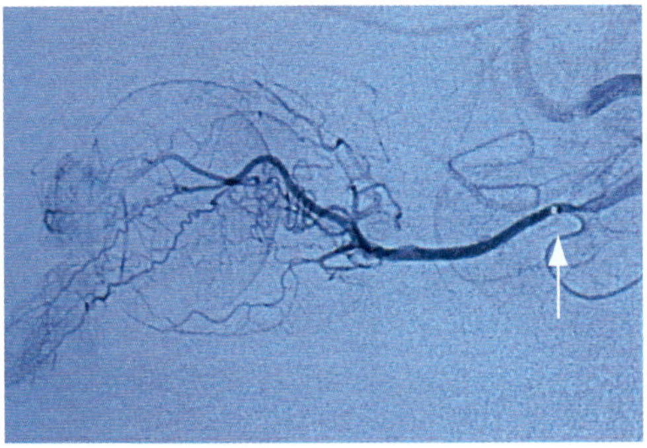

Figure 19-14 Angiogram of eye with retinoblastoma under fluoroscopy undergoing treatment with intra-arterial chemotherapy. *Arrow* demonstrates the location of the microcatheter injection into the ophthalmic vasculature. *(Courtesy of Dan S. Gombos, MD.)*

purpose, most commonly melphalan. Studies suggest that this drug is highly effective for subretinal seeds. Direct intravitreal injection of agents such as melphalan is gaining acceptance for the management of persistent or recurrent vitreous seeds. Given the potential for significant complications associated with local therapy, these approaches should be used only by clinicians well trained in the management of retinoblastoma to avoid potential extraocular extension.

Laser Therapy Including Transpupillary Thermotherapy

Various lasers have been employed to treat retinoblastoma; most experts use the 810-nm infrared diode laser. Lasers can either be used as a primary modality or serve as an adjuvant therapy after systemic or local chemotherapy.

Cryotherapy

Cryotherapy is an effective treatment for tumors with an apical thickness of up to 3 mm. It is applied under direct visualization with a triple freeze–thaw technique. Typically, laser photoablation is chosen for posteriorly located tumors and cryoablation for more anteriorly located tumors. Repetitive tumor treatments are often required for both techniques, in addition to close monitoring for tumor growth or treatment complications.

External-Beam Radiation Therapy

Because retinoblastoma tumors are responsive to radiation, external-beam radiation has become a salvage technique, used only when chemotherapy has failed.

Two major concerns have limited the application of external-beam radiotherapy using standard techniques:

1. the association between germline mutations of the *RB1* gene and a lifelong increase in the risk of second, independent primary malignancies (eg, osteosarcoma) that is exacerbated by exposure to external-beam radiotherapy
2. the potential for radiation-related sequelae, which include midface hypoplasia, radiation-induced cataract, and radiation optic neuropathy and retinopathy

Plaque Radiotherapy (Brachytherapy)

Radioactive plaque therapy may be used both as a salvage therapy for eyes in which globe-conserving therapies have failed to destroy all viable tumor and as a primary treatment for eyes with relatively small to medium-sized tumors. This technique is generally applicable for tumors less than 16 mm in basal diameter and 8 mm in apical thickness. The most commonly used isotopes are iodine-125 and ruthenium-106. Intraoperative localization with ultrasound enhances local tumor control for plaque brachytherapy. When compared with external-beam radiotherapy, this radiotherapy modality may be associated with a greater likelihood of radiation optic neuropathy or retinopathy. Limiting the radiation dose to periocular structures may lower the incidence of radiation-induced second malignancies.

Prospective Trials

The Children's Oncology Group (COG) has begun a series of international, multicenter prospective trials to improve the outcomes and clarify the toxicities associated with the modern treatment of retinoblastoma. These studies are assessing various aspects of care, including the role of adjuvant systemic chemotherapy in high-risk histopathology, treatment of extraocular retinoblastoma with intensive chemotherapy, and the efficacy of intra-arterial chemotherapy in unilateral group D disease.

Spontaneous Regression

In rare instances, retinoblastoma can undergo complete and spontaneous necrosis (although this is seldom recognized with active disease). Spontaneous regression is recognized clinically after involutional changes such as phthisis have occurred. The incidence of spontaneous regression is unknown. Although the mechanism by which spontaneous regression occurs is not understood, its histologic appearance is diagnostic. The vitreous cavities of these phthisical eyes are filled with islands of calcified cells embedded in a mass of fibroconnective tissue. Close inspection of the peripheral portion of these calcified islands reveals the ghosted contours of fossilized tumor cells. The process is often accompanied by exuberant proliferation of retinal pigment and ciliary epithelia.

Prognosis

Children with intraocular retinoblastoma who have access to modern medical care have a very good prognosis for survival; survival rates are greater than 95% for children in industrialized countries. The most important risk factor associated with death is extraocular extension of tumor, either directly through the sclera or, more commonly, by invasion of the optic nerve, especially to the surgically resected margin (see Chapter 11, Fig 11-45). The impact of choroidal invasion on survival rates is unclear. Although a multivariate analysis of a large case series showed that choroidal invasion is not predictive of metastases, the significance of this pathologic finding remains controversial and is still under investigation. Some evidence suggests, however, that bilateral tumors may increase the risk of death because of their association with primary intracranial tumors (see the section Primitive Neuroectodermal Tumor in this chapter).

Children who survive bilateral retinoblastoma have an increased incidence of nonocular malignancies later in life. The mean latency for second tumor development is approximately 9 years from management of the primary retinoblastoma. The *RB1* mutation is associated with an approximately 25% incidence of second tumor development within 50 years in patients treated without exposure to radiation therapy. External-beam radiation therapy decreases the latency period, in turn increasing both the incidence of second tumors in the first 30 years of life and the proportion of tumors in the head and neck. The most common type of second cancer in these patients is osteogenic sarcoma. Other relatively common second malignancies include pinealoblastomas, brain tumors, cutaneous melanomas, soft-tissue sarcomas, and primitive unclassifiable tumors (Table 19-4). Estimates suggest that up to 20% of patients who have bilateral retinoblastoma will present with an apparently unrelated neoplasm within 20 years and that up to 40% will present with a third malignancy within 30 years. The prognosis for survival in patients with retinoblastoma who later present with sarcomas is lower than 50%.

Table 19-4 Associated Malignancies in Retinoblastoma Survivors

Tumors Arising in the Field of Radiation of the Eye		Tumors Arising Outside the Field of Radiation of the Eye	
Pathologic Type	**Percent**	**Pathologic Type**	**Percent**
Osteosarcoma	40	Osteosarcoma	36
Fibrosarcoma	10	Cutaneous melanoma	12
Soft-tissue sarcoma	8	Primitive neuroectodermal tumor	9
Anaplastic and unclassifiable	8	Ewing sarcoma	6
Squamous cell carcinoma	5	Papillary thyroid carcinoma	6
Rhabdomyosarcoma	5	Assorted other	30
Assorted other	24		

Data from Moll AC, Imhof SM, Schouten-Van Meeteren AY, Kuik DJ, Hofman P, Boers M. Second primary tumors in hereditary retinoblastoma: a register-based study,1945–1997: is there an age effect on radiation-related risk? *Ophthalmology.* 2001;108(6):1109–1114. Also Abramson DH, Frank CM. Second nonocular tumors in survivors of bilateral retinoblastoma: a possible age effect on radiation-related risk. *Ophthalmology.* 1998;105(4):573–579. Also Abramson DH, Ellsworth RM, Kitchin FD, Tung G. Second nonocular tumors in retinoblastoma survivors. Are they radiation-induced? *Ophthalmology.* 1984;91(11):1351–1355.

CHAPTER 20

Ocular Involvement in Systemic Malignancies

Secondary Tumors of the Eye

Metastatic Carcinoma

Since the first description in 1872 of a metastatic tumor in the eye of a patient with carcinoma, a large body of literature has indicated that the most common type of intraocular or orbital tumor in adults is metastatic. Several comprehensive studies of ocular metastatic tumors have been conducted: some have reported the incidence of tumor metastases in a consecutive series in autopsies, some have dealt with tumor incidence in patients with generalized malignancy, and others have used a clinicopathologic approach. As long-term survival from systemic primary malignancy continues to increase, the ophthalmologist will be confronted with a growing incidence of intraocular and orbital metastatic disease requiring prompt recognition and appropriate diagnostic and therapeutic management.

Metastases to the eye are being diagnosed with increasing frequency for various reasons:

- increased incidence of certain tumor types that metastasize to the eye (eg, breast, lung)
- prolonged survival of patients with certain cancer types (eg, breast cancer)
- increased awareness among medical oncologists and ophthalmologists of the pattern of metastatic disease

Primary tumor sites

The majority of metastatic solid tumors to the eye are carcinomas from various organs. Cutaneous melanoma rarely metastasizes to the eye. Table 20-1 shows the most common primary tumors that metastasize to the choroid.

Mechanisms of metastasis to the eye

The mechanism of intraocular metastasis depends on the hematogenous dissemination of tumor cells. The anatomy of the arterial blood supply to the eye dictates the predilection of tumor cell deposits within the eye. The posterior choroid, with its rich vascular supply, is the most favored site of intraocular metastases; it is affected 10–20 times as frequently as is the iris or ciliary body. The retina and optic nerve head, which are supplied by the single central retinal artery, are rarely the sole site of involvement. Bilateral ocular involvement has

Table 20-1 Primary Sites of Choroidal Metastasis (in Decreasing Order of Frequency)

Males ($n = 137$)	Females ($n = 287$)
Lung (40%)	Breast (70%)
Unknown (30%)	Lung (10%)
Gastrointestinal (10%)	Unknown (10%)
Kidney (5%)	Others (<5%)
Prostate (5%)	Gastrointestinal (<5%)
Skin (<5%)	Skin (1%)
Others (<5%)	Kidney (<1%)
Breast (1%)	

Modified from Shields CL, Shields JA, Gross NE, et al. Survey of 520 eyes with uveal metastases. *Ophthalmology.* 1997;104:1265–1276.

been reported in approximately 25% of cases, and multifocal deposits are frequently seen within the involved eye. Many patients with ocular metastases also have concurrent central nervous system (CNS) and pulmonary metastases (Fig 20-1). Ocular metastatic lesions are sometimes found before a primary tumor is detected.

Clinical evaluation

The clinical features of intraocular metastases depend on the site of involvement. Metastases to the iris and ciliary body usually appear as white or gray-white gelatinous nodules (Figs 20-2, 20-3, 20-4). The clinical features of anterior uveal metastases may include

- iridocyclitis
- secondary glaucoma
- rubeosis iridis
- hyphema
- irregular pupil

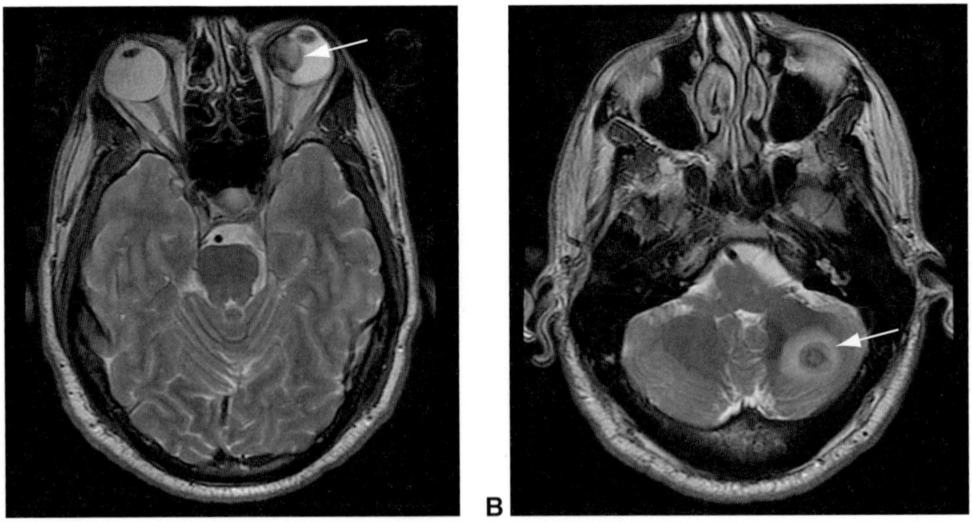

A B

Figure 20-1 Magnetic resonance imaging (MRI) studies of central nervous system (CNS) metastases. **A,** Metastatic intraocular tumor in the left eye *(arrow)*. **B,** Concurrent CNS malignancy in the brain *(arrow)*. *(Courtesy of Dan S. Gombos, MD.)*

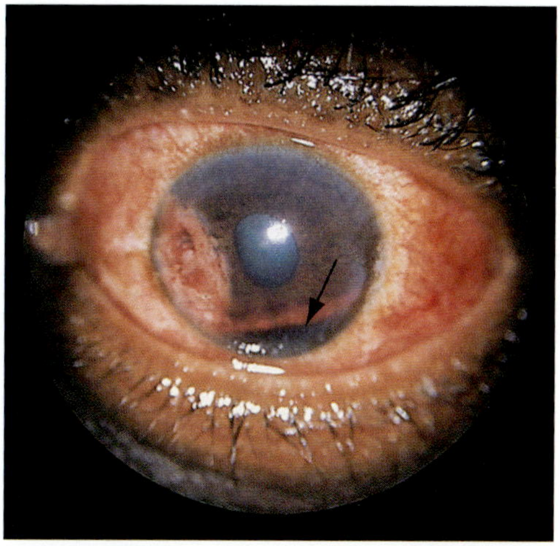

Figure 20-2 Metastasis to the iris with associated hyphema *(arrow).*

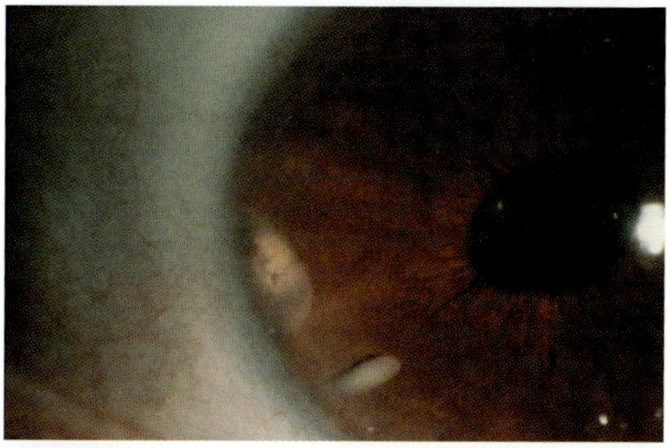

Figure 20-3 Metastasis from breast carcinoma to the iris. *(Courtesy of Timothy G. Murray, MD.)*

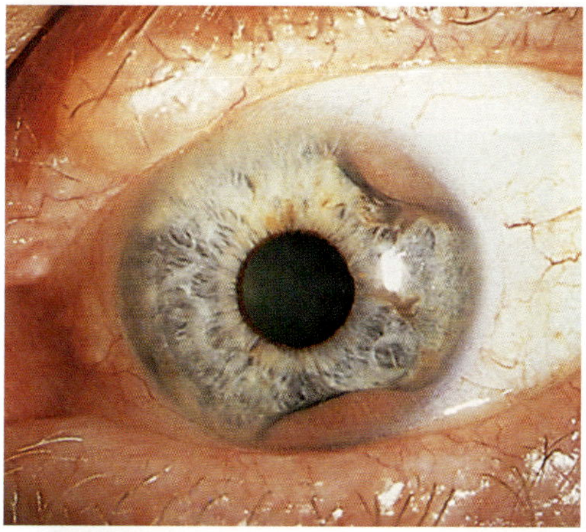

Figure 20-4 Metastatic cutaneous melanoma to the iris. Note both lesions at periphery.

Anterior segment tumors are best evaluated with slit-lamp biomicroscopy coupled with gonioscopy. High-resolution ultrasound imaging may quantify tumor size and anatomical relationships.

Patients with a tumor in the posterior pole commonly report painless loss of vision. Indirect binocular ophthalmoscopy may reveal a nonrhegmatogenous (ie, exudative) retinal detachment associated with a placoid amelanotic tumor mass (Figs 20-5, 20-6, 20-7). These lesions are usually relatively flat and ill-defined, often gray-yellow or yellow-white, with secondary alterations at the level of the retinal pigment epithelium (RPE) presenting as clumps of brown pigment ("leopard spots"; Fig 20-8).

The mushroom configuration seen in primary choroidal melanoma from breakthrough of Bruch membrane is rarely present in uveal metastases. The retina overlying the metastasis may appear opaque and become detached. Rapid tumor growth with necrosis and uveitis are occasionally observed. Dilated epibulbar vessels may be seen in the quadrant overlying the metastasis. For a differential diagnosis of choroidal metastasis, see Table 20-2.

Ancillary tests

Although *fluorescein angiography* may be helpful in defining the margins of a metastatic tumor, it is typically less useful in differentiating a metastasis from a primary intraocular neoplasm. The double circulation pattern and prominent early choroidal filling often seen in choroidal melanomas are rarely found in metastatic tumors.

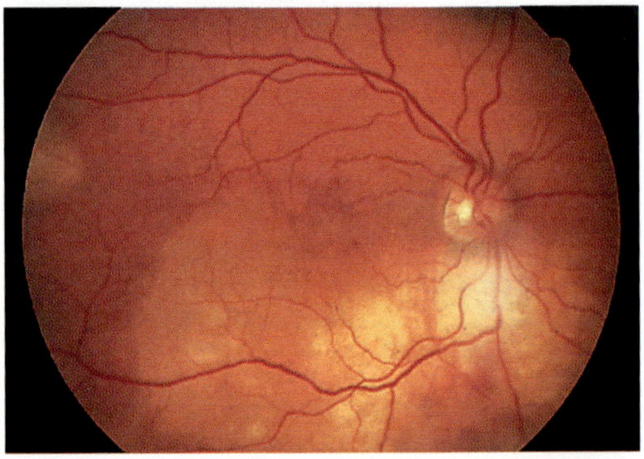

Figure 20-5 Multiple metastatic lesions to the choroid. Note the pale yellow color and relative flatness.

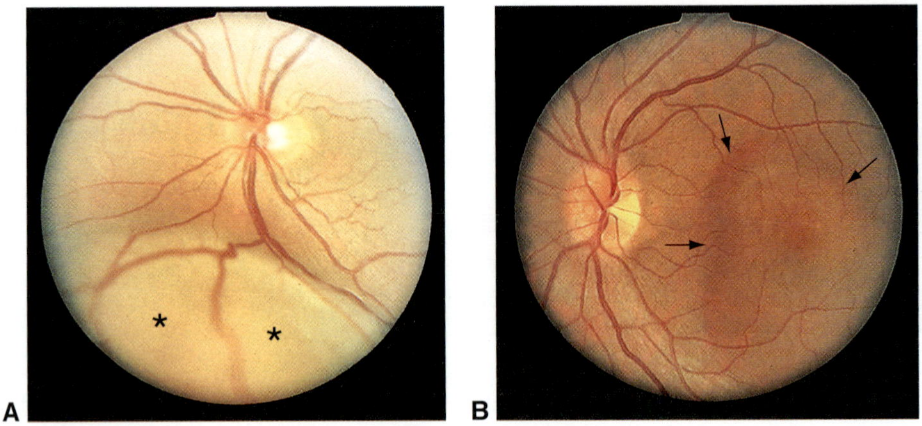

Figure 20-6 Choroidal metastasis. **A,** Metastatic lesion to the choroid inferiorly, associated with bullous retinal detachment *(asterisks).* **B,** Subtle metastatic lesion to the choroid *(arrows),* near the fovea, associated with serous effusion.

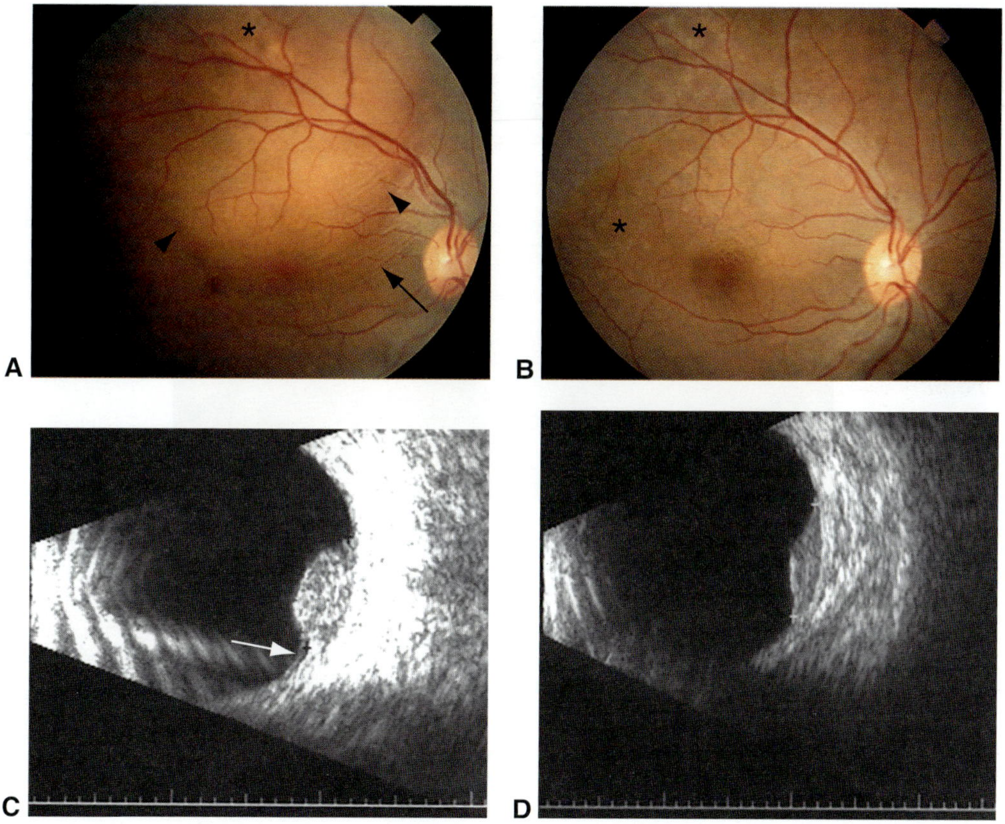

Figure 20-7 Metastatic breast carcinoma to the choroid before and after radiation therapy. **A,** Clinical photograph of metastatic breast carcinoma to the choroid. Note the yellowish choroidal lesion *(between arrowheads)* with focal retinal striae *(arrow)* and pigmentary change *(asterisk)*. **B,** Postradiation, note the focal drusenlike yellowish lesions *(asterisks)* and resolution of the retinal striae in the macular region. **C,** A B-scan ultrasonography shows a choroidal mass demonstrated in part **A** with shallow exudative retinal detachment *(arrow)*. **D,** A B-scan ultrasound shows reduction in the size of the choroidal mass after radiation therapy and resolution of the exudative retinal detachment, corresponding to part **B.** *(Courtesy of Dan S. Gombos, MD.)*

Ultrasonography is diagnostically valuable in patients with a metastatic tumor. B-scan ultrasonography shows an echogenic choroidal mass with an ill-defined, sometimes lobulated, outline (see Fig 20-7C, D). Overlying secondary retinal detachment is commonly detected in these cases. A-scan ultrasonography demonstrates irregular reflectivity.

Enhanced depth imaging optical coherence tomography (EDI-OCT) may demonstrate a “lumpy, bumpy” contour, choriocapillaris compression, and photoreceptor loss.

Fine-needle aspiration biopsy may be helpful in rare cases when the diagnosis cannot be established by noninvasive procedures. Although metastatic tumors may recapitulate the histology of the primary tumor, they are often less differentiated. Special histochemical and immunohistochemical stains assist in the diagnosis of metastatic tumors.

Metastases to the optic nerve may produce edema of the optic nerve head, decreased vision, and visual field defects. Because metastases may involve the parenchyma or the

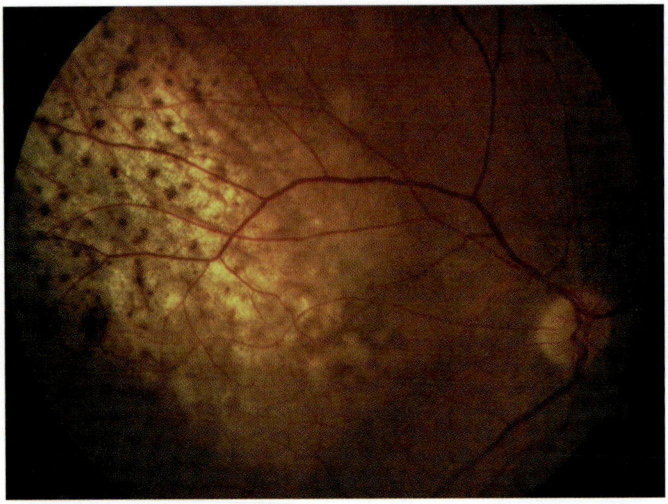

Figure 20-8 Breast carcinoma metastasis to the choroid, clinical appearance. Note the amelanotic infiltrative choroidal mass with secondary overlying retinal pigment epithelial changes accounting for the characteristic "leopard spots." *(Courtesy of Matthew W. Wilson, MD.)*

Table 20-2 Differential Diagnosis of Choroidal Metastasis

Amelanotic nevus	Vogt-Koyanagi-Harada syndrome
Amelanotic melanoma	Central serous retinopathy
Choroidal hemangioma	Infectious lesions
Choroidal osteoma	Organized subretinal hemorrhage
Choroidal detachment	Extensive neovascular membranes
Posterior scleritis	Rhegmatogenous retinal detachment

optic nerve sheath, magnetic resonance imaging (MRI) and ultrasonography may be valuable in detecting the presence of additional lesions and identifying their location.

Metastases to the retina, which are very rare, appear as white, noncohesive lesions, often distributed in a perivascular location suggestive of cotton-wool spots (Fig 20-9). Because of secondary vitreous seeding of tumor cells, these metastases sometimes resemble retinitis more than they do a true tumor. Vitreous aspirates for cytologic studies may confirm the diagnosis.

Other diagnostic factors

One of the most important diagnostic factors in the evaluation of suspected metastatic tumors is a history of systemic malignancy. More than 90% of patients with uveal metastasis from carcinoma of the breast, for example, have a history of treatment prior to the development of ocular involvement. In the remaining 10% of patients, the primary tumor can usually be diagnosed by breast examination at the time the suspicious ocular lesion is detected. For other patients, however, often there is no prior history of malignancy. This is especially true of patients with ocular metastasis from the lung. A complete systemic

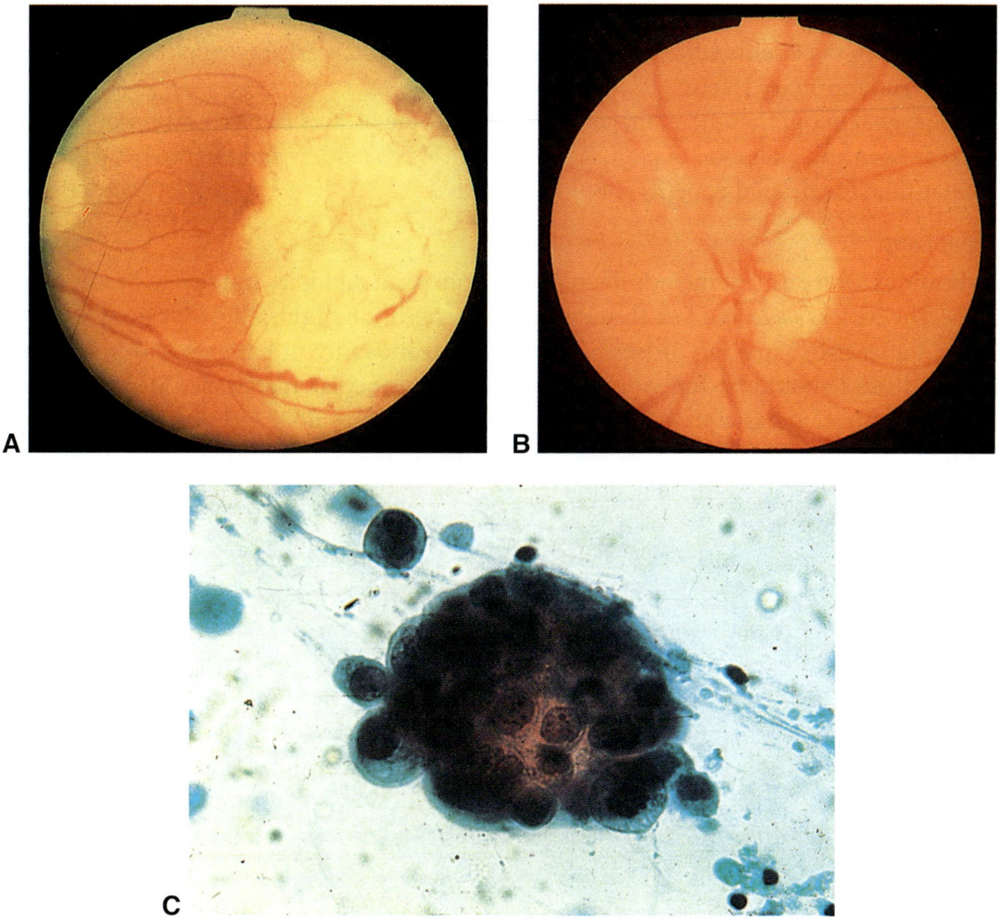

Figure 20-9 Lung carcinoma metastasis to the retina. **A,** Metastatic lung carcinoma involving the macula. Vision was reduced to finger counting. **B,** Same eye, showing characteristic perivascular distribution of metastases. **C,** Vitreous aspirate from the same eye, showing an aggregate of tumor cells, characteristic of adenocarcinoma of the lung.

evaluation, a family history, and a history of smoking may alert the ophthalmologist to the suspected site of an occult primary tumor. Any patient with an amelanotic fundus mass suspected of being a metastatic focus should undergo a thorough systemic evaluation, including imaging of the breast, chest, abdomen, and pelvis.

Prognosis

The diagnosis of tumor metastatic to the uvea implies a poor prognosis, because widespread dissemination of the primary tumor has usually occurred. In one report, the survival time following the diagnosis of metastasis to the uvea ranged from 1 to 67 months, depending on the primary cancer type. Metastatic carcinoid is associated with long survival times. Historically, patients with breast carcinoma metastatic to the uvea survived an average of 9–13 months after the metastasis was recognized, but the number of patients who survive for many years after initial diagnosis is increasing. Shorter survival time is typically seen in patients with lung carcinoma or carcinomas arising from the gastrointestinal or genitourinary tracts.

The goal in ophthalmic management of ocular metastases is preservation or restoration of vision and palliation of pain. Radical surgical procedures and treatments with risks greater than the desired benefits should be avoided.

Treatment

Indications for treatment include decreased vision, pain, diplopia, and severe ocular proptosis. The patient's age and health status and the condition of the fellow eye are also critical in the decision-making process. The treatment modality in patients with metastatic ocular disease should be individually tailored. When ocular metastases are concurrent with widespread metastatic disease, systemic chemotherapy alone or in combination with local therapy is reasonable. In patients manifesting metastases in the eye alone, local therapy modalities may be sufficient, allowing conservation of visual function with minimal systemic morbidity.

Chemotherapy or hormonal therapy for sensitive tumors (eg, breast cancer) may induce a prompt response. In such patients, no additional ocular treatment may be indicated. However, when vision is endangered by choroidal metastases in spite of chemotherapy, additional modalities of local therapy, such as external-beam radiation, brachytherapy, photodynamic therapy, or transpupillary thermotherapy, may be necessary. Radiotherapy is frequently associated with rapid improvement of the patient's symptoms, along with resolution of exudative retinal detachment and, often, direct reduction in tumor size. Possible adverse effects of the radiation include cataract, radiation retinopathy, and radiation optic neuropathy. In rare cases, enucleation is performed because of severe, unrelenting pain.

Amer R, Pe'er J, Chowers I, Anteby I. Treatment options in the management of choroidal metastases. *Ophthalmologica.* 2004;218(6):372–377.

Ferry AP, Font RL. Carcinoma metastatic to the eye and orbit. I. A clinicopathologic study of 227 cases. *Arch Ophthalmol.* 1974;92(4):276–286.

Ghodasra DH, Demirci H. Photodynamic Therapy for Choroidal Metastasis. *Am J Ophthalmol.* 2016;161:104–109.

Jardel P, Sauerwein W, Olivier T, et al. Management of choroidal metastases. *Cancer Treat Rev.* 2014;40(10):1119–1128.

Shields CL, Shields JA, Gross NE, Schwartz GP, Lally SE. Survey of 520 eyes with uveal metastases. *Ophthalmology.* 1997;104(8):1265–1276.

Direct Intraocular Extension

Direct extension of extraocular tumors into the eye is rare; the sclera is usually an effective barrier against intraocular invasion. Intraocular extension occurs most commonly with conjunctival squamous cell carcinoma and less frequently with conjunctival melanoma and basal cell carcinoma of the eyelid. Only a small minority of carcinomas of the conjunctiva penetrate the globe, and these are often variants of squamous cell carcinoma: mucoepidermoid carcinoma or spindle cell variant. These more aggressive neoplasms usually recur several times after local excision before they invade the eye.

Lymphomatous Tumors

Intraocular lymphomas may arise in different parts of the eye, expressing various clinical manifestations. *Primary intraocular lymphoma* (also known as *large cell lymphoma, vitreoretinal lymphoma,* or *retinal lymphoma*) is the most common and most aggressive type of lymphoma involving the eye and is often associated with primary central nervous system lymphoma (PCNSL). In these cases, the vitreous and retina are involved. Less frequently, the eye is involved in *systemic lymphoma (also called visceral or nodal lymphoma).* In systemic lymphoma, the uveal tract is more commonly involved, usually in a pattern of metastatic disease. In advanced cases, the intraocular findings of the 2 types may overlap. In recent decades, the incidence of PCNSL has increased significantly in both immunocompetent and immunocompromised individuals.

Primary Intraocular Lymphoma

Clinical evaluation

Ocular signs and symptoms may occur before CNS findings. In such cases, the disease may masquerade as a nonspecific uveitis. The onset of bilateral posterior uveitis in patients older than 50 years is suggestive of large cell lymphoma, as is "chronic" uveitis in patients in their fifth to seventh decade. Although 30% of patients present with unilateral involvement, delayed involvement of the second eye occurs in approximately 85% of patients.

Diffuse vitreous cells may be associated with deep subretinal and/or sub-RPE yellow-white infiltrates (Fig 20-10). Often, fine details of the retina are obscured by the density of the vitritis ("headlight in the fog"). Retinal vasculitis and/or vascular occlusion may be observed. The RPE may reveal characteristic clumping overlying the sub-RPE infiltrates (see Fig 10-14 and the discussion of histologic findings in Chapter 10). Anterior chamber reaction may be minimal.

Photographic and fluorescein angiographic studies document baseline clinical findings but are rarely helpful in defining a differential diagnosis. Ultrasonographic examination

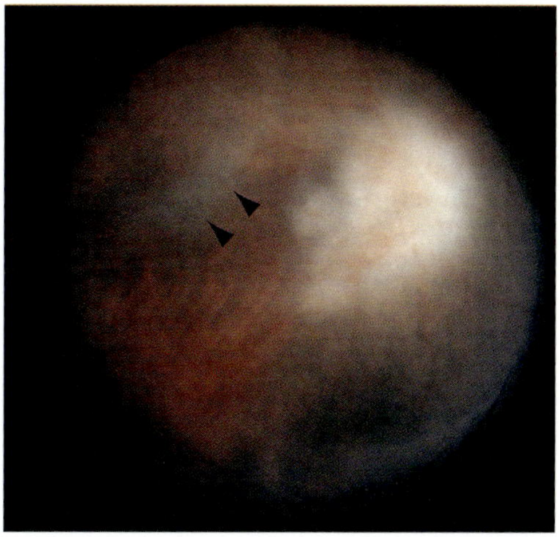

Figure 20-10 Fundus picture from a patient with vitreoretinal lymphoma. Note the vitreous haze, optic nerve head involvement, and subretinal infiltrate *(arrowheads)*. *(Courtesy of Jacob Pe'er, MD.)*

may reveal discrete nodular or placoid infiltration of the subretinal space, associated retinal detachment, and vitreous syneresis with increased reflectivity. Clinical history and neurologic evaluation reveal neurologic deficits in up to 10% of patients, and 60% of patients show concomitant CNS involvement at the time of presentation. If the diagnosis is suspected, neurologic consultation coupled with CT or MRI studies and lumbar puncture should be coordinated with diagnostic vitrectomy.

Pathologic studies

Diagnostic confirmation of ocular involvement requires sampling of the vitreous and, when appropriate, the subretinal space. Coordinated presurgical planning with the ophthalmic pathologist regarding sample handling is critical. The ophthalmic pathologist should be skilled in the handling of small-volume intraocular specimens and experienced in the evaluation of vitreous samples.

The best approach to pathologic evaluation of the specimen remains controversial. Diagnostic pars plana vitrectomy is indicated to obtain an undiluted vitreous specimen. If a subretinal nodule is accessible in a region of the retina unlikely to compromise visual function, subretinal aspiration of the lesion can be performed. A single vitrectomy biopsy may not be adequate; a second biopsy may be required. Evaluation of the vitreous and subretinal specimen may be performed using cytopathology (see Chapter 10, Fig 10-15), including immunohistochemical studies for subclassification of the cells, flow cytometry, and polymerase chain reaction (PCR) and fluorescence in situ hybridization (FISH) analysis for gene rearrangements and the ratio of interleukin-10 (IL-10) to IL-6 (see Chapters 3, 4, and 10).

Preferably, a pathologist familiar with the diagnosis of intraocular large cell lymphoma evaluates the specimen. If an adequate specimen is obtained, multiple pathologic approaches may be employed. Cytologic evaluation is essential in establishing the diagnosis; with flow cytometry, PCR, and cytokine levels (ratio of IL-10 to IL-6) serving as ancillary studies. Specimens that reveal malignant lymphocytic cells establish the diagnosis (Fig 20-11), and evaluation of cell surface markers may allow for subclassification of the tumor.

Treatment

Because the blood–ocular barriers may limit penetration of chemotherapeutic agents into the eye, irradiation of the affected eye using fractionated external-beam radiation has remained popular in some centers for treatment of intraocular lymphoma. However, although radiotherapy may induce ocular remission, the tumor can recur, and further irradiation places the patient at risk for vision loss caused by radiation retinopathy. Radiotherapy to the eye is often given with systemic or intrathecal chemotherapy. Some centers use systemic chemotherapy alone, mainly high-dose methotrexate, for the treatment of vitreoretinal lymphoma. However, studies have shown that drug penetration into the retina and vitreous is limited with systemic administration, and recurrence is common. Because of concern about the disadvantages of ocular irradiation and systemic chemotherapy, centers use intraocular chemotherapy, injecting methotrexate or rituximab into the vitreous, with very good responses and low recurrence rates. Parallel to the treatment

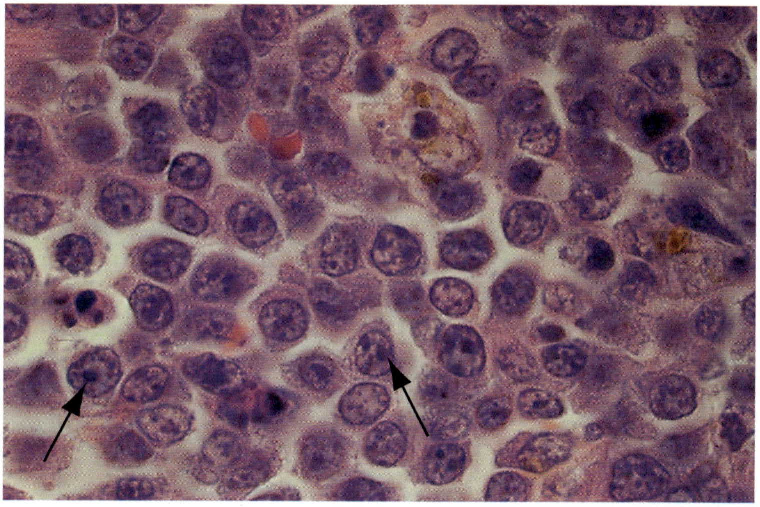

Figure 20-11 Large cell lymphoma, cytology. Note the cytologic atypia including prominent nucleoli *(arrows)* of these neoplastic lymphoid cells, which were obtained by fine-needle aspiration biopsy.

of the intraocular disease, the CNS and/or systemic lymphoma should be treated by a medical oncologist.

Prognosis

The prognosis for patients with large cell lymphoma is poor, but advances in early diagnosis have produced a cohort of long-term survivors. Serial follow-up with consultative management by an experienced medical oncologist is critical in the management of this disease. Patients with PCNSL should be observed carefully by an ophthalmologist for possible ocular involvement, even after remission of the CNS disease.

Kim MM, Dabaja BS, Medeiros J, et al. Survival outcomes of primary intraocular lymphoma: a single-institution experience [epub ahead of print January 2, 2014]. *Am J Clin Oncol.* doi:10.1097/COC.0000000000000028.

Sagoo MS, Mehta H, Swampillai AJ, et al. Primary intraocular lymphoma. *Surv Ophthalmol.* 2014;59(5):503–516.

Uveal Lymphoproliferative Lesions

Many cases of uveal lymphoid infiltration, formerly known as *reactive lymphoid hyperplasia,* are now recognized as low-grade lymphomas. These lesions, which typically present in patients in the sixth decade of life, can occur at any uveal site. Similar lymphoid proliferation can occur in the conjunctiva and orbit (see also Chapter 5 for conjunctival involvement, Chapter 12 for uveal involvement, and Chapter 14 for orbital involvement).

Clinical evaluation

Patients typically notice painless, progressive vision loss. Ophthalmoscopically, a diffuse or, in rare cases, nodular amelanotic thickening of the choroid is noted. On CT/MRI or ocular echography imaging, an adjacent episcleral component may be seen. Exudative retinal detachment and secondary glaucoma may be present in up to 85% of eyes. Frequently, delay between the onset of symptoms and diagnostic intervention is significant.

This rare disorder is characterized pathologically by localized or diffuse infiltration of the uveal tract by lymphoid cells. The etiology is unknown. Clinically, this condition can simulate posterior uveal melanoma, metastatic carcinoma to the uvea, sympathetic ophthalmia, Vogt-Koyanagi-Harada syndrome, and posterior scleritis. Proptosis of the affected eye may occur in up to 15% of patients who develop simultaneous orbital infiltration with benign lymphoid cells. Ultrasonographic testing reveals a diffuse, homogeneous choroidal infiltrate with associated secondary retinal detachment. Extraocular extension or orbital involvement may be best detected with ultrasonography.

Pathologic studies

Biopsy confirmation should be targeted to the most accessible tissue. If extraocular involvement is present, biopsy of the involved conjunctiva or orbit may be considered. Fine-needle aspiration biopsy or pars plana vitrectomy with biopsy may be indicated for isolated uveal involvement. Coordination with the ophthalmic pathologist is crucial, as it increases the likelihood of confirmation with appropriate cell marker studies.

Treatment

Historically, eyes with this type of lymphoid infiltration were generally managed by enucleation due to presumed malignancy. Current management emphasizes globe-conserving therapy aimed at vision preservation. Early intervention with low-dose ocular and orbital fractionated external-beam radiotherapy may definitively manage the disease.

Prognosis

The prognosis for survival is excellent for patients with uveal lymphoid infiltration, with the rare exception of patients with systemic lymphoma. Preservation of visual function appears related to primary tumor location and secondary sequelae, including exudative retinal detachment or glaucoma. Early intervention appears to enhance the likelihood of vision preservation.

Secondary Involvement of Systemic Lymphoma

Ocular lymphoma may represent secondary spread from systemic disease.

Clinical evaluation

Secondary ocular involvement of systemic lymphoma has a variable presentation. Features may include uveitis, infiltration of any portion of the uveal tract, or a discrete mass of the conjunctiva, eyelid, or orbit. Diagnostic biopsy is directed to the most accessible region of the eye where a large amount of tissue can be accessed.

Treatment

Treatment is dictated by the type of lymphoma and extent of disease. Therapy may include systemic chemotherapy, orbital radiation, or bone marrow transplantation. Such cases are best managed in coordination with a medical oncologist.

Ocular Manifestations of Leukemia

Ocular manifestations of leukemia are common, occurring in as many as 80% of the eyes of patients examined at autopsy. Clinical studies have documented ophthalmic findings in as many as 40% of patients at diagnosis. Patients may be asymptomatic, or they may report blurred or decreased vision. Clinically, the retina is the most commonly affected intraocular structure. Leukemic retinopathy is characterized by intraretinal and subhyaloid hemorrhages, hard exudates, cotton-wool spots, and white-centered retinal hemorrhages (pseudo–Roth spots)—all of which are usually the result of associated anemia, hyperviscosity, and/or thrombocytopenia (Fig 20-12). True leukemic infiltrates are less common and appear as yellow deposits in the retina and the subretinal space. Perivascular leukemic infiltrates produce gray-white streaks in the retina. Vitreous involvement by leukemia is rare and most often results from direct extension via retinal hemorrhage. If necessary, a diagnostic vitrectomy can be performed to establish a diagnosis.

Although clinically, the retina is the most commonly affected ocular structure, histologic studies have shown that the uvea is more commonly affected than the retina. The uveal tract may serve as a "sanctuary site," predisposing the eye to be the structure in which recurrent disease first manifests clinically. Choroidal infiltrates may be difficult to detect with indirect ophthalmoscopy; they may be better detected on ultrasonography as diffuse thickening of the choroid. Serous retinal detachments may overlie these infiltrates. Leukemic involvement of the iris manifests as a diffuse thickening with loss of the iris crypts, and, in some cases, small nodules may be seen at the margin of the pupil. Leukemic cells may invade the anterior chamber, forming a pseudohypopyon. Infiltration of the angle by these cells can give rise to secondary glaucoma.

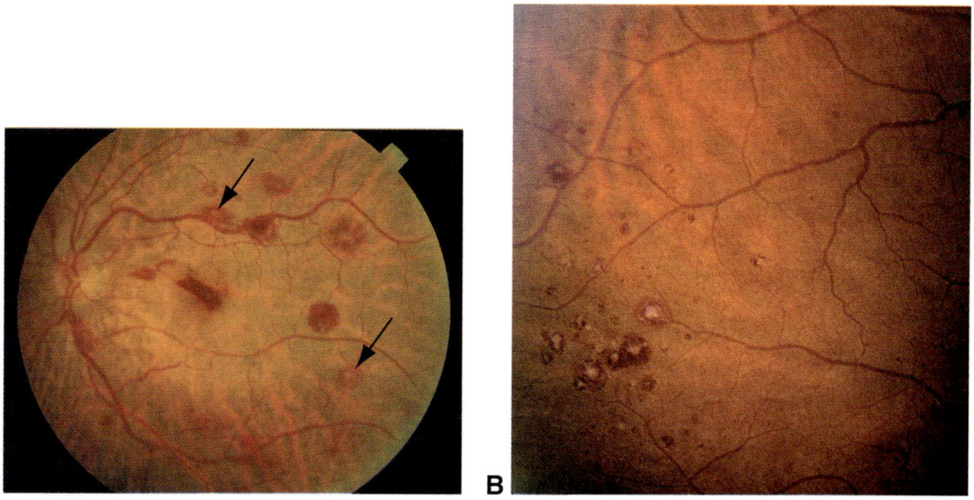

A B

Figure 20-12 Retinal involvement in leukemia. **A,** Clinical photograph of leukemic retinopathy demonstrates scattered intraretinal hemorrhages, some of which have white centers *(arrows)*. **B,** White-centered hemorrhages. *(Part A courtesy of Robert H. Rosa, Jr, MD; part B courtesy of Jacob Pe'er, MD.)*

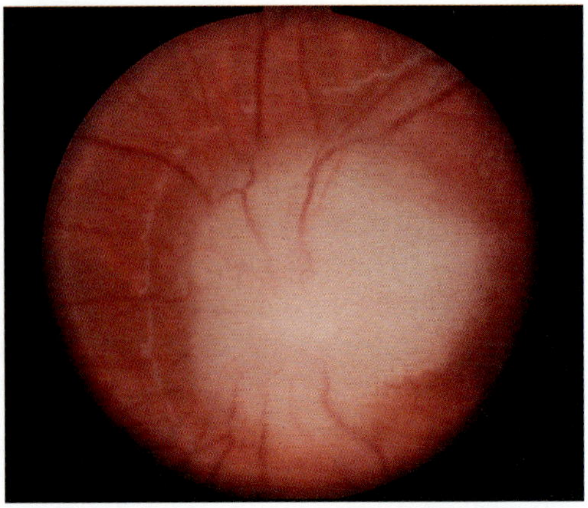

Figure 20-13 Leukemic infiltration of the optic nerve. *(Courtesy of Robert H. Rosa, Jr, MD.)*

A patient with leukemic infiltration of the optic nerve (Fig 20-13) may present with severe vision loss and optic nerve edema. One or both eyes may be affected. This is an ophthalmic emergency and requires immediate treatment to preserve as much vision as possible. Systemic and CNS assessment including lumbar puncture with cytology is necessary to confirm the diagnosis. Systemic and intrathecal combination chemotherapy is needed, with or without radiation.

Leukemic infiltrates may also involve the orbital soft tissue, with resultant proptosis. These tumors, which are more common with myelogenous leukemias, are referred to as *granulocytic sarcomas* or *chloromas.* They have a predilection for the lateral and medial walls of the orbit.

Treatment of leukemic involvement of the eye generally consists of low-dose radiation therapy to the eye and systemic chemotherapy. The prognosis for vision depends on the type of leukemia and the extent of ocular involvement.

Basic Texts

Ophthalmic Pathology and Intraocular Tumors

Cummings TJ. *Ophthalmic Pathology: A Concise Guide.* New York: Springer-Verlag; 2013.

Dutton JJ. *Atlas of Clinical and Surgical Orbital Anatomy.* 2nd ed. Philadelphia: Elsevier/Saunders; 2011.

Eagle RC. *Eye Pathology: An Atlas and Text.* 2nd ed. Philadelphia: Lippincott Williams & Wilkins; 2011.

Font RL, Croxatto JO, Rao NA. *Tumors of the Eye and Ocular Adnexa.* Annapolis Junction, Maryland: American Registry of Pathology; 2006.

Grossniklaus HE, Bergstrom C, Baker Hubbard G, Wells JR, Singh AD, eds. *Pocket Guide to Ocular Oncology and Pathology.* Berlin Heidelberg: Springer-Verlag; 2012.

Karcioglu ZA, ed. *Orbital Tumors: Diagnosis and Treatment.* 2nd ed. New York: Springer-Verlag; 2015.

McLean IW, Burnier MN, Zimmerman LE, Jakobiec FA. *Tumors of the Eye and Ocular Adnexa.* Washington: Armed Forces Institute of Pathology; 1995.

Roberts F, Thum CK. *Lee's Ophthalmic Histopathology.* 3rd ed. London: Springer-Verlag; 2014.

Shields JA, Shields CL. *Eyelid, Conjunctival, and Orbital Tumors: An Atlas and Text.* 2nd ed. Philadelphia: Lippincott Williams & Wilkins; 2007.

Shields JA, Shields CL. *Intraocular Tumors: An Atlas and Textbook.* 3rd ed. Philadelphia: Lippincott Williams & Wilkins; 2015.

Singh AD, Dolan B, Biscotti CV, eds. *FNA Cytology of Ophthalmic Tumors.* Switzerland: Karger Publishers; 2012.

Spencer WH, ed. *Ophthalmic Pathology: An Atlas and Textbook.* 4th ed. Philadelphia: Elsevier/Saunders; 1996.

Steffen H, Grossniklaus H, eds. *Eye Pathology: An Illustrated Guide.* Berlin Heidelberg: Springer-Verlag; 2015.

Yanoff M, Sassani JW. *Ocular Pathology.* 7th ed. Philadelphia: Elsevier/Saunders; 2015.

Related Academy Materials

The Academy is dedicated to providing a wealth of high-quality clinical education resources for ophthalmologists.

Print Publications and Electronic Products

For a complete listing of Academy products related to topics covered in this BCSC Section, visit our online store at http://store.aao.org/clinical-education/topic/comprehensive-ophthalmology.html. Or call Customer Service at 866.561.8558 (toll free, US only) or +1 415.561.8540, Monday through Friday, between 8:00 AM and 5:00 PM (PST).

Online Resources

Visit the Ophthalmic News and Education (ONE®) Network at http://www.aao.org/clinical-education to find relevant videos, online courses, journal articles, practice guidelines, self-assessment quizzes, images, and more. The ONE Network is a free Academy-member benefit.

Access free, trusted articles and content with the Academy's collaborative online encyclopedia, EyeWiki, at www.aao.org/eyewiki.

Requesting Continuing Medical Education Credit

The American Academy of Ophthalmology is accredited by the Accreditation Council for Continuing Medical Education to provide continuing medical education for physicians.

The American Academy of Ophthalmology designates this enduring material for a maximum of 10 *AMA PRA Category 1 Credits*™. Physicians should claim only the credit commensurate with the extent of their participation in the activity.

The American Medical Association requires that all learners participating in activities involving enduring materials complete a formal assessment before claiming continuing medical education (CME) credit. To assess your achievement in this activity and ensure that a specified level of knowledge has been reached, a posttest for this Section of the Basic and Clinical Science Course is provided online. A minimum score of 80% must be obtained to pass the test and claim CME credit.

To take the posttest and request CME credit online:

1. Go to www.aao.org/cme-central and log in.
2. Click on "Claim CME Credit and View My CME Transcript" and then "Report AAO Credits."
3. Select the appropriate Academy activity. You will be directed to the posttest.
4. Once you have passed the test with a score of 80% or higher, you will be directed to your transcript. *If you are not an Academy member, you will be able to print out a certificate of participation once you have passed the test.*

CME expiration date: June 1, 2019. *AMA PRA Category 1 Credits*™ may be claimed only once between June 1, 2016, and the expiration date.

For assistance, contact the Academy's Customer Service department at 866-561-8558 (US only) or +1 415-561-8540 between 8:00 AM and 5:00 PM (PST), Monday through Friday, or send an e-mail to customer_service@aao.org.

Study Questions

Please note that these questions are not part of your CME reporting process. They are provided here for your own educational use and identification of any professional practice gaps. The required CME posttest is available online (see “Requesting CME Credit”). Following the questions are a blank answer sheet and answers with discussions. Although a concerted effort has been made to avoid ambiguity and redundancy in these questions, the authors recognize that differences of opinion may occur regarding the “best” answer. The discussions are provided to demonstrate the rationale used to derive the answer. They may also be helpful in confirming that your approach to the problem was correct or, if necessary, in fixing the principle in your memory.

1. Langhans giant cells are typically observed in histologic specimens obtained from patients with what disorder?
   a. bacterial infection
   b. lymphoma
   c. sarcoidosis
   d. orbital pseudotumor

2. Touton giant cells are typically observed in histologic specimens obtained from patients with what disorder?
   a. bacterial keratitis
   b. juvenile xanthogranuloma
   c. *Acanthamoeba* keratitis
   d. follicular cell lymphoma

3. Commotio retinae corresponds to what histologic change?
   a. presence of subretinal fluid (localized neurosensory detachment)
   b. disruption in the architecture of the inner and outer segments of the photoreceptors
   c. ischemia of the nerve fiber layer
   d. disruption of myelin in the nerve fiber layer (NFL)

4. What clinical feature typically leads to phthisis bulbi?
   a. low intraocular pressure (IOP)
   b. high IOP
   c. vitreous hemorrhage
   d. intraocular ossification

5. When glaucoma occurs in association with angle recession, what is the cause of the glaucoma?
   a. damage to the trabecular meshwork
   b. associated lens subluxation
   c. iridodialysis
   d. a tear in the ciliary body muscle

6. During gross examination, which extraocular muscle is the most helpful in determining the laterality of a globe?
   a. superior oblique muscle
   b. inferior rectus muscle
   c. inferior oblique muscle
   d. superior rectus muscle

7. A patient who was diagnosed with sebaceous carcinoma of the right lower eyelid at an outside institution has been referred to your institution for further management. What would be the most appropriate next step in the managing the patient?
   a. Schedule the patient for surgical excision with frozen sections within the next 3 days.
   b. Request pathology slides from the outside institution for review.
   c. Refer the patient for Mohs excision of the residual lesion.
   d. Schedule the patient for another incisional biopsy to confirm the diagnosis.

8. A patient presents with an eyelid mass. What is an appropriate indication for a frozen section?
   a. to surgically control the margins of a neoplasm
   b. to render a formal diagnosis
   c. to interpret a melanocytic cutaneous lesion
   d. to make a diagnosis more expediently

9. An immunohistochemical stain for desmin may be an important adjunct in the diagnosis of what neoplasm?
   a. rhabdomyosarcoma
   b. melanoma
   c. carcinoma
   d. lymphoma

10. How should tissue be prepared in order to submit it for flow cytometry?
    a. fixed with 5% or 10% buffered formaldehyde
    b. fixed with glutaraldehyde
    c. frozen at –70° Celsius
    d. kept fresh or immersed in RPMI media

11. A 65-year-old woman presents with bilateral cicatrizing conjunctivitis. What method of analysis would be most informative in establishing a diagnosis?
    a. flow cytometry
    b. direct immunofluorescence
    c. immunohistochemistry
    d. fluorescence in situ hybridization

12. A conjunctival pigmented lesion is biopsied. Which histologic feature is indicates a risk of malignancy?
    a. epithelial cysts in the substantia propria surrounded by pigmented cells
    b. increased pigmentation in conjunctival epithelial cells
    c. epithelioid melanocytes in the superficial epithelium
    d. intensely pigmented dendritic melanocytes in the episclera

13. A mutation in which gene has been found to manifest with high frequency in nevi of Ota, blue nevi, and uveal melanoma?
    a. *PAX6*
    b. *BAP1*
    c. *BRAF*
    d. *GNAQ*

14. A corneal scraping in the setting of keratitis demonstrates double-walled cysts. What is the etiology of this keratitis?
    a. *Pseudomonas*
    b. herpesvirus
    c. *Acanthamoeba*
    d. *Fusarium*

15. Mutations in which gene have been associated with several epithelial–stromal corneal dystrophies?
    a. *TGFBI*
    b. *GNAQ*
    c. *CHST6*
    d. *COL8A1*

16. Penetrating keratoplasty is performed on a patient with suspected granular dystrophy. What histochemical stain may aid in accurate interpretation of the deposits characterizing this dystrophy?
    a. Congo red
    b. Masson-trichrome
    c. periodic acid–Schiff (PAS)
    d. alcian blue

17. What anterior segment histological findings are characteristic of primary congenital glaucoma (PCG)?
    a. hypoplastic scleral spur and an anomalous insertion of the ciliary muscle
    b. hypertrophy of the ciliary muscle, trabecular meshwork, and Schlemm canal
    c. endothelialization of the trabecular meshwork and anterior iris surface
    d. neovascularization of the trabecular meshwork and anterior iris surface

18. What anterior segment finding(s) are characteristic of Axenfeld-Rieger syndrome?
    a. corectopia and polycoria
    b. abnormal endothelial cells
    c. peripheral anterior synechiae
    d. fibrillar material in the anterior chamber angle

19. Hemolytic glaucoma is characterized by the accumulation of what material in the trabecular meshwork?
    a. rigid hemolyzed erythrocytes
    b. pigmented epithelioid melanocytes
    c. hemosiderin-laden macrophages
    d. eosinophilic protein-laden histiocytes

20. Polymorphisms in what gene are associated with pseudoexfoliation syndrome?
    a. *LOXL1*
    b. *BRCA2*
    c. *PAX6*
    d. *TGFBI*

21. Nanophthalmos is associated with what morphologic feature?
    a. normal lens
    b. iris hypoplasia
    c. scleral thinning
    d. optic atrophy

22. Epibulbar dermoids are examples of what type of lesion?
    a. choristoma
    b. hamartoma
    c. neoplasia
    d. reactive

23. What histochemical stain would be useful in confirming a diagnosis of senile calcific plaque?
    a. alizarin red
    b. alcian blue
    c. calcofluor white
    d. acridine orange

24. Nodular fasciitis is considered what type of process?
    a. reactive
    b. neoplastic
    c. degenerative
    d. infectious

25. What is the location in the lens where new lens cortical fibers are produced?
    a. nucleus
    b. anterior capsule
    c. equator
    d. posterior capsule

26. Embryologically, from which germ cell layer is the lens derived?
    a. surface ectoderm
    b. mesoderm
    c. endoderm
    d. neuroectoderm

27. What is 1 of the typical histologic features of posterior subcapsular cataract?
    a. posterior migration of lens epithelial cells
    b. disorganization of posterior lens fibers
    c. infiltration of the posterior lens by inflammatory cells
    d. retention of lens fiber nuclei

28. Proliferative vitreoretinopathy (PVR) may be a complication of rhegmatogenous retinal detachment. What primary cellular element is observed histologically in periretinal membranes that have been excised during vitrectomy for PVR?
    a. retinal pigment epithelium (RPE) cells
    b. amacrine cells
    c. bipolar cells
    d. choroidal melanocytes

29. Gardner syndrome, which is a subtype of familial adenomatous polyposis, is associated with a mutation in the *APC* gene. Patients with this genetic mutation have an increased lifetime risk of developing colon polyps, benign tumors, and cancer. The ophthalmologist may identify affected family members prior to the development of cancer with ophthalmoscopy screening. What ocular fundus finding identifies the carriers?
    a. combined hamartoma of the retina and RPE
    b. adenoma of the RPE
    c. congenital hypertrophy of the RPE
    d. osseous metaplasia of the RPE

30. What determines iris color?
    a. melanin granules in anterior stromal melanocytes
    b. melanin granules in the posterior pigment epithelium
    c. thickness of posterior pigment epithelial layer
    d. thickness of anterior stromal layer

31. Aniridia is associated with what other ocular finding?
    a. corneal pannus
    b. optic atrophy
    c. coloboma
    d. staphyloma

32. Vogt-Koyanagi-Harada (VKH) syndrome is associated with what finding?
    a. Dalen-Fuchs nodules
    b. choriocapillaris sparing
    c. fundus autofluorescence
    d. optic nerve head atrophy

33. Orbital extension of choroidal melanomas most often occurs by what mechanism?
    a. invasion through intact sclera posteriorly
    b. growth through scleral emissary canals
    c. extension through the lamina cribrosa
    d. scleromalacia resulting from radiation

34. An 85-year-old man presents with erythema and madarosis on clinical examination. Incisional biopsy reveals foamy cells and pagetoid spread. A complete surgical excision is planned. What is the best histochemical stain to highlight these cells?
    a. PAS
    b. Sudan black B
    c. hematoxylin-eosin
    d. von Kossa

35. A 13-year-old boy presents with redness of the right eye, constant epiphora, and umbilicated, nodular, waxy lesions on the lid margin. What kind of conjunctivitis does this patient have?
    a. bacterial
    b. follicular
    c. pseudomembranous
    d. giant papillary

36. A 7-year-old boy presents with rapid left-sided proptosis. Imaging reveals an orbital tumor with bony destruction. Translocation in what gene is likely implicated in this tumor?
    a. *PITX1*
    b. *FOXO1*
    c. *PAX6*
    d. *GLC1*

37. A 62-year-old man presents with a lateral orbital mass that has been progressing over 3 years. He denies pain or diplopia. A computed tomography (CT) scan reveals that the mass is well circumscribed. What is the best next step in the management of this patient?
    a. incisional biopsy
    b. fine-needle aspiration biopsy
    c. observation
    d. lateral orbitotomy with excisional biopsy

38. What combination of material and histochemical stain in cystic spaces seen microscopically would help characterize a patient with cavernous optic atrophy of Schnabel?
    a. mucopolysaccharides, alcian blue stain
    b. vitreous, alcian blue stain
    c. mucopolysaccharides, Prussian blue stain
    d. amyloid, Congo red stain

39. An 8-year-old girl presents with flat, light brown spots on the skin, benign skin growths, and an optic nerve glioma. Her father has similar findings. What feature would a biopsy of her optic nerve tumor most likely reveal?
    a. Rosenthal fibers
    b. psammoma bodies
    c. staghorn vascular spaces
    d. Verocay bodies

40. In a patient with a central nervous system (CNS) hemorrhage, which cell types would stain positive for hemosiderin?
    a. oligodendrocytes
    b. microglial cells
    c. astrocytes
    d. bipolar cells

41. At the time a choroidal melanoma is diagnosed, which test is recommended to help rule out metastasis?
    a. lumbar puncture
    b. brain magnetic resonance imaging (MRI)
    c. bone marrow biopsy
    d. abdominal imaging

42. What is the most important histologic risk factor for mortality in an enucleated globe with retinoblastoma?
    a. the presence of anterior segment involvement
    b. the presence of subretinal seeds
    c. the extent of optic nerve and choroidal invasion
    d. the presence of vitreous seeds

43. Which clinical characteristic is typical of Coats disease?
    a. unilateral
    b. presents between the ages of 40 and 65
    c. more common in women
    d. associated with cerebellar hemangioblastoma

44. Intraocular calcification in the eye of a child is most diagnostic of what disease?
    a. retinoblastoma
    b. toxocariasis
    c. persistent fetal vasculature
    d. Coats disease

45. What is the most common secondary tumor in retinoblastoma survivors?
    a. fibrosarcoma
    b. melanoma
    c. pinealoblastoma
    d. osteosarcoma

46. If a parent has bilateral retinoblastoma, what is the child's risk of developing retinoblastoma?
    a. 45%
    b. 50%
    c. 90%
    d. 100%

47. A 3-month-old infant presents with a single 2- × 2-mm retinoblastoma tumor in the maculopapillary bundle of the right eye, located within1 mm from the fovea. There are no other retinal lesions and no vitreous or subretinal seeds. Using the International Classification for Intraocular Retinoblastoma, what is the correct grouping for this eye?
    a. group I
    b. group II
    c. group A
    d. group B

48. What is the most common initial therapy for medulloepithelioma?
    a. systemic chemotherapy
    b. intravitreal chemotherapy
    c. plaque radiation therapy
    d. enucleation

49. What is the treatment of choice for a patient with metastatic carcinoma to the choroid?
    a. systemic chemotherapy
    b. external-beam radiation therapy
    c. laser therapy
    d. individually tailored therapy

50. What is the most common finding on eye examination in patients with leukemia?
    a. retinal hemorrhages
    b. aqueous cells
    c. retinal perivascular sheathing
    d. vitreous cells

Answer Sheet for Section 4 Study Questions

Question	Answer	Question	Answer
1	a b c d	26	a b c d
2	a b c d	27	a b c d
3	a b c d	28	a b c d
4	a b c d	29	a b c d
5	a b c d	30	a b c d
6	a b c d	31	a b c d
7	a b c d	32	a b c d
8	a b c d	33	a b c d
9	a b c d	34	a b c d
10	a b c d	35	a b c d
11	a b c d	36	a b c d
12	a b c d	37	a b c d
13	a b c d	38	a b c d
14	a b c d	39	a b c d
15	a b c d	40	a b c d
16	a b c d	41	a b c d
17	a b c d	42	a b c d
18	a b c d	43	a b c d
19	a b c d	44	a b c d
20	a b c d	45	a b c d
21	a b c d	46	a b c d
22	a b c d	47	a b c d
23	a b c d	48	a b c d
24	a b c d	49	a b c d
25	a b c d	50	a b c d

Answers

1. **c.** Multinucleated giant cells, including the Langhans giant cell, are characteristic of granulomatous inflammation and often observed in histologic specimens of sarcoid granulomas. Bacterial infections are characterized by acute inflammation and the presence of neutrophils. Lymphoma is a malignant lymphoproliferative process in which dense tissue infiltration of a monoclonal population of lymphocytes is typically present. The inflammatory infiltrate seen in orbital pseudotumor, also called nonspecific orbital inflammation, is composed of a mixture of acute and chronic inflammatory cells, including eosinophils, neutrophils, macrophages, lymphocytes, and plasma cells.
2. **b.** The Touton giant cell can be distinguished by the presence of several nuclei in a distinct pattern: a ring of nuclei surrounds a central homogeneous, eosinophilic cytoplasm; foamy cytoplasm surrounds the nuclei. Touton giant cells are seen in lesions with high lipid content, such as fat necrosis, xanthomas, and xanthogranulomas. Both bacterial keratitis and *Acanthamoeba* keratitis are characterized histologically by a dense infiltrate of neutrophils with variable tissue necrosis. Follicular cell lymphoma is characterized histologically by closely packed follicles that contain atypical lymphoid cells.
3. **b.** The changes resulting from contusion injury to the retina manifest clinically as areas of retinal whitening. For many years, it was believed that this indicated a possible diagnosis of retinal edema or focal ischemia, both of which demonstrate retinal opacification clinically. The advent of optical coherence tomography showed that retinal whitening can also correspond to disruption in the architecture of the retinal photoreceptor inner and outer segments. The presence of subretinal fluid does not significantly change the color of the ocular fundus. Microinfarcts of the nerve fiber layer (NFL), or cotton-wool spots, are located in the superficial retina. Myelin is not typically present in the retinal NFL; ganglion cell axons acquire myelin sheaths posterior to the lamina cribrosa.
4. **a.** Phthisical globes demonstrate *s*hrinkage, *a*trophy, and *d*isorganization (called "SAD eyes"). Loss of adequate intraocular pressure (IOP) leads to shrinkage of the eye. A formerly hypertensive eye will often demonstrate normal or low IOP as it becomes phthisical. Phthisical eyes may demonstrate vitreous hemorrhage or hemorrhage in other ocular structures. Intraocular ossification occurs late; it is a typical histologic finding in phthisis bulbi.
5. **a.** Recession of the anterior chamber angle is due to a tear in the face of the ciliary body, between the longitudinal and circular muscles, with posterior displacement of the iris root. Concurrent damage and eventual scarring of the trabecular meshwork may lead to glaucoma. Lens subluxation and iridodialysis may occur in addition to angle recession after blunt ocular trauma; however, the glaucoma that occurs in association with angle recession is most commonly caused by damage to the trabecular meshwork.
6. **c.** When trying to determine laterality of the globe, the inferior oblique muscle is a very helpful landmark. This muscle inserts temporally over the macula, with its fibers running inferiorly. Because of the posterior location of the inferior oblique insertion, the inferior oblique muscle is not typically cut flush with the sclera at the time enucleation. The rectus muscles usually are cut flush with the sclera during enucleation in order to attach them to the prosthetic orbital implant. Therefore, the rectus muscles are not easy to visualize on the surface of an enucleated globe. The superior oblique is only present as a tendon at its insertion on the globe. This tendon, which

is more anterior than the inferior oblique muscle, may be cut short surgically, making it less likely to be easily identified on an enucleated globe.

7. **b.** It is considered the standard of care to forward the slides from the original biopsy to the institution where the patient is being treated prior to any definitive treatment for malignancy. At most hospitals, this is written policy, in order to: (1) insure that the diagnosis is accurate prior to treatment, and (2) provide the pathologist with an example of the histologic features of the tumor so that the tumor can be identified in subsequent biopsies or excisions. Mohs excision and frozen section margin control are not recommended for sebaceous carcinoma because of the difficulty in identifying pagetoid spread on frozen sections.
8. **a.** Frozen sections are appropriate to ensure complete resection of the neoplasm. Frozen sections are generally not recommended on melanocytic lesions because of the potential for artifact. A formal diagnosis should be made on permanent sections. Frozen sections should not be used as means to expedite a diagnosis.
9. **a.** Because desmin is a marker of striated muscle differentiation, it may be useful in the diagnosis of rhabdomyosarcoma. Cytokeratin is appropriate in the workup of carcinoma. S100, Melan-A, and HMB45 immunohistochemical stains are useful in the diagnosis of melanocytic tumors. A panel of immunohistochemical stains, including CD20 (a marker of B-cell differentiation), is important in the workup of ocular adnexal and intraocular lymphomas.
10. **d.** Flow cytometry requires fresh tissue. The tissue can be submitted in gauze moistened with saline, or in a special nutrient or tissue culture medium, such as RPMI.
11. **b.** Direct immunofluorescence is the gold standard for diagnosis of ocular cicatricial pemphigoid. The tissue must be submitted fresh or in a special transport medium (Michel or Zeus).
12. **c.** Epithelioid morphology and migration into the superficial epithelium are consistent with atypical melanocytic proliferation and indicate a risk of malignancy. Epithelial cysts in the stroma are suggestive of a compound nevus. Increased pigmentation in the epithelial cells may be seen in complexion-associated melanosis or conjunctival hypermelanosis/primary acquired melanosis without atypia. Intensely pigmented dendritic melanocytes in the episclera are a feature of oculodermal melanocytosis (nevus of Ota).
13. **d.** Mutations in the *GNAQ* and *GNA11* genes have been found in 50%–85% of blue nevi and uveal melanomas and in a smaller percentage of nevi of Ota. They are considered founding mutations in the development of uveal melanoma. *PAX6* mutations are associated with congenital eye malformations, including aniridia (WAGR syndrome = Wilms tumor, aniridia, genitourinary malformations, and mental retardation); congenital cataract; ectopia pupillae; Peters anomaly; morning glory disc anomaly; optic nerve hypoplasia; and colobomas of the optic nerve, retina, and choroid. *BAP1* gene mutations have been identified in about 80% of uveal melanomas with a poor prognosis (class 2 tumors). Almost half of the tumors from patients with cutaneous melanoma have mutations in the *BRAF* gene. Mutations in the *BRAF* gene are only found in uveal melanoma in rare cases.
14. **c.** *Acanthamoeba* protozoa have a double-walled cyst morphology, and these cysts are difficult to eradicate from the corneal stroma. Less commonly, trophozoite forms may also be identified. Epithelial cells infected with herpesvirus may display intranuclear inclusions; these are rarely seen histologically, because corneal grafting is not generally performed

during the acute phase of infection. *Pseudomonas* is a gram-negative bacterium and is rod shaped (bacillus).

15. **a.** *TGFBI* mutations have been found in Reis-Bücklers, Thiel-Behnke, lattice, and granular corneal dystrophies.
16. **b.** Masson-trichrome highlights deposits of hyaline material that characterize granular corneal dystrophy. Congo red stains amyloid deposits in lattice and granular-lattice dystrophies. Alcian blue stains nonsulfated glycosaminoglycan deposits in macular dystrophy.
17. **a.** Primary congenital glaucoma (PCG) is believed to be the result of arrested development of the anterior chamber elements. Histologically, the anterior chamber retains an immature conformation that is characterized by anterior insertion of the iris root, mesenchymal tissue in the anterior chamber angle, and a poorly developed scleral spur in which the ciliary muscle inserts directly into the trabecular meshwork. Hypertrophy of the ciliary muscle, trabecular meshwork, and Schlemm canal is not associated with PCG. Endothelialization of the trabecular meshwork and anterior iris surface is seen in iridocorneal endothelial syndrome. Neovascularization of the trabecular meshwork and anterior iris surface is present in many diseases associated with ischemia, including diabetes, central retinal vein occlusion, intraocular tumors, and ocular ischemic syndrome.
18. **a.** Axenfeld-Rieger syndrome is part of the spectrum of developmental anomalies termed anterior segment dysgenesis. Ocular manifestations include corectopia and polycoria, posterior embryotoxon, iris strands adherent to Schwalbe line, iris hypoplasia, and a maldeveloped anterior chamber angle. Abnormal endothelial cells are seen in iridocorneal endothelial syndrome. Peripheral anterior synechiae are associated with other diseases, such as chronic angle closure and rubeosis iridis. Fibrillar material in the anterior chamber angle is seen in pseudoexfoliation syndrome.
19. **c.** Hemolytic glaucoma is characterized by the accumulation of hemosiderin-laden macrophages in the trabecular meshwork. Rigid hemolyzed erythrocytes are seen following intraocular hemorrhage in ghost cell glaucoma. Pigmented epithelioid melanocytes may invade the trabecular meshwork in the setting of uveal melanomas. In phacolytic glaucoma, eosinophilic protein-laden macrophages are seen within the trabecular meshwork.
20. **a.** Polymorphisms in *LOXL1* are associated with pseudoexfoliation syndrome. *BRCA1* mutations are associated with many cancers, including breast cancer and ovarian cancer. *PAX6* mutations are associated with developmental abnormalities, such as aniridia and Peters anomaly. *TGFBI (BIGH3)* mutations are associated with corneal dystrophies.
21. **a.** Nanophthalmos is a rare disorder characterized by a short axial length (15–20 mm), a normal or slightly enlarged lens, and thickened sclera. Nanophthalmic eyes are predisposed to uveal effusion and glaucoma. Iris hypoplasia, scleral thinning, and optic atrophy are not associated with nanophthalmos.
22. **a.** An epibulbar dermoid is an example of a choristoma, a lesion composed of normal mature tissue in an abnormal location. A hamartoma is an exaggerated hypertrophy and hyperplasia of mature tissue in a normal location; an example of a hamartoma is a capillary. Neoplasia describes unregulated growth of cells that results in a tumor; neoplasia can be benign or malignant. Reactive lesions occur in response to a stimulus, such as inflammation or trauma. For example, chronic inflammation can lead to reactive fibrosis.
23. **a.** Alizarin red stains calcium and is therefore useful in identifying lesions containing calcium, such as senile calcific plaques. Alcian blue, which stains mucopolysaccharides, is

often used to identify the composition of corneal deposits in macular dystrophy. Calcofluor white and acridine orange can be employed for the identification of *Acanthamoeba*.

24. **a.** Nodular fasciitis is a reactive process that may lead to tumefaction in rare cases. It is a rapidly growing, usually self-limited process. Neoplastic processes (eg, basal cell carcinoma) are characterized by unregulated growth that does not resolve spontaneously. Degenerative processes (eg, senile calcific plaques) result from aging. Infectious processes (eg, corneal ulcers) are the result of infectious agents such as bacteria, viruses, and fungi.

25. **c.** The lens epithelium produces the crystalline proteins that become new lens cortical fibers. The outer edge of the epithelial layer at the lens equator, also known as the "lens bow," is the active area of production of these new lens fibers. The nucleus is formed embryologically and grows throughout life as cortical fibers become compacted; the outer layers of the cortex represent the newest lens cortical fibers. The anterior capsule is lined by a monolayer of lens epithelial cells. The posterior capsule normally does not have any epithelium associated with it; therefore lens cortical fibers cannot be produced there.

26. **a.** The lens is embryologically derived from the surface ectoderm. The lens plate of the surface ectoderm invaginates toward the underlying neuroectoderm and becomes the lens vesicle at around 30 days of gestation. The underlying neuroectoderm simultaneously migrates and proliferates, becoming the optic cup from which neuroepithelium and neurosensory retina are derived. The lens vesicle eventually loses its connection to the surface ectoderm and migrates into the center of the optic cup. Structures such as the sphincter and dilator muscle of the iris, iris stroma, and ciliary muscle are derived from mesoderm. The endoderm does not contribute to the structures of the eye or orbit.

27. **a.** Normally, lens epithelial cells are present along the inner surface of the anterior lens capsule and terminate at the lens equator. When the equatorial lens epithelial cells migrate posteriorly onto the posterior lens capsule, they swell 5–6 times their normal size and become bladder cells (also called Wedl cells), resulting in the clinical appearance of posterior subcapsular cataract.

28. **a.** Proliferative vitreoretinopathy (PVR) membranes form as a result of proliferation of retinal pigment epithelium (RPE) cells and other cellular elements, including Müller cells, fibrous astrocytes, macrophages, fibroblasts, and myofibroblasts. Amacrine and bipolar cells, which are found in the inner nuclear layer of the retina, are not a major constituent of PVR membranes. Unless there is rupture of Bruch membrane, choroidal melanocytes do not have access to the subretinal space or vitreous cavity, and therefore are not typically observed in PVR membranes.

29. **c.** RPE lesions that mimic congenital hypertrophy of the RPE (CHRPE) may be present in Gardner syndrome. The presence of 4 or more of these lesions in each eye of a patient with a family history of Gardner syndrome or the *APC* mutation identifies that patient as a carrier of the gene mutation. These patients have a significantly increased risk for the development of colon cancer. In combined hamartoma of the retina and RPE, the RPE is hyperplastic and frequently migrates into the retina in a perivascular location. Vitreous condensation and fibroglial proliferation may be present on the surface of the tumor. Neoplasia (adenoma and adenocarcinoma) of the RPE is very rare. Osseous metaplasia of the RPE with bone formation may be a prominent feature in phthisis bulbi.

30. **a.** Iris color is determined by the size and number of melanin pigment granules in the anterior stromal melanocytes. Melanin granules in the posterior pigment epithelium, the thickness of posterior pigment epithelial layer, and the thickness of the anterior stromal layer do not determine iris color.

31. **a.** Aniridia is associated with cataract, corneal pannus, and foveal hypoplasia. Optic atrophy, colobomas, and staphylomas are not usually associated with aniridia.

32. **a.** Dalen-Fuchs nodules are collections of epithelioid histiocytes and lymphocytes between Bruch membrane and the RPE. They can be seen in sympathetic ophthalmia and Vogt-Koyanagi-Harada (VKH) syndrome. In VKH syndrome, the entire choroid, including the choriocapillaris, is typically involved by the inflammatory process; relative sparing of the choriocapillaris is characteristic of sympathetic ophthalmia. Fundus autofluorescence and optic nerve head atrophy are not usually associated with VKH syndrome.

33. **b.** Choroidal melanomas may extend through scleral emissary canals into the orbit. Superficial invasion of the sclera is often seen, but extension through intact sclera into the orbit is extremely rare. Retinoblastoma may invade the lamina cribrosa, extending into the optic nerve and brain; however, uveal melanoma does not typically invade the optic nerve or brain. The irradiation (eg, brachytherapy) used to treat choroidal melanomas does not usually lead to scleromalacia.

34. **b.** Histologically, well-differentiated sebaceous carcinomas are readily identified by the microvesicular foamy nature of the tumor cell cytoplasm. Because they reveal lipid within the cytoplasm of tumor cells, special stains, such as oil red O or Sudan black B, can be used to diagnose sebaceous carcinomas. Tissue staining for lipids should be performed on frozen or cryostat sections, because the lipid constituents are often removed during paraffin processing. Another common histologic feature of sebaceous carcinoma is pagetoid spread, which involves the dissemination of individual tumor cells and/or clusters of tumor cells within the epidermis or conjunctival epithelium. The PAS reagent, which stains glycogen and proteoglycans, is useful for identifying basement membranes (eg, Descemet membrane, lens capsule) and mucin-producing cells (eg, conjunctival goblet cells) in ocular tissues. Hematoxylin-eosin is a general tissue stain that stains the nucleus blue and the cytoplasm pink-red. Calcium phosphate salts are stained black with the von Kossa stain, as in band keratopathy.

35. **b.** Molluscum contagiosum, which is caused by a member of the poxvirus family, is characterized by dome-shaped, waxy epidermal nodules with a central umbilication. If present on the eyelid margin, these nodules may cause a secondary follicular conjunctivitis. Histologically, the epithelial nuclei are displaced peripherally by large eosinophilic (pink) viral inclusions known as molluscum or Henderson-Patterson bodies. As the infected cells migrate to the surface, the viral inclusions become more basophilic (blue/dark purple). Bacterial conjunctivitis is associated with a papillary reaction and purulent discharge. In pseudomembranous conjunctivitis, the fibrin network is easily peeled off, leaving the conjunctiva intact; pseudomembranes form on the conjunctiva. Giant papillary conjunctivitis (GPC) occurs in primary and secondary forms, all of which are at least partially caused by chronic ocular allergy. Primary forms of GPC include vernal and atopic keratoconjunctivitis. Secondary GPC is caused by contact lenses, ocular prostheses, or exposed sutures.

36. **b.** In rhabdomyosarcoma, which is the most common orbital malignant tumor in childhood, proptosis is often sudden and progresses rapidly, requiring emergency treatment. Rhabdomyosarcomas arise from primitive mesenchymal cells that differentiate toward skeletal muscle. There are 3 recognized histologic types of orbital rhabdomyosarcoma: embryonal (most common), alveolar (worst prognosis), and pleomorphic (best prognosis). Histologically, spindle cells are arranged in a loose syncytium with occasional cells bearing cross-striations. These cross-striations are found in approximately 60% of embryonal rhabdomyosarcomas. Cytogenetic studies are important for identifying translocations such

as *FOXO1,* which has prognostic implications. *PITX1* mutations are associated with upper and lower limb deformities (club foot, Liebenberg syndrome). *PAX6* mutations are associated with developmental ocular malformations (aniridia, Peters anomaly). *GLC1* mutations are associated with primary open-angle glaucoma.

37. **d.** The most common epithelial tumor of the lacrimal gland is pleomorphic adenoma (benign mixed tumor). This tumor is pseudoencapsulated and grows slowly by expansion. Typically, the patient experiences no pain. Histologically, pleomorphic adenoma has a fibrous pseudocapsule and comprises a mixture of ductal-derived epithelial and stromal elements. Transformation into a malignant mixed tumor may take place in a long-standing or incompletely excised pleomorphic adenoma, with relatively rapid growth after a period of relative quiescence. Carcinomas, including adenocarcinoma (carcinoma ex pleomorphic adenoma) and adenoid cystic carcinoma, may also develop in recurrent pleomorphic adenomas. In order to avoid recurrence and potential malignant transformation, the most appropriate management for this patient is lateral orbitotomy with excisional biopsy. When a pleomorphic adenoma is suspected, incisional biopsy and fine-needle aspiration biopsy should be avoided. Observation is not the best management because long-standing pleomorphic adenomas may undergo malignant transformation.

38. **a.** Cavernous optic atrophy of Schnabel is characterized microscopically by large cystic spaces that are posterior to the lamina cribrosa and contain mucopolysaccharide material, which stains with alcian blue stain.

39. **a.** Optic nerve gliomas, which are frequently associated with neurofibromatosis 1 (NF1), most commonly present in the first decade of life and are low-grade juvenile pilocytic astrocytomas. Enlarged, deeply eosinophilic filaments known as Rosenthal fibers, which represent degenerating cell processes, may be found in these low-grade tumors. Psammoma bodies may be found in meningiomas. Staghorn vascular spaces are observed in hemangiopericytomas and related solitary fibrous tumors. Verocay bodies are collections of fibrils that resemble sensory corpuscles in the Antoni A spindle cell pattern observed in schwannomas (also called neurilemomas).

40. **b.** The cells of the supportive tissue of the central nervous system (CNS), oligodendrocytes, astrocytes, and microglial cells, are glial cells. Oligodendrocytes produce and maintain the myelin sheath of the optic nerve, astrocytes are involved with support and nutrition, and microglial cells (CNS histiocytes) have a phagocytic function. Thus, the "macrophages" of the CNS, or microglial cells, would engulf hemosiderin after a CNS or retinal hemorrhage. Bipolar cells, which are neuronal cells found in the inner nuclear layer of the retina, are not phagocytic cells.

41. **d.** The liver is the most frequent site of metastasis from uveal melanoma. Metastasis to other organs, such as the lungs, skin, and bones, is rarely found without liver involvement.

42. **c.** Invasion of the optic nerve increases the risk of CNS metastasis, either by direct access in or along the nerve, or by seeding of the subarachnoid space. Massive deep invasion of the choroid increases the risk of hematogenous spread.

43. **a.** Coats disease is a unilateral retinal vasculopathy (retinal telangiectasis with exudative maculopathy and/or retinopathy) that occurs more commonly in boys younger than 10 years.

44. **a.** Intraocular calcifications are the hallmark of retinoblastoma; they signify retinoblastoma until proven otherwise. In rare instances, intraocular calcifications may be seen in toxocariasis, persistent fetal vasculature, and Coats disease. In these cases, calcifications

are usually focal and discrete, occurring within granulomas (toxocariasis) or a retrolental membrane (persistent fetal vasculature) or at the level of the RPE (Coats disease).

45. **d.** Osteosarcomas represent 40% of tumors arising within the field of radiation and 36% outside the field of radiation in patients previously treated for retinoblastoma.

46. **a.** A parent with retinoblastoma likely has a somatic mutation of at least 1 allele of the retinoblastoma gene *(RB1)*. Thus, there is a 50% chance that the parent will pass the mutated allele to each of his or her children. If the abnormal allele is inherited, there is a 90% chance of penetration. Therefore, the child's risk of developing retinoblastoma is the sum of 0.50 × 0.90, which is 0.45, or 45%.

47. **d.** The International Classification for Intraocular Retinoblastoma, which has replaced the Reese-Ellsworth Classification for Intraocular Tumors in grouping eyes with retinoblastoma, progresses from group A to group E. Any retinal lesion of any size within 3 mm of the fovea without focal or diffuse vitreous seeds is classified as group B.

48. **d.** Medulloepithelioma often presents in an advanced state, with erosion into the anterior chamber and iris root, as well as neovascular glaucoma. In addition, these tumors may harbor malignant features. Because of this, management of medulloepithelioma usually consists of enucleation. Unlike its highly malignant counterpart in the CNS, as long as the tumor has not spread beyond the eye, intraocular medulloepithelioma has a good prognosis. Treatment options for ciliary body medulloepithelioma may also include cryotherapy, local resection, and plaque or external-beam radiation therapy. The role of systemic or intravitreal chemotherapy in the treatment of ciliary body medulloepithelioma is not well established. Cryotherapy can be used for smaller or recurrent tumors. Local resection of medulloepithelioma is associated with tumor recurrence in 50%–100%. Standard-dose external-beam radiotherapy shows a mild response, but plaque radiation therapy is an alternative for smaller tumors. For larger tumors, enucleation is the preferred method of treatment.

49. **d.** The clinician should individually tailor the treatment of a patient with choroidal metastasis after consulting with the patient's oncologist and radiation therapist. Prior and current chemotherapy and radiation administration as well as tumor focality, laterality, and proximity to critical visual structures are all factors that affect treatment.

50. **a.** Retinal hemorrhages, typically white-centered hemorrhages, are the most common ocular manifestation of leukemia. Patients with leukemia and retinal hemorrhages typically have anemia and thrombocytopenia. The other findings listed are much less common.

Index

(*f* = figure; *t* = table)